Cutaneous Manifestations of DIABETES

Cutaneous Manifestations of DIABETES

Emilia Noemí Cohen Sabban MD
Deputy Chief of the Dermatology Division
Instituto de Investigaciones Médicas Lanari
Ciudad Autónoma de Buenos Aires
Buenos Aires, Argentina
Associate Professor of Dermatology
Buenos Aires University
Buenos Aires, Argentina

Foreword

Ana Kaminsky MD

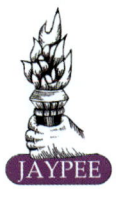

JAYPEE *The Health Sciences Publisher*
New Delhi | London | Panama

Jaypee Brothers Medical Publishers (P) Ltd

Headquarters
Jaypee Brothers Medical Publishers (P) Ltd
4838/24, Ansari Road, Daryaganj
New Delhi 110 002, India
Phone: +91-11-43574357
Fax: +91-11-43574314
Email: jaypee@jaypeebrothers.com

Overseas Offices

J.P. Medical Ltd
83 Victoria Street, London
SW1H 0HW (UK)
Phone: +44 20 3170 8910
Fax: +44 (0)20 3008 6180
Email: info@jpmedpub.com

Jaypee-Highlights Medical Publishers Inc
City of Knowledge, Bld. 235, 2nd Floor, Clayton
Panama City, Panama
Phone: +1 507-301-0496
Fax: +1 507-301-0499
Email: cservice@jphmedical.com

Jaypee Brothers Medical Publishers (P) Ltd
17/1-B Babar Road, Block-B, Shaymali
Mohammadpur, Dhaka-1207
Bangladesh
Mobile: +08801912003485
Email: jaypeedhaka@gmail.com

Jaypee Brothers Medical Publishers (P) Ltd
Bhotahity, Kathmandu, Nepal
Phone: +977-9741283608
Email: kathmandu@jaypeebrothers.com

Website: www.jaypeebrothers.com
Website: www.jaypeedigital.com

© 2017, Jaypee Brothers Medical Publishers

The views and opinions expressed in this book are solely those of the original contributor(s)/author(s) and do not necessarily represent those of editor(s) of the book.

All rights reserved. No part of this publication may be reproduced, stored or transmitted in any form or by any means, electronic, mechanical, photocopying, recording or otherwise, without the prior permission in writing of the publishers.

All brand names and product names used in this book are trade names, service marks, trademarks or registered trademarks of their respective owners. The publisher is not associated with any product or vendor mentioned in this book.

Medical knowledge and practice change constantly. This book is designed to provide accurate, authoritative information about the subject matter in question. However, readers are advised to check the most current information available on procedures included and check information from the manufacturer of each product to be administered, to verify the recommended dose, formula, method and duration of administration, adverse effects and contraindications. It is the responsibility of the practitioner to take all appropriate safety precautions. Neither the publisher nor the author(s)/editor(s) assume any liability for any injury and/or damage to persons or property arising from or related to use of material in this book.

This book is sold on the understanding that the publisher is not engaged in providing professional medical services. If such advice or services are required, the services of a competent medical professional should be sought.

Every effort has been made where necessary to contact holders of copyright to obtain permission to reproduce copyright material. If any have been inadvertently overlooked, the publisher will be pleased to make the necessary arrangements at the first opportunity.

Inquiries for bulk sales may be solicited at: jaypee@jaypeebrothers.com

Cutaneous Manifestations of Diabetes

First Edition: **2017**

ISBN 978-93-5270-039-4

Printed at Sanat Printers

Dedicated to
My father

Contributors

Roberto Arenas MD
Chief of the Mycology Section
'Dr Manuel Gea Gonzalez' General
Hospital
México City, Mexico

Anahí Belatti MD
Dermatologist Physician at Wound
Healing
Department of Dermatology Service
Italian Hospital
Buenos Aires, Argentina

Horacio Antonio Cabo MD PhD
Head Professor of Dermatology
Universidad de Buenos Aires (UBA)
Buenos Aires, Argentina
Specialist in Dermatology
Universidad de Buenos Aires (UBA)
Buenos Aires, Argentina
Head of Dermatology
Institute of Medical Research
Universidad de Buenos Aires (UBA)
Buenos Aires, Argentina

Noelia Capellato MD
Family Physician and Attending
Physician at Wound Healing
Dermatology Service
Italian Hospital
Buenos Aires, Argentina

Emilia Noemí Cohen Sabban MD
Deputy-Chief of the Dermatology Division
Instituto de Investigaciones
Médicas Lanari
Ciudad Autónoma de Buenos Aires
Buenos Aires, Argentina
Associate Professor of Dermatology
Buenos Aires University
Buenos Aires, Argentina

Judith Dominguez-Cherit MD
Chair of Dermatology
Instituto Nacional de Ciencias Médicas y
Nutrición Salvador Zubirán
Mexico City, Mexico

César Iván Eugenio-González MD
Resident
Department of Dermatology
'Dr Manuel Gea Gonzalez' General Hospital
Mexico City, Mexico

Michelle Gatica-Torres MD
Dermatopathology Fellow
Montefiore Medical Center/Albert
Einstein College of Medicine
Bronx, New York, USA

Lucrecia Juárez MD
Specialist in Dermatology
La Plata University
Buenos Aires, Argentina

Marina Luz Margossian MD
Visiting Doctor of the Diabetes Division
of the Hospital de Clínicas 'José
de San Martín'
Ciudad Autónoma de Buenos Aires
University of Buenos Aires
Buenos Aires, Argentina

Félix Miguel Puchulu MD
Chief of the Diabetes Division of the
Hospital de Clínicas 'José de San Martín'
Ciudad Autónoma de Buenos Aires
University of Buenos Aires
Buenos Aires, Argentina

María Gala Santini-Araujo MD
Attending Physician at Foot and Ankle
Service
Department of Orthopedic Surgery
Hospital Italiano de Buenos Aires
Buenos Aires, Argentina

Denise Steiner MD
Medical Dermatologist
Professor of Dermatology
University of Mogi das Cruzes
São Paulo, Brazil
Head of Dermatology Service
University of Mogi das Cruzes
São Paulo, Brazil

Patricia Troielli MD
Dermatologist
Faculty of Dermatology
University of Buenos Aires
Buenos Aires, Argentina

Foreword

When an author gives us the privilege of presenting his book, we are certainly honored; but we also know that he/she proposes a challenge that must be faced with academic responsibility and all the critical judgment that experience allows us to play.

This book has been conceived as a compendium of skin manifestations that may arise in patients with diabetes. But it is also a call to professional reflection about the importance and impact of diabetes in its broad spectrum, from the pathophysiology of the skin to each of its components, including the appendages. In 14 profusely illustrated chapters, written by renowned specialists from Argentina and other countries, the reader begins a path from the most basic concepts—definition, classification and diagnosis of diabetes—continues with its cutaneous manifestations, infections and skin alterations due to vasculopathy and neuropathy. Skin markers have also been described which alert us that there is something beyond what we see. The course culminates with the treatment and the problems induced by antidiabetic treatment, emphasizing the attention and the multidisciplinary approach and management.

I have no doubt that this contribution of Dr Emilia Noemí Cohen Sabban is the result of an arduous and complex task: to gather in a book the experience of many years of exercise of the medical profession and teaching. For this reason, I consider that this work is of great value not only for the dermatologists but also for the internist doctors and for those who work in other specialties of the art of curing, since medicine covers the organism as a whole.

Ana Kaminsky MD
Assistant Professor of Dermatology
School of Medicine
Buenos Aires' University
Argentina

Preface

I started in 1992 as Assistant of the Section of Internal Medicine and Skin at the Dermatology Division of the Hospital de Clínicas José de San Martín, University of Buenos Aires, Buenos Aires, Argentina.

Diabetes, as a disease that can affect all ages, all races, any sex, but fundamentally every organ of the body, caught me right away.

We have worked multidisciplinary since then, examining, diagnosing and treating diabetic patients.

I've come a long way, which inspired me to dump in this book, all that I have received over the years.

I hope the gratitude I feel is reflected in the usefulness this book has for all those health care professionals, who work with diabetic patients to whom we can benefit.

Emilia Noemí Cohen Sabban

Acknowledgments

To all of my teachers for transmitting their knowledge with generosity.
To my patients for trusting me.
To all the contributors for helping me to bring out the book.

Contents

1. **Definition, Classification and Diagnosis of Diabetes Mellitus**   1
   Félix Miguel Puchulu

2. **Introduction to Cutaneous Manifestations of Diabetes Mellitus**   11
   Emilia Noemí Cohen Sabban

3. **Cutaneous Barrier and Diabetes**   15
   Patricia Troielli, Lucrecia Juárez

4. **Cutaneous Markers of Diabetes Mellitus**   31
   Emilia Noemí Cohen Sabban

5. **Skin-Thickening Syndrome**   53
   Emilia Noemí Cohen Sabban, Horacio Antonio Cabo

6. **Acanthosis Nigricans and Other Cutaneous Manifestations of Insulin Resistance and Metabolic Syndrome**   73
   Emilia Noemí Cohen Sabban

7. **Cutaneous Infections in Diabetics**   83
   Part 7A: Fungal Infections in Diabetics   83
   Roberto Arenas, César Iván Eugenio-González

   Part 7B: Bacterial Infections in Diabetics   92
   Emilia Noemí Cohen Sabban

8. **Dermatoses Most Frequently Related to Diabetes**   105
   Emilia Noemí Cohen Sabban

9. **Cutaneous Manifestations Induced by Antidiabetic Treatment**   137
   Emilia Noemí Cohen Sabban, Marina Luz Margossian

10. **Cutaneous Manifestations due to Vasculopathy, Neuropathy and Diabetic Foot Syndrome**   149
    Emilia Noemí Cohen Sabban

11. **Diabetes, Non-Enzymatic Glycation and Aging**   167
    Emilia Noemí Cohen Sabban, Denise Steiner

12. **Nail Alterations in Diabetic Patients** 177
   Judith Dominguez-Cherit, Michelle Gatica-Torres

13. **Ulcers and Wound Healing in Diabetics** 187
   Patricia Troielli, Lucrecia Juárez

14. **Multidisciplinary Approach in Managing Wound Healing** 201
   Anahi Belatti, Noelia Capellato, Maria Gala Santini Araujo

Index *221*

CHAPTER 1

Definition, Classification and Diagnosis of Diabetes Mellitus

Félix Miguel Puchulu

INTRODUCTION

Diabetes mellitus (DM) is a syndrome characterized by hyperglycemia and impaired metabolism of carbohydrates, proteins and fats due to an absolute or relative deficiency of the secretion and/or insulin action.

Its prevalence is 7–8% approximately, of which 90% corresponds to type 2 diabetes and the rest is distributed among the different types of diabetes.

DIAGNOSIS OF DIABETES MELLITUS

The DM is defined by blood glucose levels. They will be considered diabetic those exceeding 126 mg/dL fasting twice or submit above 200 mg/dL values at any time of day or at two hours of testing glucose tolerance.

Normal values are below 100 mg/dL or fasting under 140 mg/dL 2 hours of testing glucose tolerance.

There are some people with glucose levels between 100 mg/dL and 126 mg/dL on the fasting state, or more than or equal to 140 mg/dL but less than 200 mg/dL after 75 g of glucose [oral glucose tolerance test (OGTT)], they are considered nondiabetic but with alterations in carbohydrate metabolism. The first alteration is impaired fasting glucose (IFG), in which insulin resistance plays the most important role; the second disturbance is called impaired glucose tolerance (IGT), in which there is a disturbance in the normal secretion of insulin to the stimulus with glucose (Table 1).

Both alterations in the same individual can also be present. The presence of IFG and IGT indicates a higher probability of evolving to type 2 diabetes

TABLE 1: Oral glucose tolerance test: Interpretation.

Glycemia	Normal	IFG	IGT	Diabetes
0 minutes	≤ 99 mg/dL	100–125 mg/dL	≤ 99 mg/dL	≥ 126 mg/dL
120 minutes	≤ 139 mg/dL	≤ 139 mg/dL	140–199 mg/dL	≥ 200 mg/dL

(IFG: Impaired fasting glucose; IGT: Impaired glucose tolerance).

mellitus (T2DM). In the case of presenting one of the alterations, it has been seen that the IGT has a higher incidence of T2DM than the IFG.

Current diagnostic criteria of the American Diabetes Association (ADA) propose adding glycosylated hemoglobin A1c (HbA1c) within them. Values above 6.5% would define the presence of disease. In Argentina, due to the lack of standardization of the method for the determination of HbA1c, Argentine Diabetes Society [Sociedad Argentina de Diabetes (SAD)] decided to exclude this criterion.

Diabetes mellitus diagnostic criteria of the ADA are as follows:
- HbA1c more than or equal to 6.5% (in laboratories with standardized methods)
- Fasting plasma glucose more than or equal to 126 mg/dL (fasting of at least 8 hours)
- Plasma glucose within 2 hours to be more than or equal to 200 mg/dL during an OGTT (according to the technique described by World Health Organization, using a glucose load of 75 g anhydrous dissolved in water)
- Classic symptoms of hyperglycemia or hyperglycemic crisis glucose more than or equal to 200 mg/dL.

CLASSIFICATION OF DIABETES MELLITUS

The former classification of DM based on dependency insulin was modified with the intention of eliminating denominations as insulin-dependent diabetes mellitus (IDDM) and non-insulin-dependent diabetes mellitus (NIDDM), taking into account the diversity of response to therapeutic. The current classification of DM is based on the etiology of the disease, considering that type 1 diabetes is the result of the destruction of pancreatic β-cells (autoimmune or unknown cause, etc.) and type 2 diabetes is related to the association of insulin resistance and insulin deficiency.

Etiologic Classification

- Type 1 diabetes (due to β-cell destruction, usually leading to absolute insulin deficiency)
- Type 2 diabetes (due to a progressive insulin secretory defect on the background of insulin resistance)
- Gestational diabetes mellitus (GDM) (diabetes diagnosed in the second or third trimester of pregnancy, that is not clearly overt diabetes)
- Specific types of diabetes due to other causes, e.g. monogenic diabetes syndromes [such as neonatal diabetes and maturity-onset diabetes of the young (MODY)], diseases of the exocrine pancreas (such as cystic fibrosis), and drug- or chemical-induced diabetes [such as in the treatment of human immunodeficiency virus (HIV) or acquired immune deficiency syndrome (AIDS), or after organ transplantation].

TYPE 1 DIABETES MELLITUS

Type 1 diabetes mellitus (T1DM) is characterized by the sudden onset of severe symptoms associated with the absolute deficiency of insulin secretion, tendency to ketosis, and dependence on exogenous insulin to sustain life.

The histopathology of T1DM is defined by a decreased β-cell mass in association with insulitis, a characteristic lymphocytic infiltration limited to the islets of Langerhans and prominent in early stage disease in children.

It has similar characteristics with autoimmune inflammatory processes found in certain thyroid diseases (thyroiditis) and adrenal (adrenalitis). Insulitis is characterized by infiltration and resulting disruption of islets with destruction of β-cells by T lymphocytes of various types.

Pancreatic deficiency of insulin secretion is clearly associated with this type of diabetes and is due to the specific loss of β-cells, with conservation within almost normal mass of α-cells (glucagon), δ-cell (somatostatin) and pancreatic polypeptide (PP cell). This can be demonstrated by measuring blood insulin (in patients who have not received the hormone exogenously), both fasting and basal, as to different stimuli for release (e.g. administration of glucose or glucagon). Also, measure the values of C-peptide, the residual product in the conversion of proinsulin to insulin, since it is not altered or masked by receiving replacement therapy.

Type 1 diabetes mellitus usually occurs abruptly, with overt signs of hyperglycemia, and sometimes with significant deterioration of clinical status.

Hyperglycemia is the result of destruction of 80–90% of the mass of β-cell functioning.

Only the clinical manifestation is acute. There is a silent preclinical period and can be recognized by different immunological markers that reveal the underlying autoimmune process.

Most cases of T1DM are due to the autoimmune process and the destruction of β-islet cells in genetically susceptible individuals. Type 1 diabetes secondary to the autoimmune process are called type 1a in the classification. It should be noted that not all type 1 diabetes have the same clinical evolution.

Not all individuals with pathogenic autoimmune process of T1DM progress to clinical T1DM or they do it slowly, with a prior relatively long period without insulin dependence.

Antibodies have been detected years before the onset of hyperglycemia. Functional studies, such as intravenous glucose tolerance test, reveal a decrease in the first phase of insulin secretion months or weeks before the clinical onset of the disease or the presence of fasting hyperglycemia, according to the magnitude and extent of damage caused in the β-cells.

It must be considered a preclinical period in the natural history of disease, which can be identified through different immunological and genetic markers.

Genetic Determinism

Autoimmune diabetes is a T-dependent specific organ disease, which is polygenic and mainly restricted by the human leukocyte antigen (HLA). HLA-DR (Human Leukocyte Antigen-antigen D Related) is a major histocompatibility complex class II cell surface receptor encoded by the HLA on chromosome 6 region 6p21.31. The complex of HLA-DR and its ligand, a peptide of nine amino acids in length or longer, constitutes a ligand for the T-cell receptor (TCR). HLA-DR molecules are upregulated in response to signaling.

While *HLA* genes are the most important genetic factors that determine predisposition or protection to T1DM, it is clear that predisposition is necessary, but is not enough.

It has been found that other important genes also confer susceptibility to T1DM. The variable number tandem repeat region which is adjacent to the 5' end of the insulin gene is also related to T1DM predisposition.

The gene encoding the protein CTLA-4 (Cytotoxic T Lymphocyte Antigen 4) also has importance in the determinism of T1DM.

The HLA region is located in the short arm of chromosome 6. The association between HLA and T1DM was initially demonstrated by Nerup. Patients with T1DM have DR3 and/or DR4 by 94% compared with 60% in the healthy population.

People with positive HLA-DR3 have a relative risk (RR) to develop diabetes of 6.4, and in the carriers of HLA-DR4, the RR is 3.7.

The presence of both markers increases the susceptibility to develop the disease, more than the sum of the RRs of DR3 and DR4.

There are also markers that express a lower chance of developing diabetes. There is a lower frequency of HLA-DR2 in patients with T1DM, determining an RR for the disease of 0.26, so is considered as a protection factor, so people who has this HLA is protected from developing T1DM.

HLA-DQB1 belongs to the HLA class II β-chain paralogs. This class II molecule is a heterodimer consisting of an alpha (DQA) and a β-chain (DQB), both anchored in the membrane. It plays a central role in the immune system by presenting peptides derived from extracellular proteins. Class II molecules are expressed in antigen-presenting cells (APC)—B lymphocytes, dendritic cells, and macrophages.

Different allelic variants of polymorphic gene DQB are circumscribed to the second exon of the gene and are encoding the amino terminal region of the antigen-presenting molecule.

Several alleles of HLA-DQB1 are associated with an increased risk of developing T1DM. The locus is the highest genetic risk for type 1 diabetes. Again, the DQB1*0201 and DQB1*0302 alleles, particularly the phenotype DQB1*0201/*0302, has a high risk of late onset type 1 diabetes. This nomenclature can individualize each allele with 4. The risk is partially shared with the HLA-DR locus (DR3 and DR4 serotypes) (Fig. 1).

FIGURE 1: Human leukocyte antigen (HLA).
Predisposition: HLA-DR3 (DQB*0201)/DR4 (DQB1*0301)
Proteccion: DR2 (DQB1*0602)

Autoimmunity

Type 1 diabetes mellitus can be induced by a process of autoimmunity directed against the insulin-producing β-cells. This mechanism could be triggered by certain environmental factors in genetically determined individuals. The suspicion of an autoimmune process came from the striking association between T1DM and other endocrine autoimmune diseases, such as those affecting thyroid and adrenal, as the high percentage of specific antibodies was present in the serum of patients. The first description of autoimmunity in diabetes was made in 1974, they are ICA antibodies (islet cell antibodies). ICAs are present in 0.5-1.7% of the general population and 15-30% in T1DM, but at the time of onset of the disease, in patients less than 30 years, this percentage rises to 60-85%, descending to lower values after 2-3 years.

They are immunoglobulin G class autoantibodies produced by activated T lymphocytes, are not specific to β-cell. They are determined by indirect immunofluorescence (IFA) and measured in JDF units, values under 10 UJDF are considered negative. Currently, this determination has been replaced by other antibodies described here.

The glutamic acid decarboxylase antibodies (GADA) are the most useful because of the ease of its determination. They are measured by radiobinding assay (RBA). There are two isoforms, 65 kD (specific for diabetes) and 67 kD. GAD antigen is not specific β-cell, participates in the formation of gamma-aminobutyric acid (GABA).

Islet antigen-2 (IA-2), previously also known as ICA-512, is a major target of islet cell autoantibodies.

They are present in 45-75% of the cases at the beginning of the disease. They are determined by RBA.

Insulin autoantibodies (IAA) are positive in 20-50% of patients with recent onset diabetes. They are positive previous the treatment with insulin. The use of insulin determines the presence of insulin antibodies (IA) to the exogenous insulin (IA instead of IAA) as they would be related of the exogenous antigen of the hormone injection. They are measured by RBA. They have inverse correlation with age, being more common at younger ages.

It has recently been discovered antibodies against the zinc transporter-8 islet (ZnT8-A) also predicts T1DM. ZnT8 is specifically expressed in the pancreatic β-cells and has been identified as a novel target autoantigen in patients with T1DM. Antibodies to ZnT8 have been detected in 60-80% of Caucasian and 33-58% of Asian population with T1DM.

The sensitivity and predictive capacity increase with the association of markers. The association of GADA, IA-2A and IAA determines a sensitivity of 90% and a positive predictive value close to 100% for the next 5 years (Table 2).

TABLE 2: Positive predictive value for the development of T1DM in a risk group.

Antibodies	3 years (%)	5 years (%)
GADA	28	52
IA-2A	40	81
IAA	33	59
GADA + IA-2A	45	86
3 Markers	49	100

(T1DM: Type 1 diabetes mellitus; GADA: Glutamic acid decarboxylase antibodies; IA-2A: Islet antigen-2; IAA: Insulin autoantibodies).

The appearance of autoantibodies does not follow a distinct pattern, the presence of multiple autoantibodies has the highest positive predictive value for type 1 diabetes. Autoantibodies may also provide prognostic information in clinically heterogeneous patient populations. Diabetes autoantibodies are now being used in studies of high-risk populations (first-degree relatives) as well as the general population. Following the antibodies prospectively in genetically at-risk subjects affords the opportunity to identify environmental triggers and introduce preventative measures.

These antibodies are informative markers of humoral immunity that aid in prediction, prevention, classification, and intervention strategies.

Environmental Factors

Given the evidence of the genetic predisposition for diabetes and autoimmune origin, is still in search those factors that act as trigger determining the process of aggression to the pancreas to generate diabetes.

The mechanism of action involved in environmental factors is not known precisely, but it is postulated that they may act in two different ways: (1) by direct toxicity against β-cell; and (2) triggering the autoimmune mechanism against β-cell.

Age is an important factor, being less common to develop T1DM in the first nine months of life, probably related to the protection provided by the maternal antibodies to the newborn. There is an increase in incidence at 5–6 years, a peak at 12–14 years, and a slight decrease between 20 years and 35 years comes later. There are also geographical variations, with significant differences between different areas; (e.g. in Finland, the incidence is 29.5/100,000 people per year while in Hokkaido, Japan, it is 1.6/100,000 per year). Migrant studies indicate that the incidence of T1DM has increased in population groups who have moved from a low incidence region to a high incidence area, also emphasizing the influence of environmental conditions.

There have been described factors as chemical agents and specific drugs (alloxan, streptozotocin, pentamidine and a rodenticide Vacor).

A large number of epidemiological studies were conducted to determine the influence of viral infections in the development of T1DM in humans, accepting its association mainly with four viruses: mumps, coxsackie, rubella and *Cytomegalovirus*, which would act as a trigger for immune process.

Currently, although genetic and immunological markers present, is not approved the use of immunosuppressants in the preclinical period, since is not demonstrated its safety and effectiveness, and that might be unnecessary in patients who undergo to a spontaneous remission without developing the disease.

TYPE 2 DIABETES MELLITUS

Type 2 diabetes mellitus is a chronic disease with a polygenic origin of variable expression, where environmental factors play an important role in its determinism.

The variable expression of genes implies that the presence of the predisposition not invariably determines an evolution towards the disease, and that their presence only involves the risk of developing T2DM. This risk is enhanced with some environmental factors as unhealthful food, refined carbohydrates, and barriers to physical activity and stress.

This accounts for 90 to 95% of all diabetes. This form encompasses individuals who have insulin resistance and usually relative (rather than absolute) insulin deficiency. Insulin resistance alone is insufficient to develop diabetes, so it requires the alteration in insulin secretion. The insulin resistance has two determining factors, the genetic and the environmental, which is influenced by lifestyle, diet, sedentary lifestyle, overweight, medication, etc. It is more common in adults; its onset is insidious by the lack of symptoms, being common to ignore the presence of the disease.

OTHER SPECIFIC TYPES

Among the other specific types of diabetes, it is worth noting the MODY diabetes, which is characterized by diabetes that appears early in life, but behaves like type 2 diabetes and not as type 1, is characterized by impaired insulin secretion with minimal or no defects in insulin action. It is inherited in an autosomal dominant pattern, so the sons of a person with MODY have a 50% chance of inheriting this type of diabetes.

It commonly appears before 25 years of age, usually occurs in three or more generations of the same family. It is monogenic type, with dominant inheritance.

There are six types of MODY whose recognition is difficult to perform, but is important to consider the presence of this type of DM because their treatment and prognosis differ from the T1DM.

MODY 1: Hepatocyte Nuclear Factor gene chromosome 20q 4α Liver (HNF 4α)

MODY 2: Glucokinase enzyme gene chromosome 7p (GCK)
MODY 3: Hepatocyte Nuclear Factor, gene chromosome 12q 1α Liver (HNF 1α)
MODY 4: Factor 1β Hepatic gene (chromosome 17)
MODY 5: Gene Insulin Promoter Factor-1 on chromosome 13q (IPF-1)
MODY 6: NeuroD1 transcription factor chromosome 2.

The diagnosis of monogenic diabetes should be considered in children with the following findings:
- Diabetes diagnosed within the first 6 months of life
- Strong family history of diabetes but without typical features of type 2 diabetes (nonobese, low-risk ethnic group)
- Mild fasting hyperglycemia (100–150 mg/dL [5.5–8.5 mmol/L]), especially if young and nonobese
- Diabetes with negative autoantibodies and without signs of obesity or insulin resistance.

GESTATIONAL DIABETES MELLITUS (GDM)

Gestational diabetes mellitus has been defined as any degree of glucose intolerance with onset or first recognition during pregnancy. Although most cases resolve with childbirth, the definition applies regardless of whether the condition persists after pregnancy, and does not exclude the possibility that glucose intolerance precede pregnancy. It has a prevalence of 7% with a range from 1 to 14%, depending on the population studied and the diagnostic criteria used. For the diagnosis of GDM, an oral glucose tolerance test is performed between 24 weeks and 28 weeks of pregnancy; if negative and there are risk factors for, is repeated between 31 weeks and 33 weeks. It is made with 75 g of anhydrous glucose dissolved in 375 mL of water, to be ingested in 5 minutes.

The diagnostic criteria are different according to different medical societies that are considered (Table 3).
Classical risk factors for developing gestational diabetes are:
- Polycystic ovary syndrome
- A previous diagnosis of gestational diabetes or prediabetes, IGT, or impaired fasting glycemia
- A family history revealing a first-degree relative with T2DM

TABLE 3: Gestational diabetes mellitus. Diagnostic criteria.		
	ADA 75 g OGTT	*Carpenter 100 g OGTT*
0 minutes	≥ 92 mg/dL	≥ 95 mg/dL
60 minutes	≥ 180 mg/dL	≥ 180 mg/dL
120 minutes	≥ 153 mg/dL	≥ 155 mg/dL
180 minutes	-	≥ 140 mg/dL

(OGTT: Oral glucose tolerance test; ADA: American diabetes association).

- *Maternal age:* A woman's risk factor increases as she gets older (especially for women over 35 years of age).
- Ethnicity (those with higher risk factors include African-Americans, Afro-Caribbeans, Native Americans, Hispanics, Pacific Islanders, and people originating from South Asia)
- Being overweight, obese or severely obese increases the risk by a factor 2.1, 3.6 and 8.6, respectively.
- A previous pregnancy which resulted in a child with a macrosomia [high birth weight: >90th centile or >4000 g (8 lb or 12.8 oz)]
- Previous poor obstetric history
- *Other genetic risk factors:* There are at least 10 genes where certain polymorphisms are associated with an increased risk of gestational diabetes, most notably TCF7L2.

Latent autoimmune diabetes in adults (LADA) in the classification of the ADA is not considered in this type of diabetes pathogenesis that could be included in type 1 diabetes. It is known as LADA for its acronym in English. It is characterized, as indicated by its name, by its autoimmune origin that occurs in adults, but with a less abrupt onset and may not require the use of insulin for at least 6 months period. It is important to consider this possibility in adult individuals (over 35 years) and who are not overweight. GADA determination is indicated in this group of patients, being important to understand the type of diabetes present because they tend to insulin dependence and must be distinguished from type 2 diabetic with failure to oral agents. Other antibodies that may be useful for diagnosis include IA-2A and ZnT8-A. The determination of IAA is not recommended (less frequent in adults).

CONSIDERATIONS

Diabetes is the generic name of a syndrome that is defined by a blood glucose value; however, it can be concluded that there are different causes of this condition, so should be identified the type of diabetes in a newly diagnosed diabetic patient, to understand the nature of the disease, since this knowledge will make a difference in the treatment, prognosis and complications.

BIBLIOGRAPHY

1. American Diabetes Association. Standards of medical care in diabetes-2016. Diabetes Care. 2016;39(suppl 1):S1-S106.
2. Caputo M, Cerrone GE, López AP, et al. Genotipificación del gen HLA DQB1 en diabetes autoinmune del adulto (LADA). En MEDICINA. 2005;65:235-40.
3. De Grijse J, Asanghanwa M, Nouthe B, et al. Predictive power of screening for antibodies against insulinoma-associated protein 2 beta (IA-2beta) and zinc transporter-8 to select first-degree relatives of type 1 diabetic patients with risk of rapid progression to clinical onset of the disease: implications for prevention trials. Diabetologia. 2010;53:517-24.
4. Diagnosis and Classification of Diabetes Mellitus. American Diabetes Association. Diabetes Care. 2015;38:s8-16.

5. Frechtel G, Poskus E. Diabetes mellitus autoinmune de inicio en edad infanto-juvenil y adulta. In: Montpellier (Ed). Bases racionales para el diagnóstico y tratamiento. Separata; 2005.
6. Frechtel G, Taverna M, López A. Genética molecular de la diabetes mellitus y sus complicaciones. In: Ruiz M (Ed). En Diabetes Mellitus Tercera Edición. Buenos Aires, Argentina: Editorial Akadia; 2004. pp. 61-84.
7. In't Veld P. Insulitis in human type 1 diabetes: The quest for an elusive lesion. Islets. 2011;3(4):131-8.
8. International Expert Committee. International Expert Committee report on the role of the A1C assay in the diagnosis of diabetes. Diabetes Care. 2009;32:1327-34.
9. Kawasaki E. ZnT8 and type 1 diabetes. Endocr J. 2012;59(7):531-7.
10. Mehers KL, Gillespie KM. The genetic basis for type 1 diabetes. Br Med Bull. 2008;88(1):115-29.
11. Pihoker C, Gilliam LK, Hampe CS, et al. Autoantibodies in diabetes. Diabetes. 2005;54 Suppl 2:S52-61.
12. Poskus E, Ermácora M. Los avances en Diabetes Mellitus impulsados por los inmunobiológicos recombinantes. En Bioquímica y Patología Clínica. 1998;62:18-32.
13. Poskus E. Autoinmunidad, marcadores inmunológicos en diabetes mellitus. In: Ruiz M (Ed). En Diabetes Mellitus Tercera Edición. Buenos Aires, Argentina: Editorial Akadia; 2004. pp. 20-55.
14. Reaven GM. Insulin resistance-how important is it to treat? Exp Clin Endocrinol Diabetes. 2000;108(Suppl 2):S274-80.
15. Recomendaciones para gestantes con diabetes. Conclusiones del Consenso reunido por convocatoria del Comité de Diabetes y Embarazo de la SAD. Octubre. 2008.
16. Ross G. Gestational diabetes. Australian Family Physician. 2006;35(6):392-6.
17. Skyler JS. Insulin therapy in type 1 diabetes mellitus. In: DeFronzo RA (Ed). Current Therapy of Diabetes Mellitus. Mosby; 1998. pp. 36-49.
18. Vaccaro O, Ruffa G, Imperatore G, et al. Risk of diabetes in the new diagnostic category of impaired fasting glucose: a prospective analysis. Diabetes Care. 1999; 22:1490-3.
19. Valdez SN, Iacono RF, Villalba A, et al. A radioligand-binding assay for detecting antibodies specific for proinsulin and insulin using 35S-proinsulin. J Immunol Methods. 2003;279:173-81.
20. Verge CF, Gianani R, Kawasaki E, et al. Prediction of type 1 diabetes mellitus in first-degree relatives using a combination of insulin, GAD and ICA512/IA-2 autoantibodies. Diabetes. 1996;45:926-33.
21. Wenzlau JM, Moua O, Sarkar SA, et al. SlC30A8 is a major target of humoral autoimmunity in type 1 diabetes and a predictive marker in prediabetes. Ann N Y Acad Sci. 2008;1150:256-9.
22. Yang L, Luo S, Huang G, et al. The diagnostic value of zinc transporter 8 autoantibody (ZnT8A) for type 1 diabetes in Chinese. Diabetes Metab Res Rev. 2010;26:579-84.

CHAPTER 2

Introduction to Cutaneous Manifestations of Diabetes Mellitus

Emilia Noemí Cohen Sabban

The term "diabetes" is derived from a Greek word that means "go through", that alludes to the rapid passage of liquid from ingestion to urination. Diabetic patients drink a lot due to excessive thirst. Formerly, doctors would taste the urine in order to examine it and hence, arises the word "mellitus" which comes from Latin meaning "honeyed" or "sweet" due to the presence of elevated urine glucose levels.[1]

Diabetes mellitus (DM) is a chronic endocrinopathy which affects almost every organ and system in our body; the skin-the most extensive organ of the body-is surely not an exception.

The number of people with DM has experienced a dramatic increase and its prevalence continues to rise. It may occur in individuals of all ages, races and socioeconomic status.

Although this disease and its complications have been the target of multiple investigations, cutaneous manifestations of DM remain in an area where much is still to be elucidated.[2] What is established is that the skin suffers an impact caused by this acute metabolic disorder and by the chronic degenerative complications of diabetes.[3]

Alike other complications of DM, i.e. retinopathy and nephropathy; skin manifestations are the result of combined effects of hyperglycemia, neuropathy, microangiopathy and immune alterations of the host.[4]

This clinical syndrome is caused by the lack or inadequate use (resistance) of (to) insulin; a multifunctional hormone involved in the regulation of many cellular processes. In fact, skin cells express an insulin receptor (IR) which is activated in the presence of the hormone, essential for differentiation and proliferation, and also for the normal skin metabolism.

Insulin increases or accelerates the process of differentiation, reason why the highest levels of activity are precisely found in the epithelium during proliferation or differentiation; while IR activation is minimal in terminally differentiated keratinocytes. Moreover, if there is no IR expression, the differentiation process cannot be normal. This is the reason why the absence of insulin has direct effects on our skin and results in abnormalities which, for example, lead to poor wound healing.[5,6]

Insulin production occurs in the pancreas and is necessary for glucose to be transported from the bloodstream to cells, providing them with energy.

The insulin deficit caused by DM generates a state of chronic hyperglycemia, responsible for glucose following other metabolic pathways and thus increasing:
- The polyol pathway and its consequences (lower antioxidant capacity)
- Sugar autooxidation with an exaggerated production of highly reactive free radicals (i.e. 3-glucosone)
- Nonenzymatic glycation (NEG) of proteins.

These insulin dependent pathways are responsible for the three chronic complications of DM; neuropathy, microangiopathy and macroangiopathy or atherosclerosis.[7]

A decrease in the oxide reduction ratio (NAD/NADH2) generates cellular pseudohypoxia that alters qualitatively and quantitatively the basal membranes which are thickened due to the increase in hydroxylysine and in the units of disaccharides and polysaccharides with imbalance of the proteoglycans (heparin sulfate vs chondroitin sulfate).

Concomitantly, a series of modifications in the microcirculation are produced by which at present define DM as a hypercoagulable state with the following features:
- High blood viscosity
- Loss of autoregulation of vessels
- Increased platelet adhesion and aggregation (due to imbalance between thromboxane and prostacyclin)
- Prothrombotic state:
    - Less fibrinolysis due to increase in plasminogen activator inhibitor and thrombin-activated fibrinolysis inhibitor
    - Higher thrombogenesis due to increase in fibrinogen, factor VII and von Willebrand factor.

Nonenzymatic glycation of proteins consist of the attachment of reducing sugars (ketones or aldehydes) to the amine groups of proteins, lipids and nucleic acids; which contributes to aging of different macromolecules as well as to the development and progression of vascular complications of diabetes and the appearance of insulin resistance. It occurs in two phases and aims to reduce the amount of sugar; therefore, the more sugar, the higher reactivity.

In the first phase or Amadori rearrangement, ketoamides or reversible products "Schiff base" are formed first and then more stable products with covalent bonds called Amadori products. In the second phase, late and irreversible Maillard reaction presents in the course of days to weeks; these early glycation products undergo complex reactions like realignment, dehydration and condensation in order to end up irreversibly crosslinked and at the same time forming heterogeneous derivatives that are brownish and fluorescent, and which accumulate inside and outside of cells in the membranes, in circulating and structural proteins (collagen), so called advanced glycation end products (AGEs).

In the case of long lifetime proteins like collagen, the result is a cross-linked collagen which is less soluble, more rigid and resistant to degradation by enzymes (collagenases).[8]

Under hyperglycemia circumstances or oxidative stress, like in the case of DM, NEG happens faster. There is enough evidence that indicates that the interaction between AGEs and their receptor (RAGE) cause oxidative stress with the subsequent vascular inflammation and thrombosis, so that they play a very important role in the development of vascular complications of DM. More recently, it was discovered that the relationship between AGE-RAGE is at the same time interconnected with the renin-angiotensin system and that both are involved in vascular damage.[9-11]

All these biochemical alterations are intimately related to many cutaneous manifestations of DM that is why it is so important to know them.[12]

It is estimated that 30% of diabetic patients show cutaneous manifestations with the disease. If we add lesions caused by frequent complications, like vasculopathy and neuropathy, this figure reaches almost 100%. Type II diabetes patients have a higher prevalence.

Generally, we can observe cutaneous changes in patients with diagnosed but poorly controlled DM; and in this case, a timely recognition by the dermatologist, besides a good metabolic control, can help to prevent some of these skin diseases and more severe complications. However, we must not forget that unfortunately, most of hypoglycemic drugs also produce side effects on the skin.[13]

Most of the skin manifestations are due to long-term effects caused by DM on skin collagen and microcirculation. Skin infections are more common in type II DM, while autoimmune changes can frequently be observed in cases of type I diabetes.

There is a correlation between the duration of the disease and the appearance of skin lesions; being long-standing diabetics the ones who develop more devastating skin lesions; although they can also appear in the short term. One of the groups of these dermatoses is called "cutaneous markers".[14,15] One of the groups of these dermatosis is called "skin markers" that forces us to rule out undiagnosed diabetes.

The classification of the cutaneous manifestations of DM includes, apart from cutaneous markers, skin infections in diabetics (*see* Chapter 7), dermatoses frequently associated with DM (*see* Chapter 8), cutaneous manifestations induced by antidiabetic treatment (*see* Chapter 9), and finally those resulting from vasculopathy and neuropathy (*see* Chapter 10) (Table 1).[16,17]

TABLE 1: Classification of skin manifestations in diabetes mellitus (DM).	
Group 1	DM cutaneous markers
Group 2	Skin infections
Group 3	Dermatoses most most frequently associated with DM
Group 4	Cutaneous alterations produced by DM treatment
Group 5	Cutaneous manifestations produced by vasculopathy
Group 6	Cutaneous manifestations produced by neuropathy

REFERENCES

1. Real Academia Española. Diccionario de la lengua española. Madrid: RAE; 2001.
2. Chatterjee N, Chattopadhyay C, Sengupta N, et al. An observational study of cutaneous manifestations in diabetes mellitus in a tertiary care Hospital of Eastern India. Indian J Endocrinol Metab. 2014;18(2):217-20.
3. Goyal A, Raina S, Kaushal SS, et al. Pattern of cutaneous manifestations in diabetes mellitus. Indian J Dermatol. 2010;55(1):39-41.
4. Ahmed K, Muhammad Z, Qayum I. Prevalence of cutaneous manifestations of diabetes mellitus. J Ayub Med Coll Abbottabad. 2009;21:76-9.
5. Wertheimer E. Diabetic skin complications: a need for reorganizing the categories of diabetes- associated complications. Isr Med Assoc J. 2004;6:287-9.
6. Wertheimer E, Trebicz M, Eldar T, et al. Differential roles of insulin receptor and insulin-like growth factor-1 receptor in differentiation of murine skin keratinocytes. J Invest Dermatol. 2000;115:24-9.
7. Braverman I, Keh-Yen A. Ultrastructural abnormalities of the microvasculature and elastic fibers in the skin of juvenile diabetics. J Invest Dermatol. 1984;82:270-4.
8. Cohen SE. La glicosilación no enzimática: una vía común en la diabetes y el envejecimiento. Med Cutan Ibero Lat Am. 2011;39:243-6.
9. Yamagishi S. Advanced glycation end products and receptor-oxidative stress system in diabetic vascular complications. Therapher Dial. 2009;13:534-9.
10. Yamagishi S. Role of advanced glycation end products (AGEs) and receptor for AGEs (RAGE) in vascular damage in diabetes. Exp Gerontol. 2011;46:217-24.
11. Yamagishi SI, Maeda S, Matsui T, et al. Role of advanced glycation end products (AGEs) and oxidative stress in vascular complications in diabetes. Biochim Biophys Acta. 2012;1820:663-71.
12. Huntley AC. Cutaneous manifestations of Diabetes Mellitus. Diabetes Metab Rev. 1993;9:161-76.
13. Van Hattem S, Bootsma AH, Thio HB. Skin manifestations of diabetes. Cleve Clin J Med. 2008;75:772-87.
14. Spravchikov N, Sizyakov G, Gartsbein M, et al. Glucose effects on skin keratinocytes: implications for diabetes skin complications. Diabetes. 2000;50:1627-35.
15. Ahmed I, Goldstein B. Diabetes mellitus. Clin Dermatol. 2006;24:237-46.
16. Cabo LA. Diabetes y piel [tesis doctoral]. Argentina: Facultad de Medicina, University of Buenos Aires; 1983.
17. American Diabetes Association. Standards of Medical Care in Diabetes-2009. Diabetes Care. 2009;32:13-61.

CHAPTER 3

Cutaneous Barrier and Diabetes

Patricia Troielli, Lucrecia Juarez

ALTERATIONS OF THE CUTANEOUS BARRIER IN DIABETES MELLITUS

Diabetes mellitus (DM) affects functional properties of the skin. The maintenance of both the integrity and the function of cutaneous barrier (CB) is crucial to ensure skin homeostasis and avoid common complications in diabetic patients.

Strategies to mitigate the altered effects of epidermal barrier functions in DM are reviewed in this chapter including the importance of daily care and the topical barrier repair therapy.

PHYSIOLOGY OF CUTANEOUS BARRIER

Cutaneous barrier is defined as a dynamic, functional and morphological structure made up of cells and noncellular components of the skin which provides an effective isolation of the individual from his environment. It prevents infections, maintains body temperature and electrolyte balance, avoids water loss, and limits the damage of oxidative stress and effects of ultraviolet radiation (Table 1).

The complex lipid structure that makes up the CB is regulated to keep homeostasis in the skin. The "brick and mortar" concept in which CB was considered inert and made up of corneocytes (brick filled with proteins, keratins and filaggrins from keratohyalin granules) has been outdated by new scientific evidence.

A disturbance of the epidermal barrier function induces a rapid response from the keratinocytes with upregulation of the inflammatory signal cytokines, adhesion molecules and growth factors. This leads to epidermal hyperplasia and an increase of lipid synthesis to restore normal function.

Several inflammatory diseases plus a variety of drugs and therapeutic options may delay repair or alter the kinetics of the self-maintaining process of the healthy barrier.[1]

Cutaneous Manifestations of Diabetes

TABLE 1: Cutaneous barrier functions.

Barrier	Role	Effector
Permeability	Prevent excess water loss Protects from harmful chemicals, allergens and microbial pathogens Maintains body temperature	Components of skin structure
Antimicrobial	Protects against multiple pathogens (bacteria, fungi and some viruses)	Acidic pH Sphingoid bases Innate immune (antimicrobial peptides)
Antioxidant	Protects skin from oxidative stress	Tocopherol Vitamin C-E Glutathione Ubiquinol Uric acid Small proline-rich region proteins Superoxide dismutase
UV	Protects skin from UV DNA damage Protects skin from oxidative stress	Urocanic acid Structure components

(UV: Ultraviolet; DNA: Deoxyribonucleic acid).

The physical barrier localized primarily in the stratum corneum (SC) is crucial in the activity of the epidermal permeability barrier.

The viable epidermis and outer nucleated layers also contribute to the physical barrier and are essential for skin function.

In the SC, the corneocytes produced from terminal keratinocyte differentiation build a platform of protein-enriched cells, the cornified envelope, formed through cross-linking of specific precursor proteins, including involucrin, loricrin, small proline-rich region (SPRR) proteins, transglutaminase, filaggrin and corneodesmosomes, surrounded by an enriched neutral lipid, covalently bonded into the extracellular space.

Filaggrin, the principal water ligand compound, is a component of the natural moisturizing factor (NMF) and cross-linked to the cornified envelope and aggregates keratin filaments into macrofibrils.

The enriched neutral lipid-lamellar membranes localized in the extracellular spaces of the SC are synthesized in the keratinocytes as lamellar bodies (LBs) during epidermal differentiation.

Lamellar bodies are secretory organelles 0.2 Å ~ 0.3 µ with a predominant role in the maintenance of cutaneous permeability and other activities such as antimicrobial, chemical defense and movement of molecules and proteins from intra- to extracellular space.

They are first observed in the upper stratum spinosum layer of the epidermis, with increasing numbers found in the stratum granulosum layer.

They contain phospholipids, glucosylceramides, sphingomyelin, cholesterol and several enzymes. These precursor lipids are converted into nonpolar lipid products by enzymes (Fig. 1).

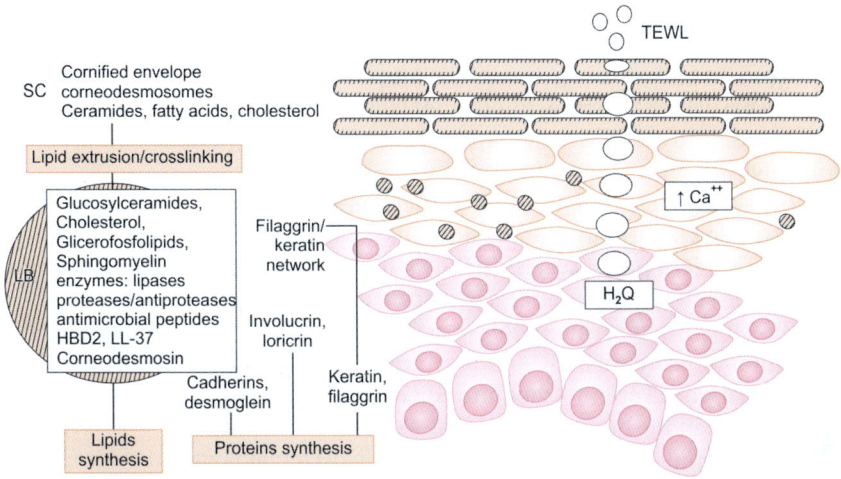

Fig. 1: Cutaneous barrier.
(LB: Lamellar bodies; SC: Stratum corneum; TEWL: Transepidermal water loss; HBD2: Human beta-defensin 2).

Beta-glucocerebrosidase converts glucosylceramides into ceramides, phospholipases convert phospholipids into free fatty acids and glycerol acidic sphingomyelinase converts sphingomyelin into ceramides.

In addition, others enzymes, proteases such as chemotryptic enzymes (kallikreins) and cathepsins, are present in LBs. Enzyme inhibitors such as the serine protease inhibitor and elafin are also packaged into LBs.

Moreover, antimicrobial peptides, such as human beta defensin 2 (HBD2) and the cathelicidin LL-37 are also present in LBs.[2-5]

The SC contains an abundance of cholesterol from the LB, and cholesterol sulfate, that is converted into cholesterol by the cholesterol sulfatase enzyme, which plays an important role in regulating SC cohesion and desquamation.

Lipids, cholesterol, ceramides and fatty acids must be present in appropriate distribution in stratum granulosum cells in order to synthesize structurally normal LB. Altered metabolism, either in excess or a deficiency of a particular lipid can result in abnormal lamellar bilayer formation and affect normal skin function.

The extracellular processing of lipids leads to a balance of 50% ceramides, 25% cholesterol, and 15% free fatty acids with very little phospholipid.

Topically applied lipids may interfere with the skin barrier function and treatment with formulations containing physiological lipids, such as cholesterol, ceramide 3, oleic acid and palmitic acid, are suggested as strategy to recover dry skin and inflammatory disorders.[6-9]

Lipids required for LB formation are derived from de novo synthesis by keratinocytes and from extracutaneous sources not as yet completely identified.

Impaired nutritional status may alter the structural integrity of the skin as well as a proper nutritional intake. The intake of Ca and vitamin C complements endogenous factors in regulating skin barrier function.[10]

The pH of the skin surface and outer layers is acidic with a pH range from 5 to 5.5 leading to a defense environment against invading organisms and allows for activity of several enzymes in the SC.

The acidic pH stimulates sphingomyelinase and beta-glucocerebrosidase activity, allowing a normal regulation of ceramide level; and blocks others enzymes such as proteases that need an optimum pH 7 or higher to increase proteolytic activity and induce corneocyte desquamation.

The increase in serine protease activity with pH 7 or higher leads to the activation of protease activated receptor 2 (PAR-2) which can increase the differentiation of keratinocytes into corneocytes and inhibit LB secretion with severe effect in the homeostasis of the skin.

The importance of preserving an acidic skin pH remains an under-recognized topic.

The pH increases and there is ceramide deficiency in skin of elderly patients.[11] This is explained by increase in levels of activity of alkaline enzymes, like alkaline ceramidase that is involved in barrier lipid degradation in aged human skin.

Alteration of pH predisposes for infectious pathologies. Candidal intertrigo is more frequent in intertriginous areas with higher pH than with other skin sites.

Diabetics are prone to develop Candidal intertrigo and has been reported that pH was significantly higher in the intertriginous zones of noninsulin-dependent diabetics compared to healthy individuals.[12,13]

Permeability Barrier

The SC functions as an outside-in barrier against foreign insults as well as an inside-out barrier to keep skin hydrated.

Draelos, in 2012, pointed out that the level of skin hydration is dependent on four factors:
1. Presence of natural hygroscopic agents, the NMF within the corneocytes
2. Presence of endogenous glycerol as a natural moisturizer and of hyaluronic acid in the epidermis and dermis
3. Ordered lamellar arrangement of intercellular lipids in the SC that form a barrier to transepidermal water loss
4. Presence of tight junctions within the stratum granulosum to further impede water loss.

There is not enough evidence to avow that diabetic patients have a specific alteration of CB.

Dry skin can be a symptom in a number of systemic diseases such as psoriasis, diabetes and renal transplantation. The mechanism of xerosis in these disorders is not yet fully understood.

Amino acids play an important role in maintaining an optimal hydration state of SC as a component of the NMF.

These groups of small hydrophilic compounds account for 5–30% of the total dry weight of SC and are the main components to which water binds directly. Small amounts of bound water is associated with the hydrophilic polar groups of intercellular lipids such as sphingomyelin and corneocytes.

Arginine, a major component of filaggrin-derived NMFs is concentrated in the middle layer of the SC, suggesting that this layer functions in skin hydration. The upper SC works like a "sponge" where solutes (e.g. ions contained in sweat or antimicrobial molecules) flow in and some are retained. The low arginine levels in the upper SC are probably due to further metabolic modification, i.e. citrullination or direct loss to the external environment.[14]

Take off sweat also contains several NMFs, lactate, urea, sodium, and potassium. Lactate and potassium significantly affect the hydration state of SC and reduced sweat delivery to the SC may cause xerosis in several chronic diseases.[15]

A case-control study found no difference in SC hydration and transepidermal water loss between diabetics and controls.[16]

On the other hand, studies such as Seirafi and colleagues suggest that patients with DM tend to show a normal hydration state with decreased sebaceous and sweat gland activity and impaired skin elasticity without impairment of the SC barrier function.[17]

It has been proven that hydration state of SC and lipids on the surface of skin of diabetics decreases with glycemic index over 110 mg/dL.

A long-standing hyperglycemia condition impairs skin barrier by accelerating skin ageing process.

Insulin plays a decisive role in homeostasis of the skin. Epidermis constitutes a glycolytic tissue. Insulin receptors of keratinocytes make up the system of insulin uptake which regulates the glycemic level in epidermal cells thus allowing to induce transitory states of hyperglycemia.[18]

The properties of the SC in patients with DM have similarities to senile xerosis. Studies show that diabetic rats have normal levels of ceramides and amino acids but show low levels of triglycerides in SC.[19]

The epidermal barrier retains moisture, regulates water flux, and modifies the rate and magnitude of transepidermal water loss (TEWL).

Nowadays, CB recovery and inflammation are instrumentally monitored as transepidermal water loss and skin blood flow using the evaporimeter and laser-Doppler flowmeter, respectively.

Pathological states of skin may be detected by measuring the TEWL rate.

The barrier has the ability to detect at an early stage homeostatic abnormalities through mild increase in the TEWL. The alteration of the Ca^{+2} gradient, the loss of elevated Ca^{+2} in the granular layer is the signal that induces in a few minutes the physiological self-repair mechanism by releasing the lipid stored in the SC. It increases the production of filaggrin and byproducts of degradation to free amino acids. These pyrrolidone carboxylic acid and urocanic acid with sugar ions form the NMF to restore hydration.

Dermatologic conditions or metabolic diseases with permeability barrier impairment diminish the capacity to adapt to different exogenous physical, infectious and chemical insults. The self-repair mechanism is not able to keep up with the magnitude or velocity to restore normal function, and without therapeutic intervention, the progression of xerosis leads to dry skin with different signs and symptoms of inflammation and infection.

Antimicrobial Barrier

Keratinocytes participate in the innate immune response of the skin. They produce lipids, peptides with antimicrobial activity, chemokines and cytokines. It also expresses receptors as toll-like receptors. Several antimicrobial peptides are extruded from the LB to the extracellular space in the SC.[3]

There are four types of β-defensins predominantly expressed in the skin that have potent antimicrobial activity against gram-positive and gram-negative bacteria, yeast, viruses and also α-cathelicidin, human cationic antimicrobial protein, the S100 protein, psoriasin and an antimicrobial RNase, RNase 7.

Recent studies demonstrated that ceramide metabolites, ceramide-1-phosphate and sphingosine-1-phosphate produced in human keratinocytes in response to subtoxic levels of endoplasmic reticulum stress stimulate production of these major epidermal innate immune elements, β-defensins and cathelicidin antimicrobial peptide via STAT1/3- or NF-κB-dependent mechanisms, respectively.

However, patients with type 2 diabetes have lower levels of *CAMP* (LL-37) and *DEFB4* (HBD-2) gene expression in peripheral blood cells which probably makes them susceptible to infectious diseases. Furthermore, it has been reported that the expression of DEFB4 is lower in diabetic foot ulcers in comparison with healthy skin suggesting that low levels of this peptide contribute to poor wound healing in diabetic patients.[20,21]

There is evidence that psychosocial stress affects the immune response, barrier function, wound healing and resistance to infection of healthy skin. Psychosocial stress results in a delay in barrier recovery and impairs the expression and the production of antimicrobial peptides, predisposing to cutaneous infection.[22]

Chronic psychosocial stress skews the immune response from a predominantly Th1 to a Th2 phenotype and disrupts barrier function via glucocorticoid-induced inhibition of epidermal lipid synthesis, which consequently impairs LB formation and decreases the size and density of corneodesmosomes.

Antioxidant Barrier

Reactive oxygen species (ROS) contribute to the processes of skin ageing and impaired skin barrier function.

The ROS are particularly harmful in that they destabilize other molecules and promote chain reactions that damage biomolecules rapidly, such as telomere shortening and deterioration, mitochondrial damage, membrane degradation and oxidation of structural and enzymatic proteins.[23,24]

The affectation of CB leads to an altered antioxidant capacity and subnormal functions.

The load of ROS in the skin is higher than in any other organ and in many cases a clear correlation between the ROS originating from internal and external insults and a proaging effect can be found.

The skin is at the interface between the body and the environment and is therefore in constant contact with pollutants, xenobiotics, and ultraviolet (UV) irradiation. These exogenous factors represent the main contributor to the formation of ROS in human skin, therefore being very specific for this organ. Additionally, alcohol intake, nutritional factors and physiological and mechanical stress are believed to contribute to this kind of ROS production. In addition, the skin is also one of the very few organs that are in direct contact with atmospheric oxygen which can contibute to ROS formation.

The sources of ROS, enzymatic as well as nonenzymatic, in the cell are manifold. Enzymes that are ROS producing, on purpose or as a byproduct, include the mitochondrial electron transport chain, NADPH oxidases, xanthine oxidoreductase, several peroxisomal oxidases, enzymes of the cytochrome P450 family, cyclooxygenases, and lipoxygenases.

To deal with the production of ROS, there are, in the skin, specific antioxidant mechanisms present at intra- and extracellular level.

Most of the antioxidants are at higher concentration in the epidermis than in the dermis. This correlates well with the fact that the ROS load is higher in the epidermis than in the dermis. Vitamin C, vitamin E, glutathione, ubiquinol, and uric acid are detectable in the SC but their concentration increases steeply towards deeper cell-layers of the SC. These comparably low concentrations of nonenzymatic and lipophilic antioxidants in the outer layers of the SC are possible because the cornified envelope itself has antioxidative capabilities. These antioxidative capabilities of the cornified envelope rely on the SPRR proteins.

The highest concentrations of enzymes and antioxidants are found in the stratum granulosum constantly declining towards the stratum basale. In this way, the suprabasal cells have lower ROS levels and are protected against UVB-induced apoptosis. The importance of the SC as an antioxidant/UV barrier is also stressed by the fact that UV can completely deplete the SC of antioxidants/vitamins. Therefore, only the remaining SC proteins (mainly SPRR2 subfamily) can exert their antioxidative properties and protect the epidermal cells.

The formation of structures known as advanced glycation end-products (AGEs) is another problematic process that can be significantly accelerated by oxidative stress. AGEs originate from the nonenzymatic glycation reaction between sugars and proteins, nucleic acids or lipids. AGEs are a very heterogeneous group of molecules and can either be ingested through food consumption or formed inside the cell. Diabetic patients have higher concentrations of AGEs.

The AGE products are implicated in the functional microangiopathy, secondary to the increased blood cell viscosity and the consecutive reduction in blood flow. The peripheral neuropathy adds its functional effects to the glycation process and the combination increases their clinical signs.

In addition, glycation alters some physicochemical characteristics of the fibrous collagen and glycation is further responsible for a yellowish hue of the skin and nails. Skin glycation creates new molecular residues and induces cross-links in the extracellular matrix of the dermis. The formation of such cross-links between macromolecules contributes to altered elasticity and the modification of other physical characteristics of the dermis in DM patients, similar to those observed during intrinsic aging and photoaging.

Some glycation inhibitors have been described. Aminoguanidine is probably the most widely used glycation inhibitor. Other compounds, including resveratrol, carnosine, and blueberry extract, exhibit some in vitro antiglycation activity. Nevertheless, studies evaluating the impact of topical products containing AGE inhibitor on the improvement of DM skin are currently missing.

Ultraviolet Barrier

Photon energy carried in UV (particularly UVB at 280-315 nm, and UVA at 315-400 nm) induces alterations that accumulate and promote the majority of the typical manifestations of skin ageing and cancer. UVB makes up only 5% of the UV radiation that reaches the surface of earth and has little penetrance but it displays great biological activity. UVA makes up the remaining 95% of incident light and is more penetrating, promoting photoaging. However, UVA carries less energy and therefore promotes carcinogenesis to a lower extent than UVB.

The main effects of acute and chronic exposure to UV radiation are DNA (deoxyribonucleic acid) damage, inflammation and immunosuppression. These effects are direct as well as indirect due to ROS production.[24]

ALTERATIONS IN CUTANEOUS BARRIER IN DIABETICS: DERMOCOSMETIC MANAGEMENT

The aim of the dermocosmetic management of the CB of diabetic patients is to prevent and improve early stage of loss of integrity of the skin and reestablish normal hydration in order to mitigate the action of internal and external factors which influence the antimicrobial, antioxidant and ultraviolet radiation protective functions. The therapeutic intervention involves a multidisciplinary approach: clinical, aesthetic and oncological dermatology.

It is essential to know the physiology of CB and skin ageing in DM in order to advise and provide proper treatments that will improve the quality of life of the patients.

Alterations of Permeability

One of the most common skin manifestations of DM is xerosis (dry skin) which varies in clinical symptoms severity.

Diabetes and dry skin is a well-documented association.[13] The presence of microvascular complications is related to its development in insulin-dependent patients.

The term "dry skin" is used to refer to clinically dehydrated, rough and scaly skin. It happens when there is an alteration in the process of cornification resulting in hyperkeratosis, scaling and abnormalities in the function of SC. It may be seen in all the cutaneous surface although it is mostly present in feet, pretibial areas and cheeks. Clinical manifestations include light roughness to major scaling with large plaques.

Xerosis is due to not only alterations innate to diabetes but to skin ageing due to old age and associated pathologies as well.[11-25] Therefore, people with diabetes have dry skin due to multifactorial origins. Some of the most ordinary causes of xerosis (also called xeroderma) are listed in Table 2.

It is important to point out the external factors that influence the degree of affectation such as use of medicines, environmental pollution, exposure to sun, diet, and smoking.

Moisturizing and keratolytic agents are useful to treat dry skin. Diabetic patients with dry skin are specially predisposed to skin infections. That is why it is sometimes necessary to prescribe topical antibiotics.[26]

Creams containing lipids and substances as urea are most commonly used.

TABLE 2: Differential diagnosis of xerosis.

Malignancy	Lymphoproliferative diseases
Autoimmune/inflammatory disease	Systemic lupus erythematosus Dermatomyositis Sarcoidosis Eosinophilic fascitis
Nutritional disease	Malnutrition Malabsorption (celiac disease/pancreatic insufficiency)
Metabolic disease	Diabetes Chronic renal failure Chronic hepatic dysfunction Hypothyroidism Hyperparathyroidism Hypopituitarism
Infectious disease	AIDS HTLV-I, HTLV-II Leprosy
Neurologic	Sympathectomy
Medications	Statins Calcium channel blockers Cimetidine Nicotinic acid

(HTLV: Human T-lymphotropic virus; AIDS: Acquired immunodeficiency syndrome).

Lipids are divided according to their way of action as physiological and nonphysiological.[7]

TOPICAL TREATMENT WITH LIPIDS

Nonphysiological Lipids

They are not usually found in LBs. They fill up extracellular spaces of SC. They are hydrophobic and block water movement and electrolytes.

These nonphysiological lipids may quickly restore normal permeability of CB but only partially and without correcting the abnormality that originated it. Petrolate (Vaseline), lanolin, bees wax, etc. are some examples of these.

Physiological Lipids

They are lipids or precursors that are usually found in LBs (cholesterol, free fatty acids and ceramides). These lipids are carried through SC to cells of granular stratum where they mix with the pool of endogenous lipids and join the LBs (Fig. 2).

Ceramides make up 50% of intercellular lipids in the epidermis and are molecules often added to moisturizing creams.[8]

Topical treatments with exogenous physiological lipids help reestablish both normal permeability of CB and antimicrobial function.[27]

Antimicrobial peptides are packed into LBs to be released later into extracellular space of SC. The availability of exogenous lipids allows for the increase of production and release of these peptides.

A particularly interesting physiological lipid present in some creams for treatment of xerosis is N-palmitoylethanolamine. It acts at a cutaneous level as agonist to cannabinoid receptor. These receptors play a role in the modulation

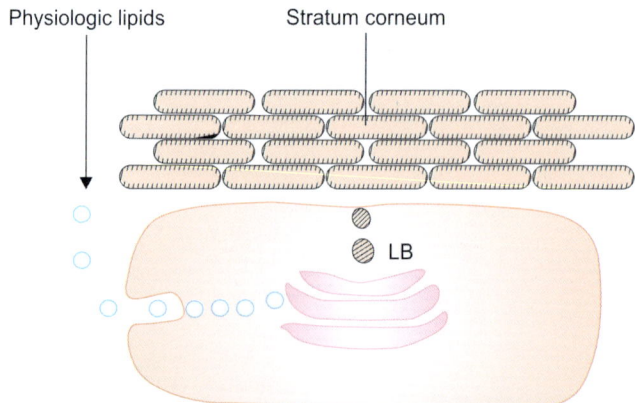

Fig. 2: Physiologic lipids traverse the stratum corneum, enter the nucleated cell layers, targeting the lamellar body (LB) secretory system.

of nociceptive symptoms. Its topical use has shown to be of great use in clinical studies to relieve chronic pruritus of various origins and in the treatment of postherpetic neuralgia.[28,29]

It may be useful to apply a mixture of physiological and nonphysiological lipids, as the response of physiological lipids is slow while nonphysiological ones, such as petrolate, result in partial improvement in permeability of CB almost at once.

TOPICAL TREATMENT WITH UREA

Urea is an organic compound whose chemical structure is made up of a carbonile group joined to two amino residues. Urea plays a very important physiological role in metabolism and excretion of nitrogenated products.

Topical urea is an effective therapeutic option in dry skin patients.[30,31]

The action mechanism of urea in skin is still not fully understood. Studies suggest that the keratolytic and moisturizing effects of urea are due to the rupture of hydrogen bridges in the SC which allows for the rupture of keratin molecules and increases the amount of sites available for the unity of water molecules. This aids restoration of altered CB and contributes to the scaling of normal skin.

There is evidence that urea also has antimicrobial properties, Grether and colleagues have shown that topical applications of urea at 20% improves the function of CB and increases the expression of antimicrobial peptides in normal skin.[30]

The urea uptake is followed by regulatory events such as expression of urea transporting elements and critical genes for the function of CB. These genes impact on the differentiation of keratinocytes, synthesis of lipids and production of antimicrobial peptides.

Urea is particularly interesting for use in diabetic patients as moisturizer and restorer. The ideal concentration is 20% and may be prescribed at 40% considering its keratolytic effect in patients with hyperkeratosis, e.g. plantar. Severe hyperkeratoses are recommended to use it under occlusion.

Urea shows excellent efficacy and safe profile although some patients may experience burning or stinging sensation in first days of use.[32]

ANTIOXIDANTS AND SUNSCREENS

Oxidative stress and action of AGEs are two processes that contribute to the impairment of CB function.[24]

Besides, they are directly and indirectly related to the mechanisms that lead to photoaging and photocarcinogenesis which impact on the physical and mental health of patients.

Photoprotection diminishes ROS generated by UV radiation, partially prevents direct damage of cellular DNA, inflammation, immunosuppression and remodeling of extracellular matrix.

There is scientific evidence showing that the use of sunscreens and topical antioxidants produce a combined effect greater than the use of one of them on its own.

Antioxidants should be applied before sunscreen. Examples of most commonly used antioxidants are detailed in Table 3.

Sunscreens should have a broad spectrum protection, higher than SPF 30, that protects against UVB and UVA rays. Dry skin can benefit from moisturizing sunscreens. These products include lanolin, oils and dimethicone and are often formulated as cream, lotions or ointments. Otherwise, advise patients to apply moisturizing cream.

Most broad spectrum formulas contain antioxidant ingredients.

Patients are motivated by the antiaging and cancer prevention benefits of daily sunscreen and antioxidant use, so explaining these advantages increases adherence to the treatment and improves the health-care setting.

PRURITUS

Pruritus is defined as an unpleasant sensation which results in scratching and may have an impact on a person's quality of life. It is a common symptom in diabetic patients caused by alteration of CB present in diabetes coupled to conditions associated to xerosis like age, nephropathy, use of medicines, etc. (Table 2). These conditions cause itching due to inflammation, dry skin, or xerosis.

Diabetic polyneuropathy is a very common cause of neuropathic pruritus. This type of pruritus flares when there is an alteration in the function of a nerve due to impairment or inflammation. Diabetic patients with neuropathy usually experience pain and/or itching in symmetrical distribution. Initially, it affects lower limbs and then extends to proximities. These symptoms have also been shown as chronic trunk pruritus and localized in scalp.

TABLE 3: Commonly used antioxidants.

Molecule	Role
Vitamin C	Suppresses ultraviolet production of free radicals Attenuates ultraviolet damage in the skin Promotes cutaneous wound healing Increase epidermal moisture content
Vitamin E	Suppresses lipid peroxidation Modulates photoaging Exhibit anti-inflammatory roles
Polyphenols (phytochemical derivatives) • Flavonoids: tea, soy, grape seed • Non-flavonoids: grape, tea, polypodium leucotomos, nuts, peanuts	Antioxidants, anti-inflammatory and immunomodulatory action

The management of this symptom is of outmost importance, preventing the itch-scratch cycle. Scratching worsens the alteration already present in CB leading to chronic inflammation and infections.

PSYCHOSOCIAL STRESS

Mental health in diabetic patients may be affected by psychological processes such as anger, denial, depression, stress, diabetic distress (stress generated by having the disease). These conditions alter the quality of life and impact the physical and mental health of the patients.[33]

The skin responds to stress in two main ways: central and peripheric. The central way corresponds to hypothalamic-pituitary-adrenal (HPA) axis, the locus ceruleus-norepinephrine sympathetic adrenomedullary system. The peripheral equivalent refers to intracutaneous HPA axis and release of mediators from peripheral sensory and autonomic nerves. Activation of these two ways affects the cutaneous immune system, the CB function, healing and susceptibility to infections.[22]

Studies carried out on animals and humans show that psychological stress alters the synthesis of epidermic lipids. Recovery of CB function from any disturbance of the skin is delayed during periods of stress compared to periods of low stress. Moreover, it has been proven that psychosocial stress decreases the expression and release of antimicrobial peptides in the epidermis, increasing the risk of infection.

DIET

A healthy diet contributes to adequate metabolic control of glycemia and several associated risk factors and may also benefit the activity and physiology of CB.

A diet rich in natural antioxidants, low in AGEs and with adequate intake of water will maximize the effects of dermatology treatments.

OVERVIEW OF MEASURES

Diabetic patients must avoid cold air, low environmental humidity, excessive contact with water (e.g. long baths) that impair xerosis, particularly in winter time.

Frequent use of soap or products for body drying such as powders or gels contribute to the onset of xerosis and associated pruritus; therefore, the use of soaps with moisturizers or soap substitutes (syndet) is highly recommended.

Baths should not be longer than 10 minutes and taken only with warm water. It is convenient to apply moisturizing cream immediately after the bath and several times during the day to ensure proper moisturizing.

Low winter temperatures, dry weather and heating worsen xerosis, so the use of humidifiers may be useful.

Adequate therapy for the correct function of CB must include, besides moisturizing creams, the use of sunscreens and topical antioxidants in areas exposed to sunlight.

CONCLUSION

- Alteration of CB in diabetes is due to diabetes per se and multiple factors such as aging, physical and mental associated diseases, use of some drugs, and environmental insults.
- It is crucial to preserve the integrity of CB of all diabetic patients, not only of those with visible xerosis.
- Patients must be taught to care for their skin and the relevance of adequate habits to avoid xerosis and mitigate damage from external factors.
- This will reduce water loss and minimize the exposure to irritating and allergenic factors.
- Symptoms such as pruritus and xerosis may alter quality of life and generate complications in the form of infections.

REFERENCES

1. Del Rosso JQ, Levin J. The clinical relevance of maintaining the functional integrity of the stratum corneum in both healthy and disease-affected skin. J Clin Aesthet Dermatol. 2011;4(9):22-42.
2. Feingold KR, Elias PM. Role of lipids in the formation and maintenance of the cutaneous permeability barrier. Biochim Biophys Acta. 2014;1841(3): 280-94.
3. Elias PM. Stratum corneum defensive functions: an integrated view. J Invest Dermatol. 2005;125(2):183-200.
4. Matsui T, Amagai M. Dissecting the formation, structure and barrier function of the stratum corneum. Int Immunol. 2015;27(6):269-80.
5. Feingold KR. Lamellar bodies: the key to cutaneous barrier function. J Invest Dermatol. 2012;132(8):1951-3.
6. Lodén M, Bárány E. Skin-identical lipids versus petrolatum in the treatment of tape-stripped and detergent-perturbed human skin. Acta Derm Venereol. 2000;80(6):412-5.
7. Feingold KR, Elias PM. Role of lipids in the formation and maintenance of the cutaneous permeability barrier.Biochim Biophys Acta. 2014;1841(3): 280-94.
8. Meckfessel MH, Brandt S. The structure, function, and importance of ceramides in skin and their use as therapeutic agents in skin-care products. J Am Acad Dermatol. 2014;71(1):177-84.
9. Piérard GE, Piérard-Franchimont C, Scheen A. Critical assessment of diabetic xerosis. Expert Opin Med Diagn. 2013;7(2):201-7.
10. Park K. Role of micronutrients in skin health and function. Biomol Ther (Seoul). 2015;23(3):207-17.
11. Garibyan L, Chiou AS, Elmariah SB. Advanced aging skin and itch: addressing an unmet need. Dermatol Ther. 2013;26(2):92-103.

12. Ali SM, Yosipovitch G. Skin pH: from basic science to basic skin care. Acta Derm Venereol. 2013;93(3):261-7.
13. Demirseren DD, Emre S, Akoglu G, et al. Relationship between skin diseases and extracutaneous complications of diabetes mellitus: clinical analysis of 750 patients. Am J Clin Dermatol. 2014;15(1):65-70.
14. Kubo A, Ishizaki I, Kubo A, et al. The stratum corneum comprises three layers with distinct metal-ion barrier properties. Sci Rep. 2013;3:1731.
15. Watabe A, Sugawara T, Kikuchi K, et al. Sweat constitutes several natural moisturizing factors, lactate, urea, sodium, and potassium. J Dermatol Sci. 2013;72(2):177-82.
16. Sakai S, Kikuchi K, Satoh J, et al. Functional properties of the stratum corneum in patients with diabetes mellitus: similarities to senile xerosis. Br J Dermatol. 2005;153(2):319-23.
17. Seirafi H, Farsinejad K, Firooz A, et al. Biophysical characteristics of skin in diabetes: a controlled study. J Eur Acad Dermatol Venereol. 2009;23(2): 146-9.
18. Park HY, Kim JH, Jung M, et al. A long-standing hyperglycaemic condition impairs skin barrier by accelerating skin ageing process. Exp Dermatol. 2011;20(12):969-74.
19. Lehman PA, Franz TJ. Effect of induced acute diabetes and insulin therapy on stratum corneum barrier function in rat skin. Skin Pharmacol Physiol. 2014;27(5):249-53.
20. Gonzalez-Curiel I, Trujillo V, Montoya-Rosales A, et al. 1,25-dihydroxyvitamin D3 induces LL-37 and HBD-2 production in keratinocytes from diabetic foot ulcers promoting wound healing: an in vitro model. PLoS One. 2014;9(10): e111355.
21. Lan CC, Wu CS, Huang SM, et al. High-Glucose Environment Inhibits p38 MAPK Signaling and Reduces Human β-Defensin-3 Expression [corrected] in Keratinocytes. Mol Med. 2011;17(7-8):771-9.
22. Hunter HJ, Momen SE, Kleyn CE. The impact of psychosocial stress on healthy skin. Clin Exp Dermatol. 2015;40(5):540-6.
23. Bosch R, Philips N, Suárez-Pérez JA, et al. Mechanisms of Photoaging and Cutaneous Photocarcinogenesis, and Photoprotective Strategies with Phytochemicals. Antioxidants (Basel). 2015;4(2):248-68.
24. Rinnerthaler M, Bischof J, Streubel MK, et al. Oxidative stress in aging human skin. Biomolecules. 2015;5(2):545-89.
25. Patel N, Spencer LA, English JC 3rd, et al. Acquired ichthyosis. J Am Acad Dermatol. 2006;55(4):647-56.
26. Piérard GE, Seité S, Hermanns-Lê T, et al. The skin landscape in diabetes mellitus. Focus on dermocosmetic management. Clin Cosmet Investig Dermatol. 2013;6:127-35.
27. Seité S, Khemis A, Rougier A, et al. Importance of treatment of skin xerosis in diabetes. J Eur Acad Dermatol Venereol. 2011;25(5):607-9.
28. Ständer S, Reinhardt HW, Luger TA. [Topical cannabinoid agonists. An effective new possibility for treating chronic pruritus]. Hautarzt. 2006;57(9):801-7.
29. Phan NQ, Siepmann D, Gralow I, et al. Adjuvant topical therapy with a cannabinoid receptor agonist in facial postherpetic neuralgia. J Dtsch Dermatol Ges. 2010;8(2):88-91.

30. Grether-Beck S, Felsner I, Brenden H, et al. Urea uptake enhances barrier function and antimicrobial defense in humans by regulating epidermal gene expression. J Invest Dermatol. 2012;132(6):1561-72.
31. Pan M, Heinecke G, Bernardo S, et al. Urea: a comprehensive review of the clinical literature. Dermatol Online J. 2013;19(11):20392.
32. Federici A, Federici G, Milani M. Use of a urea, arginine and carnosine cream versus a standard emollient glycerol cream for treatment of severe xerosis of the feet in patients with type 2 diabetes: a randomized, 8 month, assessor-blinded, controlled trial. Curr Med Res Opin. 2015;31(6):1063-9.
33. American Diabetes Associaton. [online] Available from www.diabetes.org [Accesssed January 2017].

CHAPTER

4

Cutaneous Markers of Diabetes Mellitus

Emilia Noemí Cohen Sabban

INTRODUCTION

Diabetes mellitus (DM) has a wide array of cutaneous manifestations which constitute, on the whole, a variety of disorders resulting mostly from long-lasting diabetes, and which impact significantly the patient's morbidity and mortality.

Many theories have been proposed to explain the way in which hyperglycemia can produce neuronal and vascular disorders which are a landmark of this disease. They can be separated into those that emphasize the direct toxic effect of hyperglycemia and its derivatives on the tissue (i.e. oxidants, hyperosmolarity or glycosylated products), where the skin would not be an exception; and those that give pathophysiological importance to a sustained disturbance of cell signaling pathways (i.e. changes in phospholipids or kinases) induced by products of the glucose metabolism.[1,2]

Cutaneous markers of DM are a heterogeneous group of skin diseases (dermatoses) that help us to rule out an underlying DM. Even though, there is still controversy in the literature regarding which of these cutaneous disorders present more frequently in one or another type of diabetes; no statistically significant differences were found between them in different studies of a wide series of cases.[3,4]

What is uniformly established is the fact that some of these cutaneous manifestations increase their incidence in longlasting DM, such as, diabetic dermopathy (DD) and spontaneous diabetic blister (DB), diabetic foot and gangrene.[5,6]

NECROBIOSIS LIPOIDICA

Necrobiosis lipoidica (NL) is a chronic granulomatous skin disease that affects 0.3–1.2% of type I and II diabetic patients. Lesions favor young women between 30 years and 40 years, are asymptomatic and are characteristically found on anterior and lateral surfaces of lower legs (i.e. pretibial region); although they may also be present on arms, on the trunk, the face and the scalp (Fig. 1). In 60% of the cases, it occurs in individuals with diagnosed DM. In case the diagnosis is not confirmed, it is necessary to follow up on a yearly basis for a DM diagnosis, since NL can be the first manifestation of this condition.

Different causative factors have been proposed for NL: microangiopathy, endarteritis obliterans, vasculitis, immunological mechanisms, delayed hypersensitivity, nonenzymatic glycation (NEG), trauma, platelet aggregation, alteration of neutrophil mobility and vascular occlusion with subsequent venous insufficiency. Vascular compromise is one of the main causative factors, with vessels thickening and occlusion due to glycoprotein deposits. The upregulation of GLUT-1 (glucose transporter of erythrocytes) receptor in fibroblasts, detected through immunohistochemistry, indicates that the abnormalities in glucose transportation in these cells could explain some NL findings.[7]

Clinically, they start as small erythematous well-defined nodules, which slowly enlarge forming plaques with elevated edges whereas the center is flattened and atrophic, through their surface, the underlying vessels are visible (Figs. 2 to 4). These lesions can be single or multiple, unilateral or bilateral (Figs. 5 to 7).[8]

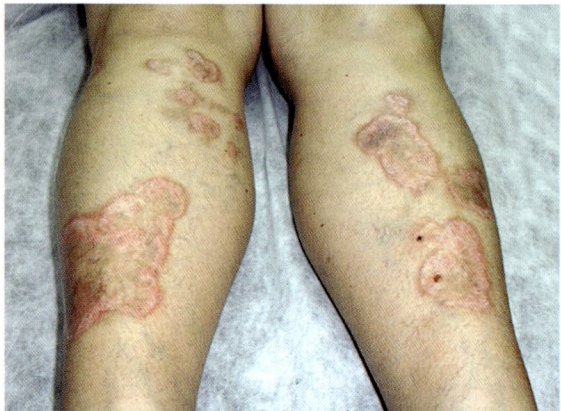

Fig. 1: Multiple plaques of necrobiosis lipoidica on pretibial region.

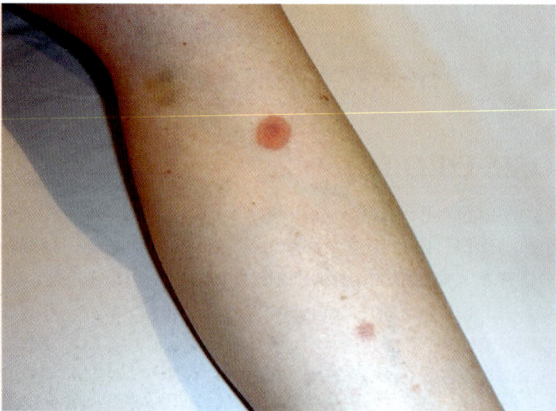

Fig. 2: Erythematous nodules. Initial form of necrobiosis lipoidica.

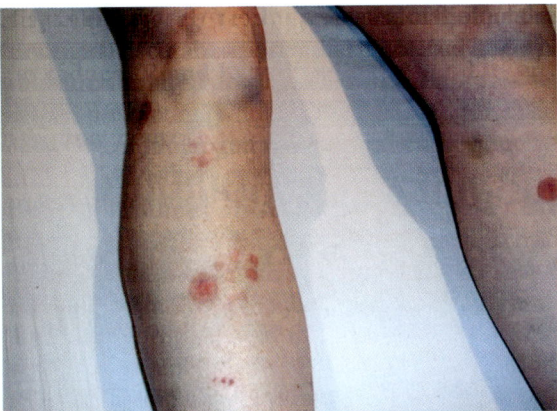

Fig. 3: Erythematous lesions and nodules of necrobiosis lipoidica.

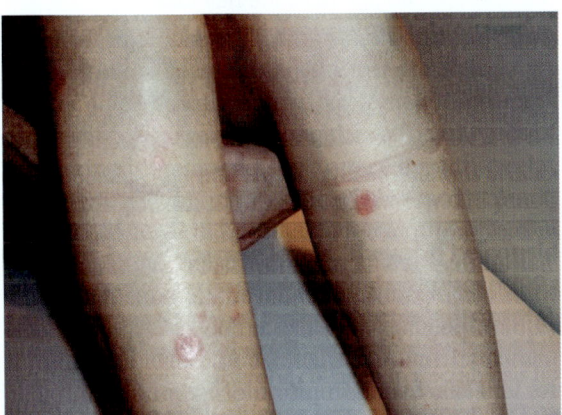

Fig. 4: On the right leg, the lesion shows an elevated edge and atrophic center; while on the left, the lesion has appeared more recently.

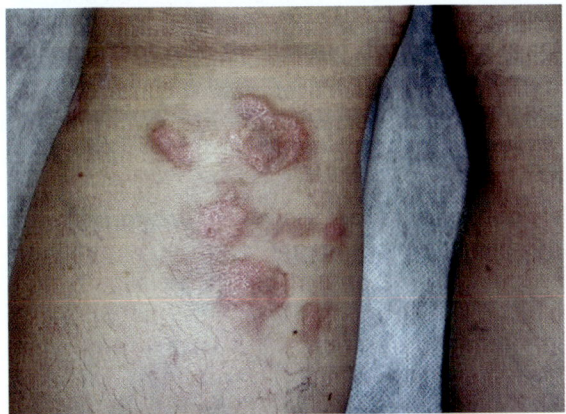

Fig. 5: Multiple plaques of necrobiosis lipoidica.

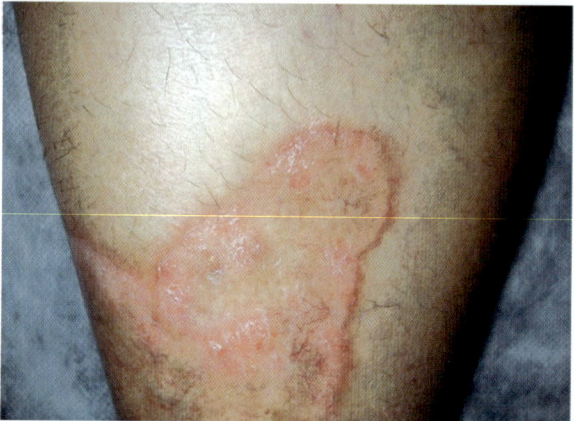

Fig. 6: Active plaque of necrobiosis lipoidica, with erythematous and elevated edges. Note the hair loss.

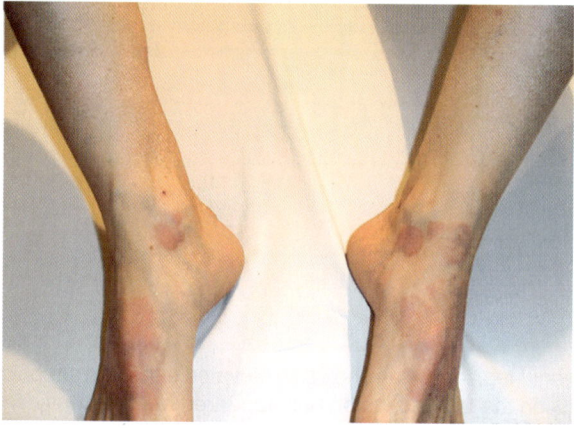

Fig. 7: Bilateral multiple plaques of necrobiosis lipoidica on both lower extremities.

Different clinical forms are described: morpheiform, ulcerated, granuloma annulare-like (GA), nodular and a transepidermal elimination variant.[9,10] The ulcerated form, spontaneous or due to trauma, comprises 15% to 35% of the cases and unlike the other variants, it is painful.[11]

Necrobiosis lipoidica can get pigmented in its essentially chronic evolution and once settled, it does not disappear (Figs. 8 and 9).

From a histological point of view (HP), a normal or atrophic epidermis is observed; in the dermis a palisade granuloma formed by a central zone with disrupted collagen bundles, spaced apart, enucleated and amorphous, surrounded by a lymphohistiocytic crown and epithelioid and giant cells (Fig. 10). The vessels present typical thickening of the base membrane distinctive of DM and endothelial cell proliferation. The histopathology helps

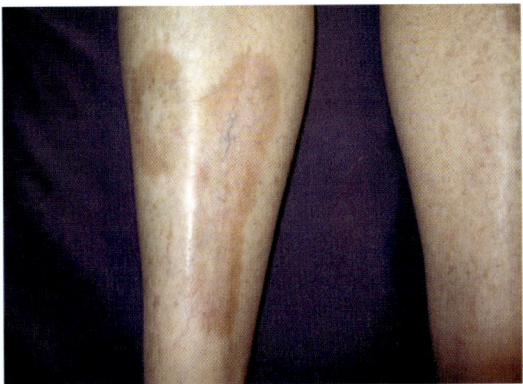

Fig. 8: Plaque of necrobiosis lipoidica with pigmented edges, while in the atrophic center the vessels are visible.

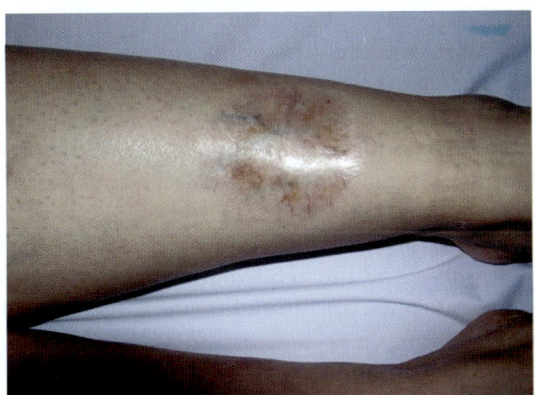

Fig. 9: Plaque of necrobiosis lipoidica with pigmented edges and atrophic center where vessels can be seen through transparency.

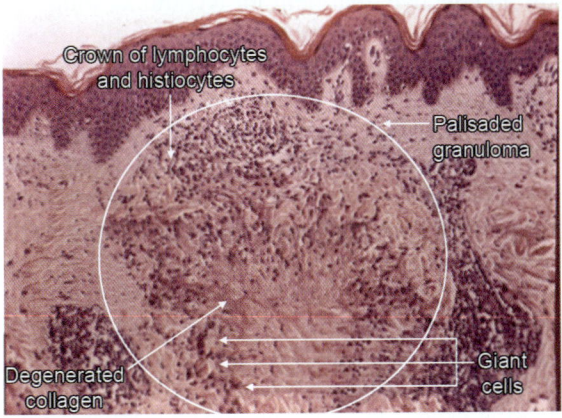

Fig. 10: Histopathology of necrobiosis lipoidica and granuloma annulare. Palisaded granuloma.

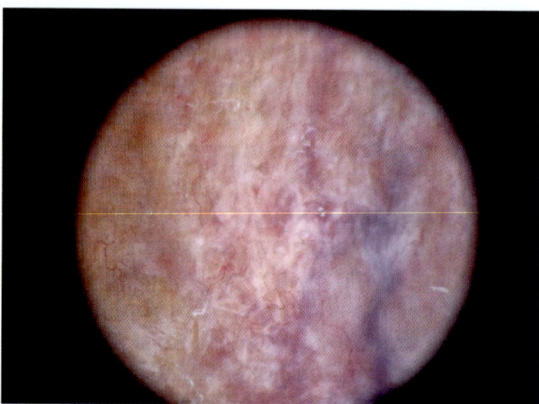

Fig. 11: Dermoscopic image of a plaque of necrobiosis lipoidica. Vascular pattern: arborizing telangiectasia on a yellowish background.

differentiate NL (where extracellular lipids are observed) from GA (where granulomas are more superficial and with abundant deposits of mucin in the central area).[12,13]

Bakos et al. revealed dermoscopic findings related to recent NL that show a vascular pattern with arborizing telangiectasias and hairpin vessels on a yellowish background (Fig. 11).[14,15]

Among differential diagnosis for NL, we cannot forget to mention GA lesions lacking atrophia and the yellowish color; sarcoidosis, necrobiotic xanthogranuloma, morphea and initial forms of leprosy (undetermined leprosy), among others.

The most important complications of NL are ulceration, which can be observed in 30% of the cases, spontaneous or due to minor trauma; an evolution towards squamos cell carcinoma is even weirder, especially in the case of chronic and ulcerated lesions.[16]

There is still no effective treatment for NL and although there are many reports on cases with diverse degrees of therapeutic success, we are still missing controlled and randomized studies that include an important amount of patients.

Due to its antiinflammatory properties, the mainstay of treatment for NL includes topical, intralesional and short courses of systemic corticosteroids. If intralesional corticosteroids are the chosen modality, the application has to be done on the edge due to two reasons. Firstly, the central part is atrophic or will evolve towards atrophy, so these agents are contraindicated. Secondly, the edge is the active part and these agents reduce inflammation and will avoid progression.

The hyperglycemic effect of corticosteroids is well known, so their indication in diabetic patients must be accompanied by a strict control of glucose blood levels, especially when applied on extensive areas or for a long period of time.[17]

Among topical therapies, the calcineurin inhibitors act inhibiting the activation of T-cells and consequently the production of interleukins (IL) and also their proliferation, resulting in an antiinflammatory and immunomodulatory effect.[18]

Another antiinflammatory therapy is phototherapy, applying both psoralen + ultraviolet A (PUVA) and UVA-1 which apparently are more beneficial in early stages of the disease.[19,20]

Other options include drugs that act on hemostasis (vascular thrombosis) like, for example, the combination of aspirin (40-80 mg a day) and dipiridamol (200 mg a day), which inhibit platelet aggregation and decrease blood viscosity; pentoxifylline, a methylated xanthine that further acts on blood cell aggregation and decrease the production of tumoral necrosis factor alpha (TNF-α), enhancing the blood flow. Dose: 400 mg, 3 times a day.[21]

Antimalarials (hydroxychloroquine and chloroquine) inhibit chemotaxis of macrophages that participate in the formation of granulomas, although their effects are not immediate. Additionally, chloroquine inhibits platelet aggregation avoiding occlusion of cutaneous blood vessels.[22,23]

Fumaric acid esters inhibit inflammatory cytokines and prevent lymphocyte-T proliferation. Even though the outcomes are encouraging, it is poorly tolerated due to nauseas, dose-dependent adverse events and lymphopenia present in almost half of the patients. Start with a dose of 30 mg of dimethyl fumarate, increasing progressively until you reach 240 mg.[24,25]

Cyclosporine, an immunosuppressive drug, is indicated in cases of refractory ulcerated NL, because it inhibits lymphocyte production of IL-2 avoiding proliferation of these cells and thus, their immune response. A dose of 2-4 mg/kg a day is responsible for a fast improvement with healing of the ulcer in 2-4 months approximately, but generally presenting recurrence when discontinued. Due to its adverse effects related to nephrotoxicity, it is contraindicated in diabetic patients with previous nephropathy. It is necessary to closely monitor blood pressure, potassium, blood count and renal function.[26] Mycophenolate mofetil is another immunosuppressant which has cytostatic effects on lymphocytes. As cyclosporine, it is effective, but recurrences are common after discontinuation of therapy.

Recently, glitazones and photodynamic therapy (PDT) have been successfully implemented. Based on the role of TNF-alpha in the formation of granulomas, biological agents like anti-TNF-alpha (etanercept and infliximab), have been used to treat cases of refractory NL.[27]

Considering that NL is a benign skin disease, it is not unreasonable to be careful anyway. In order to avoid complications and promote wound healing in ulcerated cases, it is important to modify certain lifestyle habits like quit smoking, avoid traumas and apply compression in case of lymphedema and venous stasis (Table 1).

TABLE 1: Group 1. Cutaneous markers of diabetes mellitus.

	NL	GGA	DD	AD	Xanthosis
Incidence	0.3–1.6%	Generally low	70%	<1%	+or- 10%
Age	Higher percentage between 25 and 40	50 years	More frequent in adult diabetic patients (its frequency increases with age).	Its frequency increases with age	Adults
Gender	80% women	2:1 Women/Men	70% men	Same	Same
Relationship with diabetes	15% precedes diabetes 25% simultaneous 60% in diabetic Patients 10% in Non-diabetic patients.	30% to 40% of the generalized form is associated with diabetes	80% in diabetic patients 20% in non-diabetic patients	Only diabetic patients	In diabetic and non-diabetic patients
Importance	An early diagnosis can contribute to therapeutic outcome	Search for association with diabetes	One of the most frequent markers and signal for the early diagnosis of complications	Indicator of poor prognosis	Related to advanced glycation products (AGEs)

GENERALIZED GRANULOMA ANNULARE

The relationship between GA and DM, especially its generalized form (GGA), is weaker if compared with other cutaneous markers. It is a skin disease which occurs more frequently in adult diabetic type 1 or 2 women.[28]

It is clinically characterized by erythematous, pink or skin colored papules, which coalesce forming annular, arcuate or polycyclic, well-defined plaques (Figs. 12 to 15). They are asymptomatic or slightly pruritic. Even though their etiology is not defined, it has been said that a delayed hypersensitivity reaction to a certain unknown antigen could be the cause.[29]

The following clinical forms have been described: localized GA (75%) (Figs. 16 and 17), generalized GA–accounts for 8.5–15% of GAs and is the one associated with DM (Figs. 18 and 19), subcutaneous nodules more common during childhood; perforating and macular erythematous, which are very rare. There also exist atypical variants: lichenoid and verrucous.

The generalized form can persist for years, unlike the localized variety, which, in general, spontaneously involves.[30,31]

In histological terms, the epidermis is normal. The upper half of the dermis is featured by degenerated collagen bands, a lymphohistiocytic infiltrate that surrounds it forming a palisade or with an intersticial distribution, and abundant mucin which is the key to distinguish it from other granulomatous diseases like NL, rheumatoid nodule, sarcoidosis, etc.[32,33]

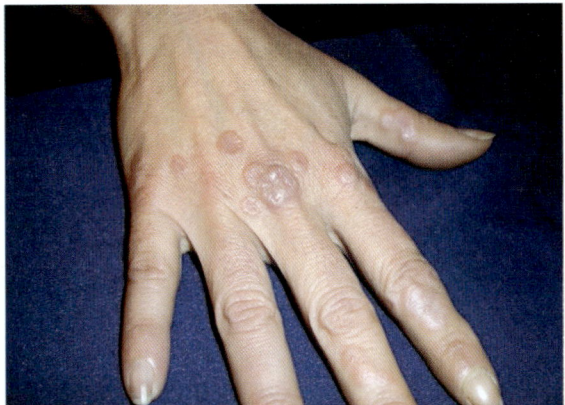

Fig. 12: Plaque formed by confluence of papules with a polycyclic or round shape.

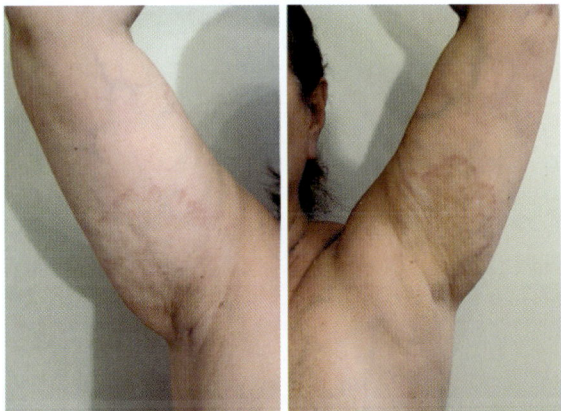

Fig. 13: Plaque of granuloma annulare on both armpits.

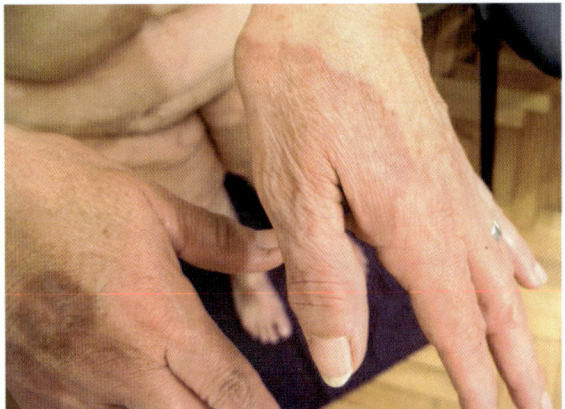

Fig. 14: Granuloma annulare. Plaques on dorsum of hands.

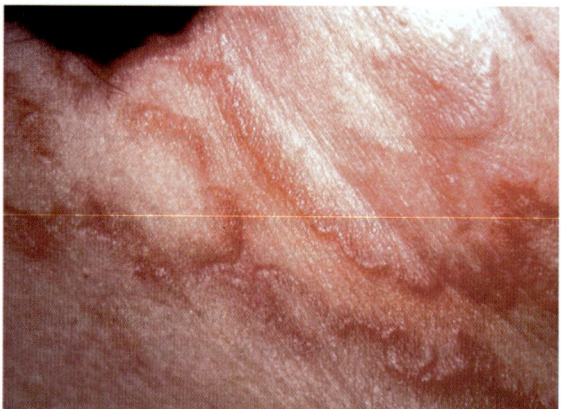

Fig. 15: Granuloma annulare on anterior side of a wrist.

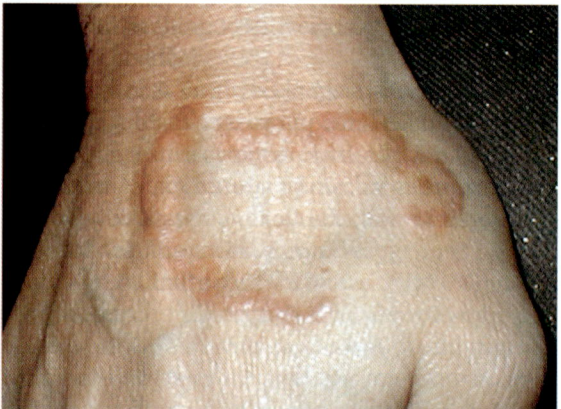

Fig. 16: Localized granuloma annulare.

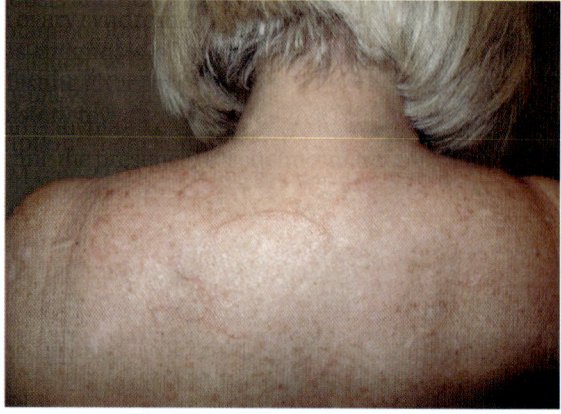

Fig. 17: Localized granuloma annulare.

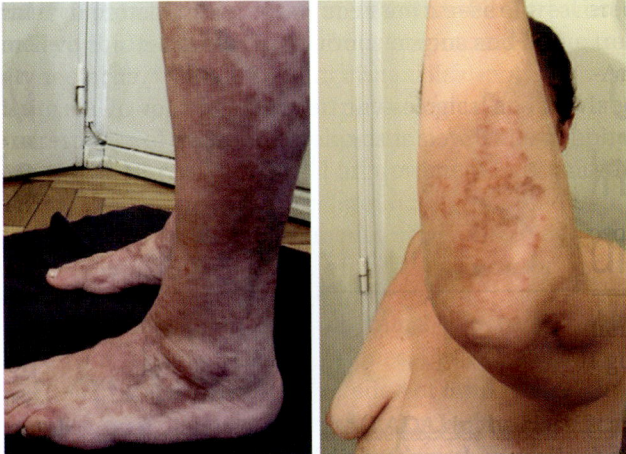

Fig. 18: Generalized granuloma annulare.

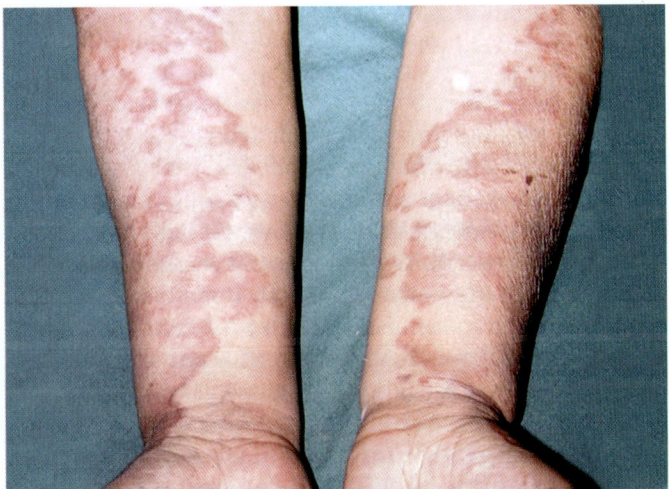

Fig. 19: Generalized granuloma annulare.

A greater incidence of DM than expected has been observed in patients with generalized and perforating GA. Other associations that have been described include alterations of lipid metabolism, malignancies and paraneoplastic syndromes (lymphomas, leukemia and solid lung and breast cancers frequently), thyroid disorders, infections (hepatitis C virus, hepatitis B virus and human immunodeficiency virus) and sarcoidosis. There are also some curious reports of cases with coexisting NL and GA.[34,35]

The chosen therapy will depend on the severity of the disease, comorbidities, possible adverse effects and the patients' preferences. Many patients with the localized form of the disease are frequently interested in getting treatment for cosmetic reasons. Both, topical corticosteroids and IL are their first option. Other therapies include calcineurin inhibitors and cryotherapy.[36]

Even if there is no successful treatment for all GGA cases, systemic corticosteroids and DAPS® (diamino-diphenyl sulfone) in a dose of 100 mg/day would be the first line of choice.[37,38]

Retinoids, pentoxifylline, antimalarials, PUVA and PDT are some of a long list of treatment options for the generalized form.[39]

Sporadically, but with a certain therapeutic success, are colchicines and potassium iodide alone or combined with nicotinamide, among others (Table 1).[40]

DIABETIC DERMOPATHY

It is also known as pretibial pigmented patches.[41] DD appears in type 1 and 2 diabetics, predominantly in males and patients around the age of 50. Present in 60% of diabetic patients, its incidence increases along with age and duration of DM. Of all the patients with pretibial patches, 80% are diabetics, 20% are not, therefore it is not considered a specific manifestation of DM. Its pathogenesis is mixed and simultaneous to the following processes: microangiopathy, inflammatory processes and fibrosis. In clinical terms, it consists of small brownish plaques with demarcated limits, round or oval in shape, with a smooth surface, without scales or crusts, organized in groups or alone, sometimes even in a linear pattern.[42]

The lesions appear preferably on lower extremities (pretibial zone), although some have been described in other areas; they are usually bilateral, but not simmetrical. They are asymptomatic, their evolution is chronic and they do not improve with diabetes control (Figs. 20 to 23).

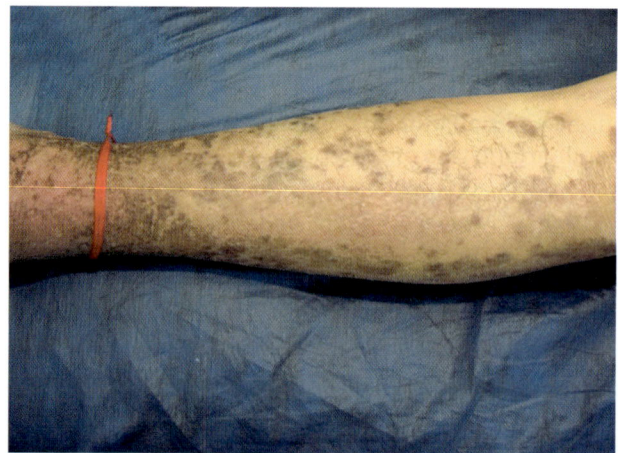

Fig. 20: Diabetic dermopathy.

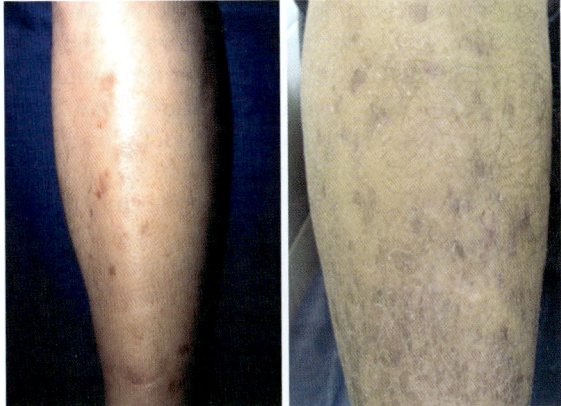

Fig. 21: Diabetic dermopathy.

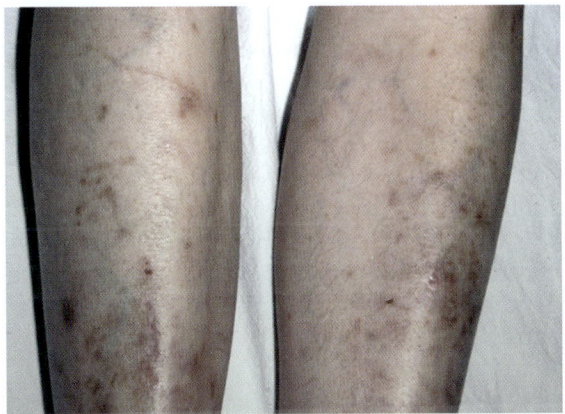

Fig. 22: Diabetic dermopathy.

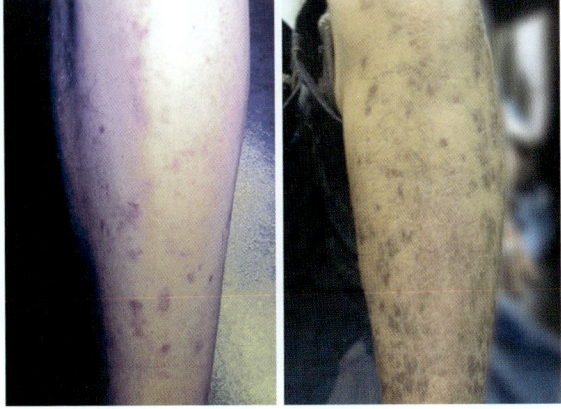

Fig. 23: Diabetic dermopathy.

Some can evolve towards a light atrophy that together with its brownish color has been given formerly the name of "circumscribed brown atrophy".[43]

Histopathologically, one can observe epidermal atrophy and thickening of the wall of microcapillary with microhemorrhage in the dermis. Its pigmentation can be explained by the hemosiderin and to a lesser extent, melanin distribution in the perivascular histiocytes.[44]

There is an unfavorable association between DD and serious microvascular complications of DM (neuropathy, retinopathy and nephropathy). Its correlation with the rise of glycosylated hemoglobin (HbA1c) and long-lasting DM has also been confirmed; therefore, the presence of DD should be considered a warning sign.[45,46]

Generally, there is no need for treatment, nor is there an effective one; some lesions resolve spontaneously (Table 1).[47]

DIABETIC BLISTER (BULLOSIS DIABETICORUM)

It happens in less than 1% of the patients, but it is the only pathognomonic marker of diabetes; that is to say, it appears only in diabetic patients and in both genders equally. Its incidence increases with age. Its pathogenesis is still to be clarified, but the following possible pathophysiological mechanisms have been considered: the skin of diabetic patients is less resistant to blister formation, in part, due to cutaneous fragility that results from diabetic angiopathy, and NEG of anchor fibers.[48,49]

Clinically, it consists in one or more tense blisters with serous or serohematic content and firm consistency, not related to trauma or friction. The blisters are painless, do not have signs of inflammation and they tend to heal spontaneously, not leaving any scars (Figs. 24 to 29).[50,51]

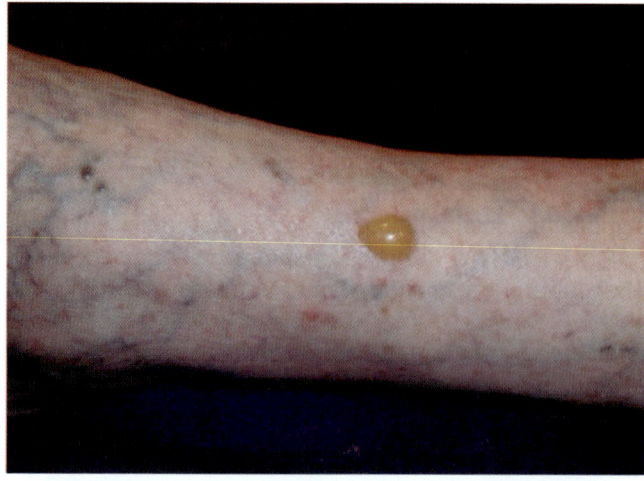

Fig. 24: Diabetic blister on normal skin of lower extremity with serous content.

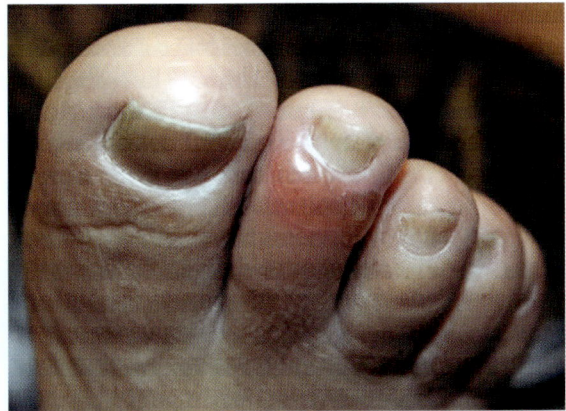

Fig. 25: Diabetic blister with serous content settled on erythematous skin.

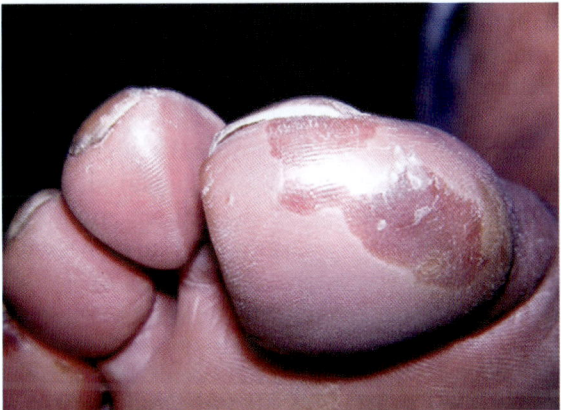

Fig. 26: Diabetic blister.

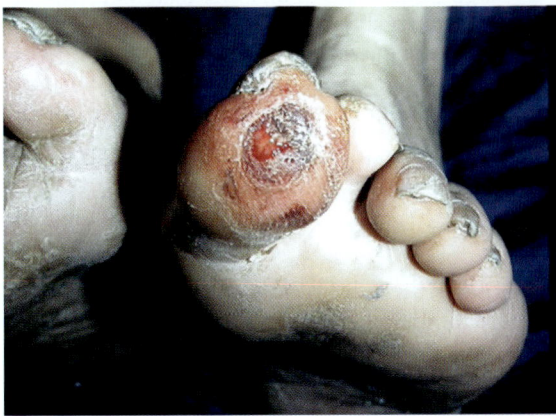

Fig. 27: Diabetic eroded blister with serohematic content.

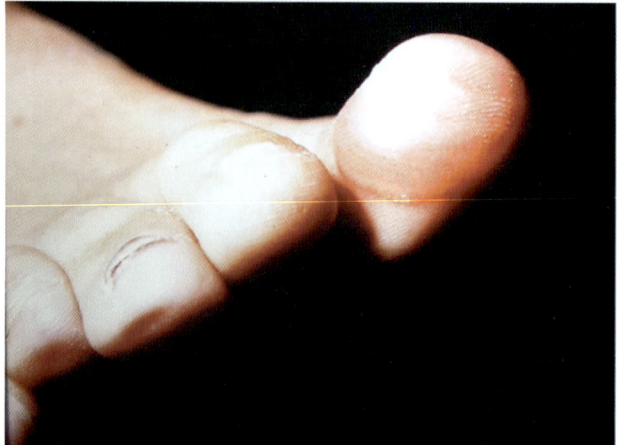

Fig. 28: Intact diabetic blister.

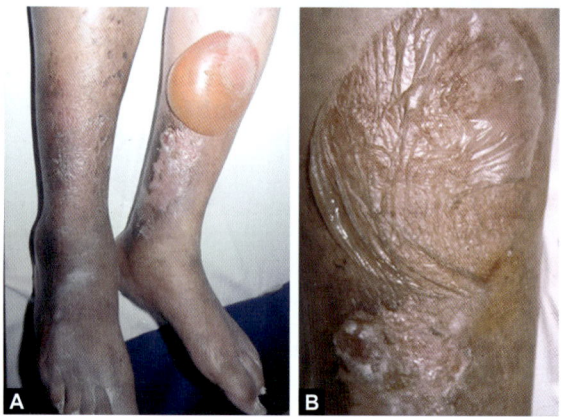

Figs. 29A and B: Large diabetic blister on lower extremity. (A) Intact blister. Note the vascular compromise on both extremities; (B) Aspiration of the content leaving the blister roof to avoid secondary infection.

Their short duration, plus their fast healing without treatment, would suggest a minor clinical situation; nevertheless, it is related to long-lasting diabetes and microvascular complications, specially peripheral neuropathy of lower extremities, so its presence is considered an indicator of poor prognosis.[52]

Histologically, most of them are intraepidermal blisters without acantholysis which explains why they heal without leaving scars (Fig. 30). In other less frequent cases, the blister appears below the dermoepidermal junction in the area of the lamina lucida. Direct or indirect immunofluorescence (IF) are negative.[53]

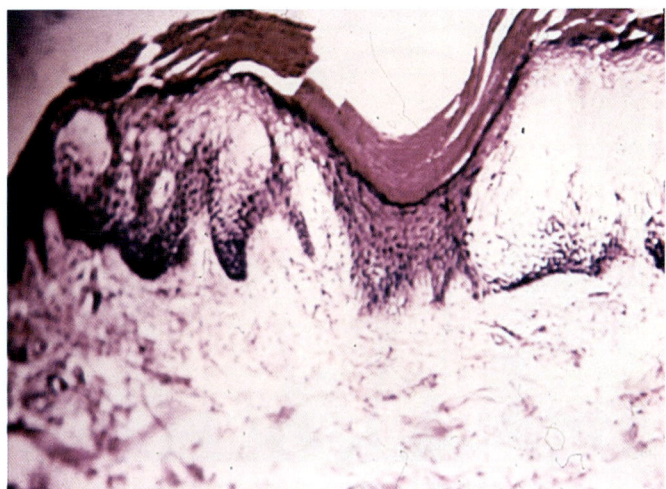

Fig. 30: Histological image of an intraepidermal diabetic blister.

Among the most feared complications are ulceration and bacterial superinfection, especially if the blisters are located on the feet—which can produce osteomyelitis, areas of necrosis and finally amputation. In case of doubt, a magnetic resonance imaging can rule out osteomyelitis.[54]

The diagnosis is suspected on a clinical basis, based on the evolution and sometimes even on histopathology to discard other bullous diseases. We should suspect of DB with the appearance of bullous lesions with direct negative IF and absence of porphyrins in urine.[55]

Taking into account that in most of the cases healing is spontaneous, the treatment should be conservative. It is important to keep the upper part of the blister intact and aspirate the fluid with a syringe to avoid superinfection. The preventive application of a topical antibiotic should not be ruled out. On the contrary, in case of ulcerated lesions, the treatment should be aggressive and supported by a multidisciplinary team (Table 1).[56]

XANTHOSIS OR YELLOW SKIN

It is characterized by yellowish skin, generally on the palms of hands, soles, nasolabial folds and armpits. The sclera allows for a differential diagnosis with jaundice. Its incidence in DM is around 10% of the cases, more frequent in adults and affecting both genders equally (Figs. 31 and 32).

It can also be observed in patients that ingest an excessive amount of vegetables rich in carotenoids, like diabetic patients.[57]

Carotenoids are deposited in the intercellular lipids of corneal cells, so the yellowish-orange color is more prominent in those areas where this layer of the epidermis is thicker.[58]

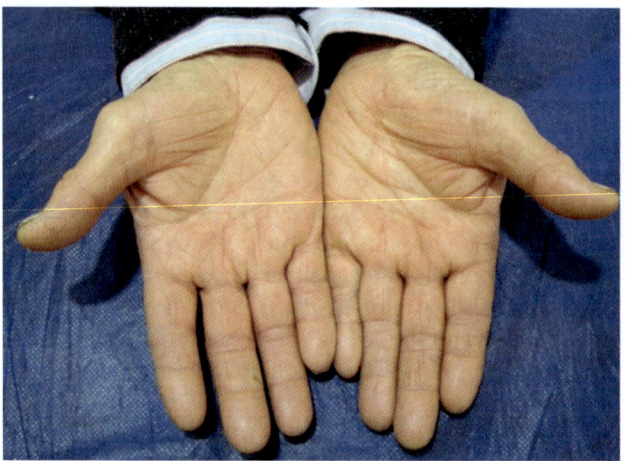

Fig. 31: Yellowish-orange coloration of the palms.

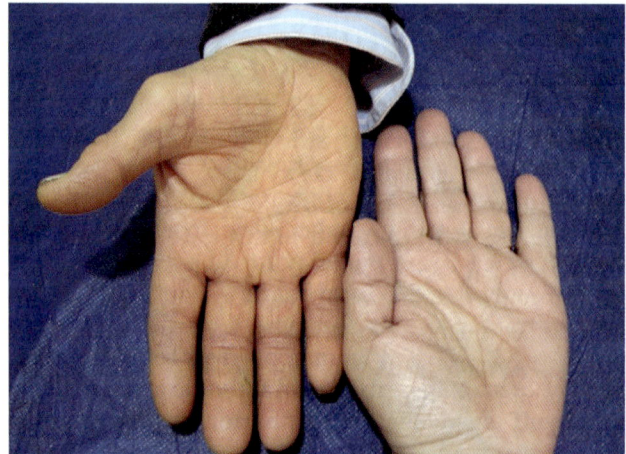

Fig. 32: Comparison of the yellowish-orange coloration of the palm of a patient (left) versus the control palm (right).

Hypercarotenemia and, in consequence, the yellowish color of the skin can be the result of the following three mechanisms:
- An increase in the intake of foods rich in carotenoids
- An increase in serum lipids
- Slowing down of the carotenoid metabolism into retinol.

In the case of diabetic patients, the yellowish color of their skin appears in spite of having normal carotenoid levels in blood and all three mechanisms previously mentioned participate; a bad conversion of beta-carotene into retinol and an increase of blood lipids, apart from a diet rich in vegetables.

That is why today it is believed that the yellow coloration of the skin of these patients, like many other cutaneous manifestations, is largely driven by the NEG process, in which delayed-release yellow-colored products are formed (AGE) (2-furoyl)-4(5)-(2-furanyl)-1H0 imidazole (6H), which accumulated in proteins like collagen, produce that characteristic color on the skin and the nails (see Table 1).[59]

Moreover, some authors confirm that diabetic patients with elevated glycemia and HbA1c levels and without a food intake rich in carotenoids ameliorate their dermatosis with a strict control of DM. This would support the theory of NEG participation in the yellow color, since it increases glucose in blood.[60]

REFERENCES

1. Sheetz MJ, King GL. Molecular understanding of hyperglycemia's adverse effects for diabetic complications. JAMA. 2002; 288(20):2579-88.
2. Farshchian M, Farshchian M, Fereydoonnejad M, et al. Cutaneous manifestations of diabetes mellitus: a case series. Cutis. 2010;86(1):315.
3. Shahzad M, Al Robaee A, Al Shobaili HA, et al. Skin manifestations in diabetic patients attending a diabetic clinic in the Qassim region, Saudi Arabia. Med Princ Pract. 2011;20(2):137-41.
4. Van Hattem S, Bootsma AH, Thio HB. Skin manifestations of diabetes. Cleveland Clinic Journal of Medicine.2008;75(1):772-87.
5. Dissemond J. Images in clinical medicine. Necrobiosis lipoidica diabeticorum. N Engl J Med. 2012;366(26):2502.
6. Kota SK, Jammula S, Kota SK et al. Necrobiosis lipoidica diabeticorum: a case-based review of literature. Indian J Endocrinol Metab. 2012;16(4):614-20.
7. Holland C, Givens V, Smoller BR. Expression of the human erythrocyte glucose transporter Glut-1 in areas of sclerotic collagen in necrobiosis lipoidica. J Cutan Pathol 2001;28:287-90.
8. Erfurt-Berge C, Seitz AT, Rehse C, et al. Update on clinical and laboratory features in necrobiosis lipoidica: a retrospective multicenter study of 52 patients. Eur J Dermatol. 2012;22(6):770-5.
9. Penny HL, Faretta M, Rifkah M, et al. Selective case study describing the use of Apligraf on necrobiosis lipoidica associated with diabetes. J Wound Care. 2014;23(2): S12-5.
10. Ianoşi SL, Tutunaru C, Georgescu CV, et al. Specific features of a rare form of disseminated necrobiosis lipoidica granuloma annulare type: a case report. Rom J Morphol Embryol. 2014; 55(4):1455-61.
11. Franklin C, Stoffels-Weindorf M, Hillen U, et al. Ulcerated necrobiosis lipoidica as a rare cause for chronic leg ulcers: case report series of ten patients. Int Wound J. 2013. doi: 10.1111/iwj.12159.
12. Alonso ML, Riós JC, González-Beato MJ, et al. Necrobiosis lipoidica of the glans penis. Acta Derm Venereol. 2011;91(1):105-6.
13. Hawryluk EB, Izikson L, English JC 3rd. Non-infectious granulomatous diseases of the skin and their associated systemic diseases: an evidence-based update to important clinical questions. Am J Clin Dermatol. 2010;11:171-81.
14. Bakos RM, Cartell A, Bakos L. Dermatoscopy of early-onset necrobiosis lipoidica. J Am Acad Dermatol. 2012;66:e143-4.

15. Conde-Montero E, Aviles-Izquierdo JA, Mendoza-Cembranos MD, et al. Dermoscopy of necrobiosis lipoidica. Actas Dermosifiliogr. 2013;104: 534-7.
16. Pătrașcu V, Giurca C, Ciurea RC, et al. Ulcerated necrobiosis lipoidica to a teenager with diabetes mellitus and obesity. Rom J Morphol Embryol. 2014;55(1): 171-6.
17. Grillo E, Rodriguez-Muñoz D, González-Garcia A, et al. Necrobiosis lipoidica. Aust Fam Physician. 2014;43(3):129-30.
18. Binamer Y, Sowerby L, El-Helou T. Treatment of ulcerative necrobiosis lipoidica with topical calcineurin inhibitor: case report and literature review. J Cutan Med Surg. 2012;16:458-61.
19. De Rie MA, Sommer A, Hoekzema R, et al. Treatment of necrobiosis lipoidica with topical psoralen plus ultraviolet A. Br J Dermatol. 2002;147:743-7.
20. Beattie PE, Dawe RS, Ibbotson SH, et al. UVA1 phototherapy for treatment of necrobiosis lipoidica. Clin Exp Dermatol. 2006;31:235-8.
21. Basaria S, Braga-Basaria M. Necrobiosis lipoidica diabeticorum: response to pentoxiphylline. J Endocrinol Invest. 2003;26:1037-40.
22. Kavala M, Sudogan S, Zindanci I, et al. Significant improvement in ulcerative necrobiosis lipoidica with hydroxychloroquine. Int J Dermatol. 2010;49: 467-9.
23. Nguyen K, Washenik K, Shupack J. Necrobiosis lipoidica diabeticorum treated with chloroquine. J Am Acad Dermatol. 2002;46:S34-6.
24. Eberle FC, Ghoreschi K, Hertl M. Fumaric acid esters in severe ulcerative necrobiosis lipoidica: a case report and evaluation of current therapies. Acta DermVenereol. 2010;90:104-6.
25. Kreuter A, Knierim C, Stucker M, et al. Fumaric acid esters in necrobiosis lipoidica: results of a prospective non controlled study. Br J Dermatol. 2005;153: 802-7.
26. Stanway A, Rademaker M, Newman P. Healing of severe ulcerative necrobiosis lipoidica with cyclosporin. Australas J Dermatol. 2004;45:119-22.
27. Reid SD, Ladizinski B, Kachiu L, et al. Update on necrobiosis lipoidica: A review of etiology, diagnosis, and treatment options JAAD. 2013;69(5):783-91.
28. Goucha S, Khaled A, Kharfi M, et al. Granuloma annulare. G Ital Dermatol Venereol. 2008;143(6):359-63.
29. Wollina U, Langner D. Treatment of disseminated granuloma annulare recalcitrant to topical therapy: a retrospective 10-year analysis with comparison of photochemotherapy alone versus photochemotherapy plus oral fumaric acid esters. JEADV. 2012;26(10):1319-21.
30. Souza FH, Ribeiro CF, Pereira MA, et al. Simultaneous occurrence of ulcerated necrobiosis lipoidica and granuloma annulare in a patient: case report. An Bras Dermatol 2011;86(5):1007-10.
31. Avitan-Hersh E, Sprecher H, Ramon M, et al. Does infection play a role in the pathogenesis of granuloma annulare? JAAD 2013; 68(2):342-3.
32. Jang EJ, Lee JY, Kim MK, et at. Erythematous granuloma annulare. Ann Dermatol. 2011;23(3):409-11.
33. Maschio M, Marigliano M, Sabbion A, et al. A rare case of granuloma annulare in a 5-year-old child with type 1 diabetes and autoimmune thyroiditis. Am J Dermatopathol. 2013;35(3):385-7.

34. Travassos AR, Soares-De-Almeida L. Residents'corner February 2014. DeRmpath& Clinic: Differential diagnosis in palisading non-infectious granulomas. Diagnosis: Case 1: Granuloma annulare. Case 2: Necrobiosis lipoidica. Eur J Dermatol. 2014;24(1):139-40.
35. Rupley KA, Ryan R, Riahi RR, et al. Granuloma annulare and necrobiosis lipoidica with sequential occurrence in a patient: report and review of literature. Dermatol Pract Concept. 2015;5(1):29-34.
36. Davison JE, Davies A, Moss C, et al. Links between granuloma annulare, necrobiosis lipoidica diabeticorum and childhood diabetes: a matter of time? Pediatr Dermatol. 2010;27(2):178-81.
37. Keimig EL. Granuloma Annulare. Dermatol Clin. 2015;33(3):315-29.
38. Martín-Sáenz E, Fernández-Guarino M, Carrillo-Gijón R, et al. Efficacy of dapsone in disseminated granuloma annulare: a case report and review of the literature. Actas Dermosifilogr. 2008;99(1):64-8.
39. Piaserico S, Zattra E, Linder D, et al. Generalized granuloma annulare treated with methylaminolevulinate photodynamic therapy. Dermatology. 2009;218(3):282-4.
40. Pătraşcu V1, Giurcă C, Ciurea RN, et al. Disseminated granuloma annulare: study on eight cases. Rom J Morphol Embryol. 2013;54(2):327-31.
41. Binkley GW. Dermopathy in diabetes mellitus. Arch Dermatol. 1965;92:106-7.
42. Murphy-Chutorian B, Han G, Cohen SR. Dermatologic Manifestations of Diabetes mellitus: a review. Endocrinol Metab Clin North Am. 2013;42(4):869-98.
43. Duhm G. Atrofia parda circunscrita pretibial y diabetes. Trabajo original 1 y 2 años de la docencia complementaria. UBA, Facultad de Medicina. 1970.
44. McCash S, Emanuel PO. Defining diabetic dermopathy. J Dermatol. 2011;38(10): 988-92.
45. Abdollahi A, Daneshpazhooh M, Amirchaghmaghi E, et al. Dermopathy and retinopathy in diabetes: is there an association?. Dermatology. 2007;214(2): 133-6.
46. Shenavandeh S, Anushiravani A, Nazarinia MA. Diabetic muscle infarction and diabetic dermopathy two manifestations of uncontrolled prolong diabetes mellitus presenting with severe leg pain and leg skin lesions. J Diabetes Metab Disord. 2014;13(1):38.
47. Morgan AJ, Schwartz RA. Diabetic dermopathy: A subtle sign with grave implications. J Am Acad Dermatol. 2008;58(3):447-51.
48. Demirseren DD, Emre S, Akoglu G, et al. Relationship between skin diseases and extracutaneous complications of diabetes mellitus: clinical analysis of 750 patients. Am J Clin Dermatol. 2014;15(1):65-70.
49. Lipsky BA, Baker PD, Ahroni JH. Diabetic bullae: 12 cases of a purportedly rare cutaneous disorder. Int J Dermatol. 2000;39(3):196-200.
50. El Fekih N, Zéglaoui F, Sioud A, et al. Bullosis diabeticorum: report of ten cases. Tunis Med. 2009;87(11):747-9.
51. Chatterjee N, Chattopadhyay C, Sengupta N, et al. An observational study of cutaneous manifestations in diabetes mellitus in a tertiary care Hospital of Eastern India. Indian J Endocrinol Metab. 2014;18(2):217-20.
52. H Riad, H Al Ansari, K Mansour, et al., "Pruritic vesicular eruption on the lower legs in a diabetic female," Case Reports in Dermatological Medicine, vol. 2013, Article ID 641416, 4 pages, 2013.

53. Murphy-Chutorian B, Han G, Cohen R. Dermatologic manifestations of diabetes mellitus: a review. Endocrinol Metab Clin N Am. 2013;42:869-98.
54. Kurdi AT. "Bullosis diabeticorum," Lancet. 2013;382(9907):e31.
55. Mota ANCM, Nery NS, Barcaui CB. Case for diagnosis. An Bras Dermatol. 2013;88(4):652-4.
56. Gupta V, Gulati N, Bhal J, et al. Bullosis Diabeticorum: rare presentation in a common disease. Case Rep Endocrinol. 2014;2014. Article ID 862912, 3 pages.
57. Hoerer E, Dreyfuss F, Herzberg M. Carotenemia, skin color and diabetes mellitus. Acta Diabetol Lat. 1975;12:202-7.
58. Haught JM, Patel S, English JC, III. Xanthoderma: a clinical review. J Am Acad Dermatol. 2007;57:1051-8.
59. Julka S, Jamdagni N, Verma S, et al. Yellow palms and soles: a rare skin manifestation in diabetes mellitus. Indian J Endocrinol Metab. 2013;17(Suppl1):S299-S300.
60. Jiun-Nong Lin. Yellow palms and soles in diabetes mellitus. N Engl J Med. 2006;355:1486.

CHAPTER
5

Skin-Thickening Syndrome

Emilia Noemí Cohen Sabban, Horacio A Cabo

INTRODUCTION

Numerous epidemiologic studies have shown that the prevalence of some rheumatologic manifestations increases in diabetic patients showing a higher incidence than in the general population.[1] Different musculoskeletal disorders observed in diabetes mellitus (DM) that involve hands and shoulders, can be painful and cause functional weakness. In the hands, it produces the so-called diabetic hand syndrome, being the limited joint mobility (LJM) the most frequent manifestation.

Its occurrence is linked to the duration of the disease, hyperglycemia, and the accumulation of advanced glycation end-products (AGEs).[2] Although many of these changes are comparable to those taking place with aging, the skin and periarticular tissue in DM behave in a unique way and differ from those occurring in nondiabetic individuals. The LJM is an example, since in DM it is of early appearance, it is associated with cutaneous changes and it is linked with microvascular disease. Within the syndrome, in addition to LJM, other rheumatologic manifestations of the diabetic patient's hands are described, including palmar flexor tenosynovitis, Dupuytren's contracture, carpal tunnel syndrome, Charcot arthropathy, and reflex sympathetic dystrophy. Adhesive capsulitis, which affects the shoulders, has also been described.[3]

Limited joint mobility is part of the skin thickening syndrome or sclerodermiform skin changes of DM, along with other cutaneous alterations that we describe in detail in this chapter (Fig. 1). It is interesting to highlight that skin thickening is very common in diabetic patients and increases with age; in contrast to the natural thinning of aged skin. It is produced due to the accumulation of collagen, a structural protein of the skin. It makes itself more resistant to collagenases degradation due to the nonenzymatic glycosylation (NEG) and the generation of advanced glycation end products that inevitably ensue in chronic hyperglycemia. Besides, in its physiopathology, vasculopathy, neuropathy or both should not be discarded.

The skin thickening syndrome includes four cutaneous manifestations: (1) Finger pebbles (FP); (2) Waxy skin (WS); (3) Limited joint mobility (LJM); and (4) Diabetic scleredema (DS) (Table 1).[4]

FINGER PEBBLES

Also known as Huntley's papules[5] (Fig. 2), FP consists of multiple tiny papules grouped on the extensor surface and side face of the fingers, on the knuckles of the metacarpophalangeal and interphalangeal joints, more frequently in the distal ones, and in the periungual region (Figs. 3 to 6).[6] It is an asymptomatic, but common finding in 60% to 70% of diabetic persons, but does not require any treatment. It can happen in 20% of nondiabetics, especially, manual workers.

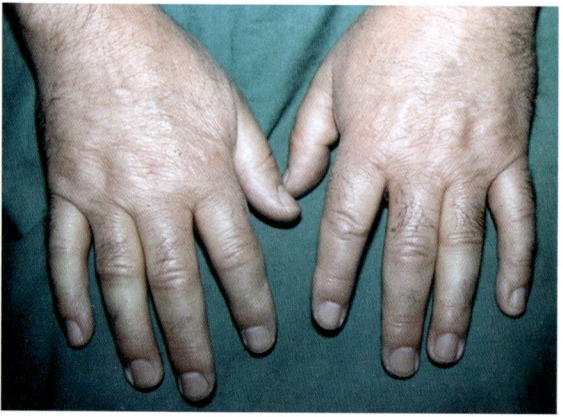

Fig. 1: Hands of a diabetic patient. Skin thickening.

TABLE 1: Skin thickening syndrome.

	Finger pebbles	Waxy skin and limited joint mobility	Diabetic scleredema
Incidence	60%	30%	2.5%
Age	Infants/youth and adults	2 variants: child and youth and the most frequent adults	> 40 years
Gender	Equal in both	Equal in both	4:1 male/female
Relationship with diabetes	80% in diabetic patients, 20% in non-diabetics	Diabetics type 1 and 2	More in type 2 obese long-standing and poorly controlled diabetics
Importance	Visual marker of skin thickening in DM	High risk of microvascular complications	Related to insulin resistance, retinopathy, HT, ischemic disease

(DM: Diabetes mellitus; HT: Arterial hypertension).

Skin-Thickening Syndrome

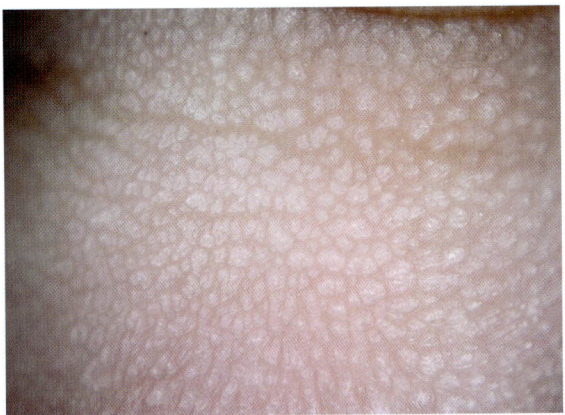

Fig. 2: Huntley's papules.

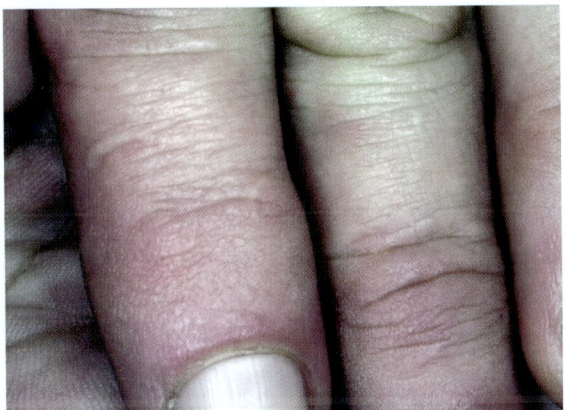

Fig. 3: Tiny papules on the interphalangeal joint and periungual region.

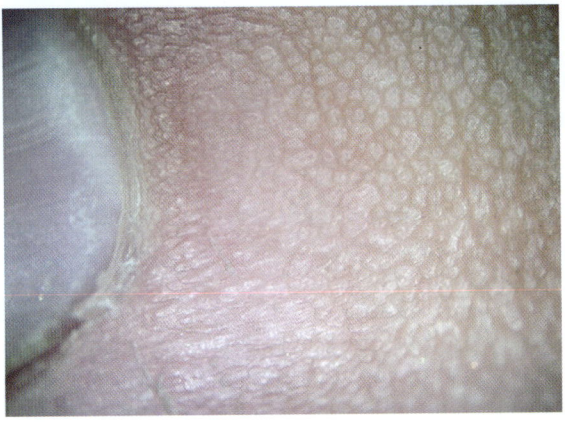

Fig. 4: Finger pebbles.

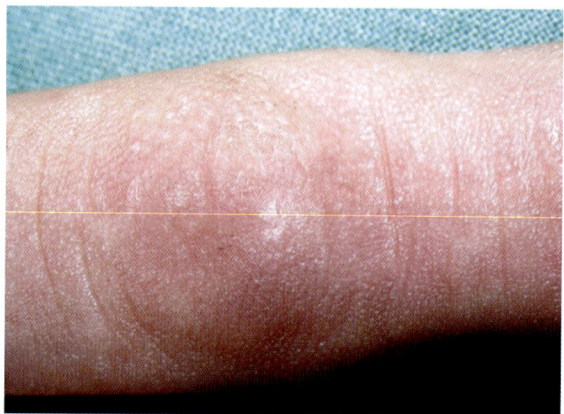

Fig, 5: Finger pebbles on interphalangeal joint.

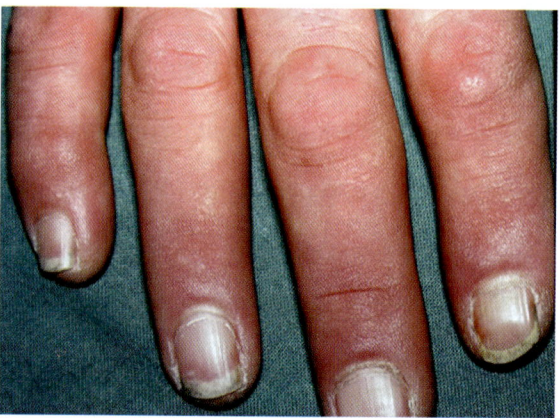

Fig. 6: Finger pebbles on periungual region and on interphalangeal joints.

When it appears in diabetic patients, it is considered a visual marker of the thickening of the dorsum of the hands (Figs. 7 and 8). It is associated with either type 1 or type 2 diabetic patients of both genders equally; although in Huntley's original description—later supported by other authors—it is more frequent in adults with DM type 2 (DM2). It has been suggested that the thickening is not only related to NEG of collagen fibers, but also to epidermal growth factors such as insulin-like growth factor (IGF-1).[7] Finger pebbles is an early signal of sclerodermiform alterations in hands.[8]

The histologic features of FP are epidermal hyperplasia with a "church tower" aspect where orthokeratotic hyperkeratosis and regular acanthosis are evident; at the dermis level, we observe changes in the collagen fibers that are located vertically, papillomatosis and areas of angiogenesis accompanied by insignificant perivascular infiltrates (Fig. 9).[9]

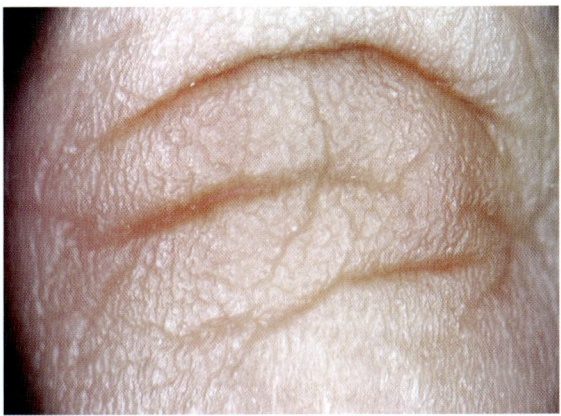

Fig. 7: Skin thickening. Note the pebbled aspect.

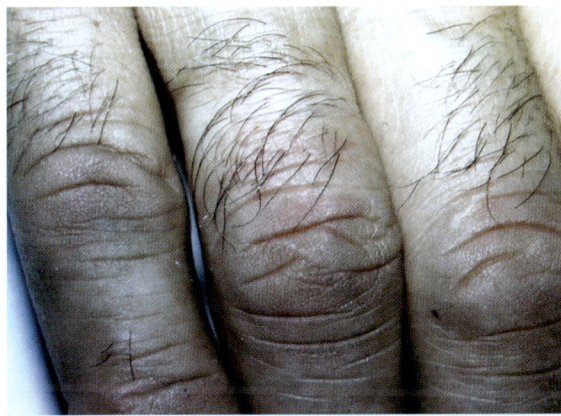

Fig. 8: Thickening on knucklebones with characteristic small papules.

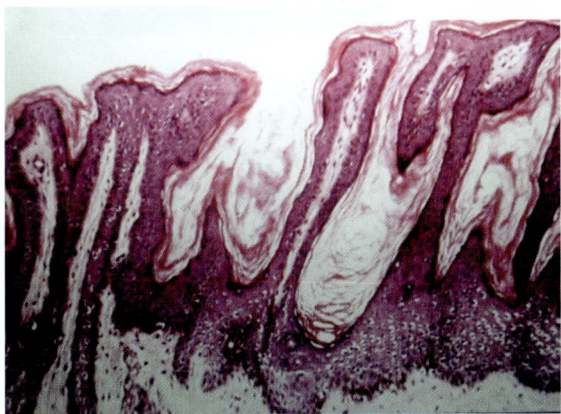

Fig. 9: Histopathology of finger pebbles.

In patients with DM2 and insulin resistance—and the consequent stimulation of insulin-like growth factor receptors (IGF)—apart from obesity, an association between FP and acanthosis nigricans and cutaneous acrochordons has been described.[10,11] It is also associated to severe obesity in the context of insulin resistance without underlying DM, as in the reported case by Granel et al., whose patient suffers from Pickwick Syndrome (severe obesity, drowsiness, excessive appetite, hypoventilation, and sleep apnea).[12]

WAXY SKIN

It is characterized by cutaneous changes over the dorsum of the hands and forearm (Fig. 10). Under physical examination the skin is shiny and tight, difficult to fold, similar to scleroderma but with its own features, different to WS, both in optical and electron microscopy. The differential diagnosis between both entities includes ulcers, the Raynaud's phenomenon, capillaroscopic alterations, autoantibodies and other laboratory data (Table 2).[13]

Waxy skin is more frequent in diabetic patients with LJM, than in diabetic individuals without that manifestation, which in turn, have thicker skin compared to nondiabetics (Figs. 11 and 12). For some authors, it is associated more to those with severe or moderate LJM.

Histopathologically, dermoepidermal thickening with accumulation of collagen and loss of cutaneous appendages are characteristic features.

LIMITED JOINT MOBILITY

Limited joint mobility (LJM) is caused by the thickening and stiffness of the periarticular connective tissue. It involves mainly the small joints of the hands and results in a severe finger contracture and the inability to fully extend fingers. It is painless and generally goes unnoticed until the deformity becomes so severe that it interferes with daily life (Figs. 13 and 14).

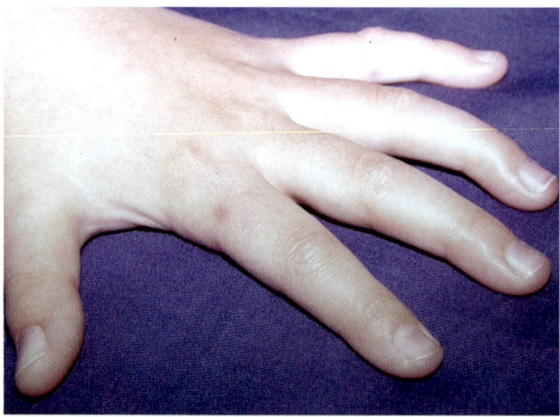

Fig. 10: Tight and shiny skin.

Skin-Thickening Syndrome

TABLE 2: Clues for the diagnosis of sclerodermiform changes in DM versus scleroderma.

	DM	Scleroderma
Age	10–20 years	40–50 years
Gender	Equal	3:1 female/male
Diabetes	Type 1 and 2	There may be an abnormal glucose tolerance.
Pain	No	Yes
Raynaud	No	Yes
Digital ulcers	No	Yes
Telangiectasia	No	Yes
Pigmentation	No	Yes
Capillaroscopy	Capillaries loss	SD pattern
Histology	Dermal collagen is thickened and hyalinized, spaces and clefts between fibers. Fat around eccrine sweat glands is preserved. No inflammatory reaction.	Epidermal atrophy Homogenization of the dermis with loss of spaces between collagen bundles. Replacement of the periglandular fat by collagen.

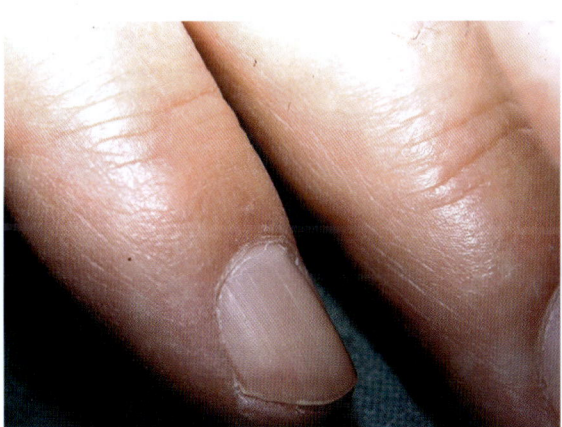

Fig. 11: Waxy skin and finger pebbles.

It is also known as cheiroarthropathy or "diabetic stiff hand syndrome" and has a prevalence of 30–40% of diabetes type 1 patients (8–50% of diabetic individuals); although it is also present in DM2, both male and female equally.[14]

Its original description dates back to the beginning of the 70s, where 3 teenagers with long-standing DM type 1 (DM1) showed a notable limited mobility of their interphalangeal and metacarpophalangeal joints of the hands, wrists, elbows and ankles and in two of them the spinal column, accompanied by a short stature, WS, a delay in sexual maturity and early microvascular

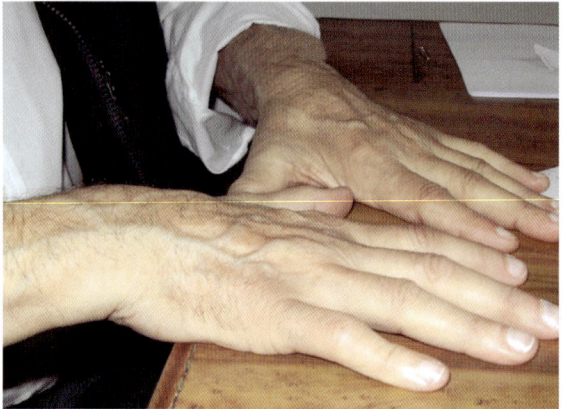

Fig. 12: Waxy skin and limited joint mobility.

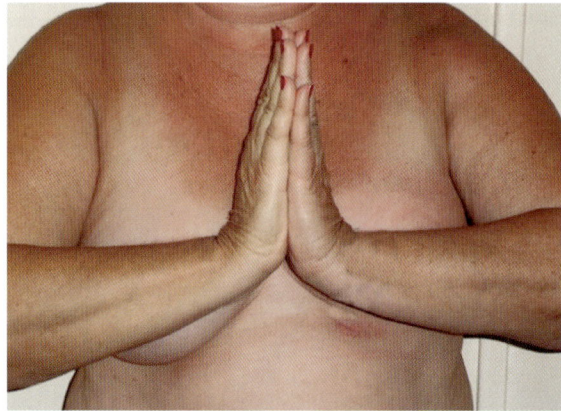

Fig. 13: Limited joint mobility, mild degree. Prayer sign.

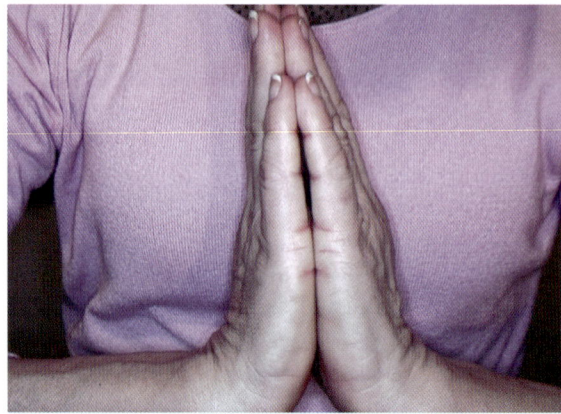

Fig. 14: Limited joint mobility, mild degree. Prayer sign.

complications. X-rays did not show any joint disorders, which confirmed that the thickening was due to the thickening and stiffnes of the periarticular tissue.[15] Despite being initially described in pediatric population, it is more prevalent in diabetic adults. Its incidence increases with age and duration of DM.

During the physical examination, the inability to extend the metacarpophalangeal and proximal and distal interphalangeal joints is observed, starting with the fifth and fourth fingers and expanding radially (Figs. 15 to 19). In the symptomatic phase there is finger stiffness, decrease of manual skills, i.e. hand mobility, especially extension. There can also be a restriction in the flection of fingers and reduction of passive and active movements. There is a notable difficulty to close the fingers into a fist, make fine movements and less grip strength (Figs. 20 and 21).

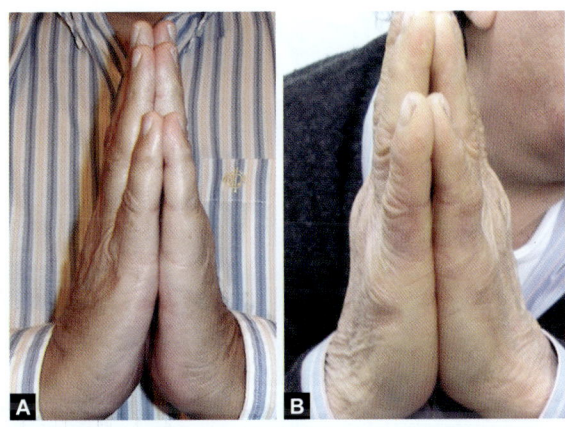

Figs. 15A and B: Limited joint mobility of the fifth finger of both hands.

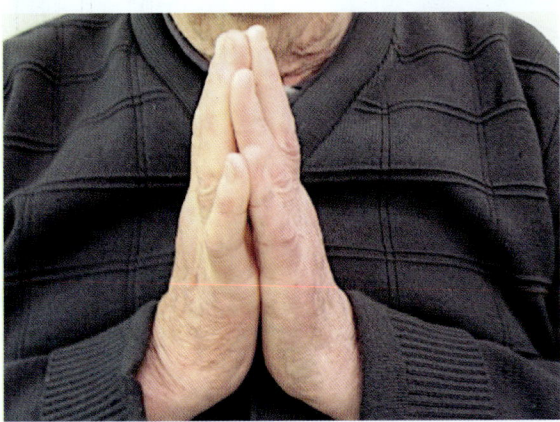

Fig.16: Limited joint mobility of the fifth finger of both hands.

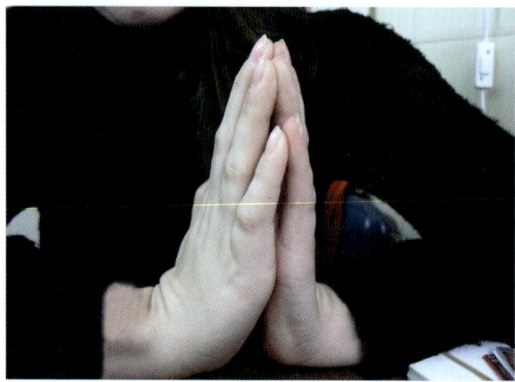

Fig. 17: Limited joint mobility of the fifth and fourth fingers of both hands.

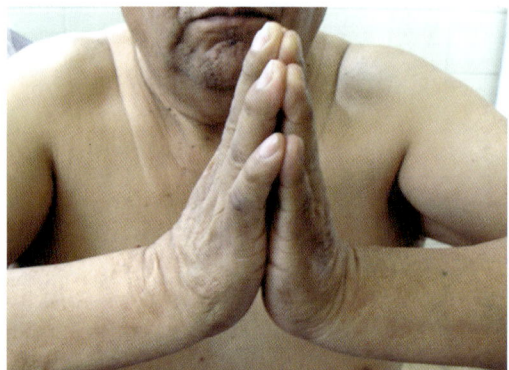

Fig. 18: Limited joint mobility of the fifth and fourth fingers of both hands.

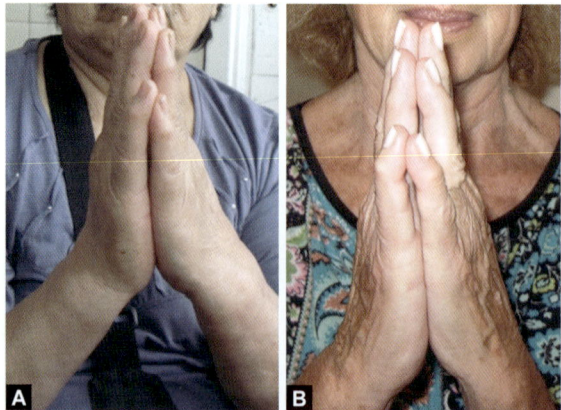

Figs. 19A and B: Limited joint mobility of the fifth and fourth fingers of both hands, moderate compromise.

The degree of involvement has been classified into *mild*, when the limitation affects one or two proximal interphalangeal joints, one large joint or only metacarpophalangeal bilateral joints. *Moderate* limitation refers to three or more proximal interphalangeal joints or the joint of one finger and one large bilateral joint. *Severe* cases are constituted by the deformity of the hand at rest or involvement of the cervical spine. The progression of changes, since the initial detection of a mild limitation to moderate or severe condition varies, starting from 3 month to 4 years, with an average of 2 years. Fifty percent of young patients with DM for more than 5 years develop moderate or severe limitation.

There are simple tests that help in its recognition. One is the "prayer sign", where it is clearly impossible for the patient to oppose the palms together completely, without leaving a gap between the two; the magnitude will depend

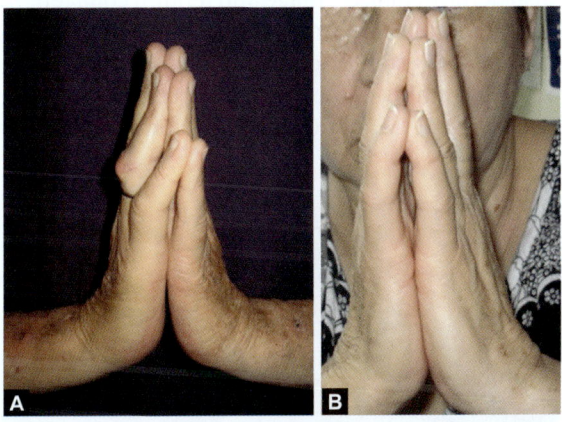

Figs. 20A and B: Limited joint mobility. Severe degree.

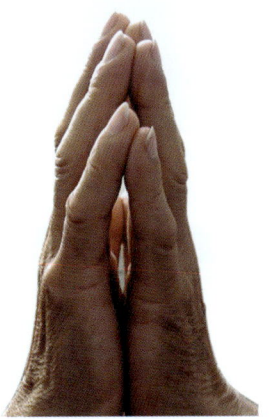

Fig. 21: Limited joint mobility, severe compromise. Prayer sign.

on the degree of affectation of the patient (Fig. 21). The other is the "tabletop sign" where the patient is not able to completely extend his/her hand on a table's surface: this makes the diagnosis of metacarpophalangeal contractures easier (Fig. 22 and Table 3).[16] If both tests turn out positive, it is recommended to make a careful examination of each joint; additionally, one should keep in mind, that these tests can have a positive result in different entities like Dupuytren's contracture and previous trauma where a comprehensive medical history will help to resolve the diagnosis.

Sometimes other joints can be affected, like wrists, elbows, ankles, shoulders, the cervical and thoracolumbar spine, and other organs (lungs). Recently, Shah et al. published LJM in shoulders, referring particularly to the limitation of the external rotation of the joint in diabetic patients compared to normal control patients.[17] The underlying cause of this syndrome appears to be multifactorial. There is a relationship between the increase non-enzymatic glycation of collagen and joint stiffness; which not only involves dermal collagen, but also periarticular, cartilage and tendon collagen, with a decrease in collagenase degradation. The importance of the glycation process for the pathogenesis of LJM was established with the proof that each increased unit of HhA1c from the beginning of the disease, corresponded to 46% of increase of the risk of developing LJM. Besides, DM can promote and even aggravate

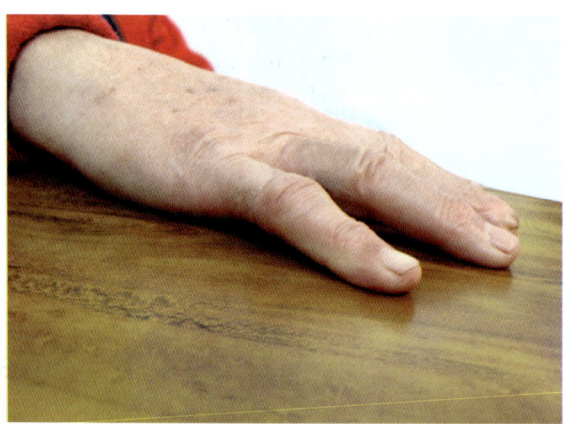

Fig. 22: Tabletop sign. Note the impossibility to extend the fingers completely.

TABLE 3: Clinical signs for limited joint mobility (LJM).	
Prayer sign	*Table top sign*
Evaluates the ability to oppose hands without leaving a space between them, allowing for the recognition of contractures in the metacarpophalangeal and interphalangeal proximal and distal joints.	Determines the ability to completely extend palms on the table's surface, allowing the recognition of metacarpophalangeal joint contractures.

anatomic and functional damage, not only because of the increase in AGEs; but also due to overweight, visceral adiposity and advanced age, where ligaments and tendons weaken naturally and are prone to brake or get injured; especially in the diabetes type 2 population, with the corresponding increase of risk. Older patients with LJM have a prolonged nerve conduction velocity (NCV) of the median and ulnar nerves when compared with those not suffering from LJM but with DM of the same duration in time, as well as less vibratory perception in the upper and lower extremities.

Patients presenting with LJM have a greater risk of developing microvascular complications, more frequently retinopathy than neuropathy and nephropathy. LJM severity is directly proportional to the frequency and severity of the microvascular disease. Rosenbloom et al. described the relationship between microvascular complications and LJM in patients with DM1 and even more in the case of the male gender, possibly due to a poor glycemic control, coronary heart and cerebrovascular disease. In women, it is related to early macrovascular disease. A recent analysis concluded that in the presence of LJM, there is an 83% increase in the risk of developing microvascular complications after 16 years of having DM, as opposed to 25% of risk in the absence of LJM. Some authors refer that LJM is an independent factor for the development of microvascular complications and increases their risk 3 to 5 times in these patients.[18]

Finally, a recent study that included 184 patients with 5 year DM, evaluated the association between LJM and the risk of accidental falls. It was concluded that the risk in patients with LJM is moderate (19-20 seconds in the assessment of balance), in comparison to a low risk in those that did not present LJM.[19]

Limited joint mobility in feet at the level of metatarsophalangeal and submetatarsal joints can cause an increase of the pressure on these plantar points with the subsequent possible occurrence of diabetic foot ulcers. LJM of the ankles with an increase in the thickness of the plantar fascia and the Achilles tendon, has also been described in patients with DM1 and DM2; more frequently in those patients with peripheral neuropathy. The thickening has been correlated positively with the body mass index (BMI).[20]

Accordingly, the presence of LJM is an important marker of subsequent microvascular disease and can constitute a useful clinical tool for the identification of a subset of patients at high risk to develop early complications.

Even though, the prayer sign and the table top sign are widely recognized in literature as diagnostic tools, they are not present in all cases as a rule. For subclinical forms of the disease, goniometry is used which in case of being positive, confirm the association between flexion restriction of small joints of the hands and microvascular complications in patients with DM 2.[21] In terms of severity assesment, the classification system of Starkman and Brink is used (Table 4).[22]

Cutaneous biopsy is rarely used for the diagnosis of this syndrome. Histopathological findings consist of a normal epidermis and an increase in collagen in the inferior dermis, with thickening and hyalinization of collagen fibers in the papillary and mid-dermis.[23]

TABLE 4: Degrees of severity of waxy skin and limited joint mobility. Brink-Starkman classification.

Degree 0	No changes
Degree I	Waxy skin, no contractures
Degree II	Contractures in the flexion of both little fingers
Degree III	Bilateral compromise of fingers and wrists
Degree IV	Bilateral compromise of other fingers
Degree V	Bilateral compromise of fingers, wrists and other joints

With regards to the natural evolution, after two decades of its acknowledgment, its incidence has experienced a substantial decrease, probably due to a better metabolic control. In 1998, the same doctors applying the same techniques they used in their description compared the initial findings and found that the frequency of LJM had decreased four times along with a dramatic decrease in other manifestations such as short stature. This important decrease in kids and teenagers with DM over time was attributed to a better glycemia and HbA1c monitoring and to new types and release systems of insulin.[24,25]

There is not a specific treatment for LJM, but the metabolic control is mandatory; although evidence over improvement with control of hyperglycemia is still controversial. Physiotherapy and occupational therapy yield variable results, with active and passive mobilization, passive extension of contractured fingers, and the use of splints that can broaden the range of movement and help stop progression.[26] Another important issue referred to in literature is smoking, that has definitely a negative influence.[27]

DIABETIC SCLEREDEMA

It is a rare disorder that affects adult diabetic patients, generally older than 40, with an approximate incidence of 2.5%. It is characterized by an increase in the thickness and diffuse, asymptomatic and symmetric induration of the skin, which confers an orange-peel appearance (Fig. 23). It affects the neck and upper back, shoulders and arms, occasionally accompanied by erythema (Figs. 24 to 26). Although less frequent, it may appear in other parts of the body like the face, abdomen, thighs, and buttocks.[28] In contrast to scleroderma, hands and feet are not involved.

Nowadays three types of scleredema are described in literature: Type 1 is the classical form or scleredema adultorum of Buschke that mainly affects women and typically starts with an infectious process of upper airways most often due to *Streptococcus* and which resolves spontaneously (Table 5); type 2 is associated with paraproteinemia including multiple myeloma; and type 3, scleredema diabeticorum that in contrast with the classical form or scleredema adultorum of Buschke has a considerable predominance in men and is not preceded by

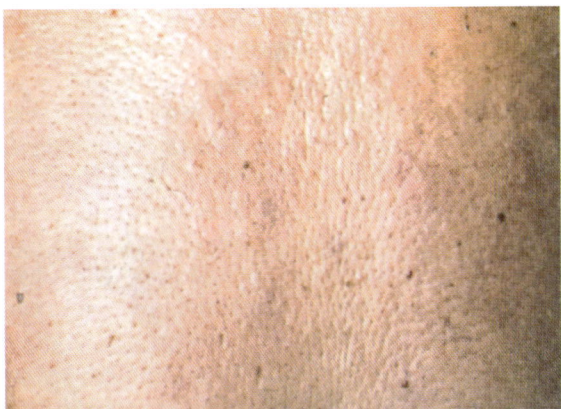

Fig. 23: Orange-peel aspect.

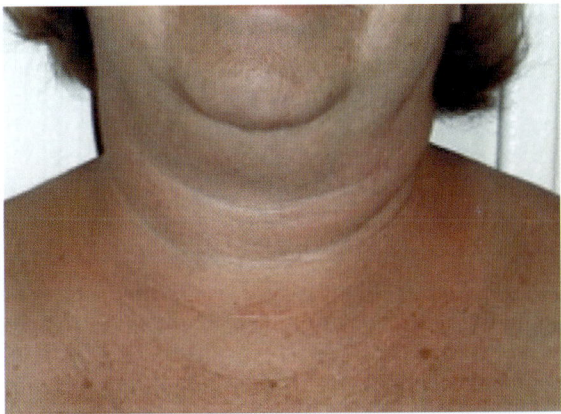

Fig. 24: Scleredema affecting the neck.

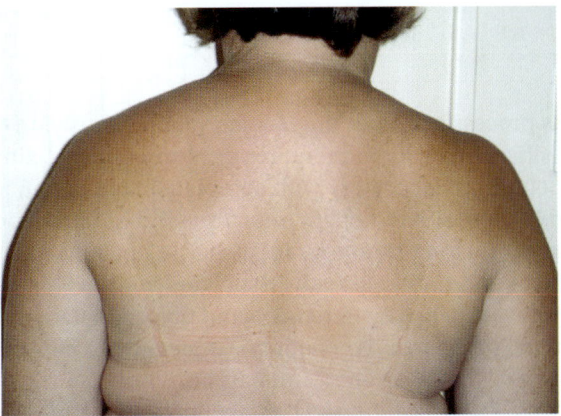

Fig. 25: Scleredema affecting the posterior neck and upper back.

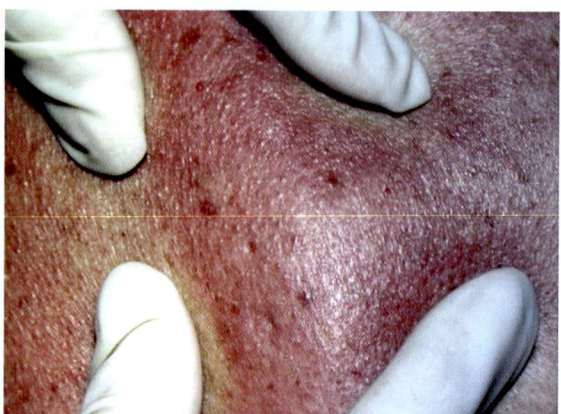

Fig. 26: Scleredema. Erythema and orange-peel aspect.

TABLE 5: Differences between scleredema diabeticorum and classical scleredema.

	Scleredema diabeticorum	Classical scleredema
Gender	4:1 male/female	2:1 female/male
Age	Adults	
Previous infection	No	Yes; upper airways due to *Streptococcus*
Clinics	Insidious onset. Affects skin of the neck and upper back, although it may extend	Sudden onset. Affects skin of neck and upper back, localized in most of the cases
Retinopathy	Yes	No
Associations	Long standing type 2 DM, poorly controlled, Obese, insulin resistant patients. HT hypertension Myocardial infarction.	Rare
Evolution	Persistent	75% resolves spontaneously
Treatment	Generally no response	None

(HT: Arterial hypertension).

any infectious process and does not involve spontaneously. In order to make a correct classification, it should requires a comprehensive clinical history of the patient including a laboratory with complete blood count, proteinogram, glycemia, HbA1c, renal and hepatic function, and autoantibodies.[29] Type 3 scleredema occurs in long-standing diabetes type 2 patients that report a poor glycemic control and it is frequently associated with insulin resistance and vascular complications like hypertension and myocardial infarction.

Even though its diagnosis is generally suspected on a clinical base, optical microscopy reveals normal epidermis and an increase in collagen at the reticular dermis. Collagen fibers are thickened and irregularly distributed, separated by clear spaces in which mucin is deposited, evidenced with stains such as Alcian Blue. Sometimes, the increase of the dermis thickness can reach up to four times its normal size. Even subcutaneous fat can be replaced by collagen fibers.[30]

Although there is considerable uncertainty about its pathogenesis, one hypothesis is a poor glycemia control that leads to an increase in NEG of the collagen fibers which in turn decrease their degradation. Another possibility is that hyperglycemia would act as a stimulant for fibroblast proliferation and synthesis of extracellular matrix components.[31-33]

Lin et al. reported the case of a female patient with long-standing DM2, 50 years of age, in which scleredema diabeticorum was associated to eccrine gland loss with the subsequent anhidrosis of the affected area. After 8 month of treatment with allopurinol 100 mg/day she noted a mild relief but without changes related to the lack of sweating.[34]

The treatment of DS continues to be a challenge, lacking a gold standard. Reports refer to series of a few cases with variable and refractory results in most of the cases. The first therapeutic step is the intensification of the metabolic control, although there is no consensus regarding the correlation between glycemia control and the improvement of DS. Colchicine has been used in cases of DS, due to its anti-inflammatory properties and to its ability to prevent collagen synthesis.[35] Immunosuppressant drugs like cyclosporine, corticosteroids and methotrexate (MTX) are other therapeutic options. It is believed that MTX, apart from interfering in the glycation process, can decrease the production of connective tissue or mucin by the fibroblasts and other cells that are involved.[36] Another therapeutic modality could be radiation therapy, psoralen combined with ultraviolet A (PUVA) (accumulative doses of UVA, 120 J/cm^3) and more recently very good results have been reported with UVA1 phototherapy,[37-39] and currently intravenous immunoglobulin G (IVIG).[40]

As mentioned previously, the diagnosis of thickening syndrome is basically clinically, and there are noninvasive methods of detection like ocular inspection, palpation, the prayer sign and the tabletop sign. There is another

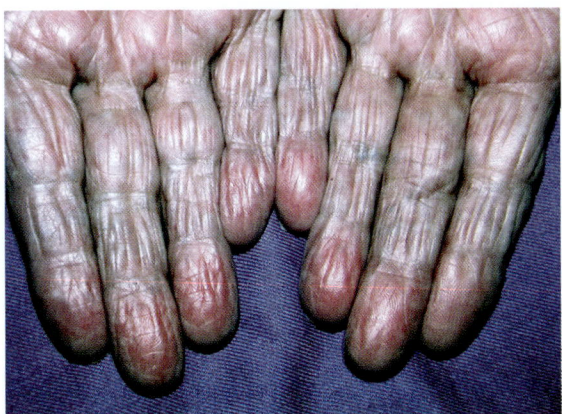

Fig. 27: Non-diabetic control patient. Wrinkles after immersion in the water.

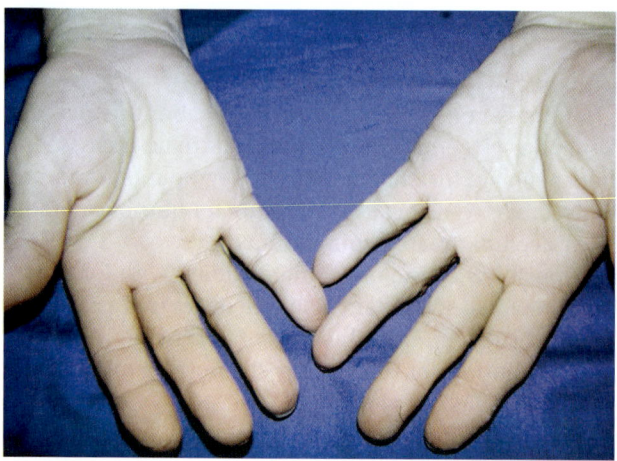

Fig. 28: Diabetic patient without wrinkles after immersion in the water.

way to check it, which is by detecting cutaneous wrinkles on the finger pads.[41] The patient's hands are submerged in warm water at 42°C for 30 minutes. In diabetic patients, no wrinkles are observed on their finger pads, contrary to what happens in the general population (Figs. 27 and 28). The mechanism by which these wrinkles diminish, is unknown, but it is thought that the cause of the thickening of the skin could be multifactorial and that sympathetic autonomic neuropathy with an increase in the deep tissue turgor, keratin NEG (epidermal protein) with an increase in the epidermal thickness and the alteration of the blood flow through the finger pads, participate.

CONCLUSION

In conclusion, the maintenance of a good metabolic control through physical exercise, an adequate diet and hypoglycemia could enhance and even prevent the development of these manifestations.

REFERENCES

1. Abate M, Schiavone C, Salini V, et al. Management of limited joint mobility in diabetic patients. Diabetes Metab Syndr Obes. 2013;6:197-207.
2. Larkin ME, Barnie A, Braffett BH, et al. Diabetes Control and Complications Trial/Epidemiology of Diabetes Interventions and Complications Research Group. Musculoskeletal complications in type 1 diabetes. Diabetes Care. 2014;37(7):1863-9.
3. Arlan L Rosenbloom. Connective tissue disorders in diabetes. In RA Defrongo, Ferrannini E, Keen H, Zimmet P (Editors). International Textbook F Diabetes Mellitus, 3rd edition. John Wiley and Sons Ltd; 2004.
4. Burner TW, Rosenthal AK. Diabetes and rheumatic diseases. Curr Opin Rheumatol. 2009;21(1):50-4.
5. Huntley C. Finger pebbles: a common finding in diabetes mellitus. J Am Acad Dermatol. 1986;14:612-7.

6. Libecco JF, Brodell RT. Finger pebbles and diabetes: a case with broad involvement of the dorsal fingers and hands. Arch Dermatol. 2001;137(4):510-1.
7. Singh R, Barden A, Mori T, et al. Advanced glycation end-products: a review. Diabetologia. 2001;44(2):129-46.
8. Cabo HA, Woscoff A, Casas JG. Empedrado digital: marcador temprano de engrosamiento cutáneo en pacientes diabéticos. Arch Argent Dermat. 1988;48: 185-9.
9. Guarneri C, Guarneri F, Borgia F, et al. Finger pebbles in a diabetic patient: Huntley's papules. International Journal of Dermatology. 2005;44:755-6.
10. Saraiya A, Al-Shoha A, Brodell RT. Hyperinsulinemia associated with acanthosis nigricans, finger pebbles, acrochordons, and the sign of Leser-Trélat. Endocr Pract. 2013;19(3):522-5.
11. Hollister DS, Brodell RT. Finger 'pebbles'. A dermatologic sign of diabetes mellitus. Postgrad Med. 2000;107(3):209-10.
12. Granel B, Serratrice J, Mohamed H, et al. Pickwickian syndrome and vanishing finger pebbles. Arch Dermatol. 2001;137(4):508-10.
13. Tyndall A, Fistarol S. The differential diagnosis of systemic sclerosis. Curr Opin Rheumatol. 2013;25(6):692-9.
14. Schiavon F, Circhetta C, Dani L. The diabetic hand. Reumatismo. 2004;56(3):139-42.
15. Rosenbloom AL, Frias JL. Diabetes, short stature and joint stiffness—a new syndrome. Clin Res. 1974;22:92A.
16. Rosenbloom AL, Silverstein JH. Connective tissue and joint disease in diabetes mellitus. Endocrinol Metab Clin North Am.1996;25:473-83.
17. Shah KM, Clark RB, McGill JB, et al. Shoulder limited joint mobility in people with diabetes mellitus. Clin Biomech (Bristol, Avon). 2015;30(3):308-13.
18. Amin R, Bahu TK, Widmer B, et al. Longitudinal relation between limited joint mobility, height, insulin like growth factor I levels, and risk of developing microalbuminuria: the Oxford Regional Prospective Study. Arch Dis Child. 2005;90:1039-44.
19. López-Martín I, Benito Ortiz L, Rodríguez-Borlado B, et al. Association between limited joint mobility syndrome and risk of accidental falls in diabetic patients. Semergen. 2015;41(2):70-5.
20. Craig ME, Duffin AC, Gallego PH, et al. Plantar fascia thickness, a measure of tissue glycation, predicts the development of complications in adolescents with type 1 diabetes. Diabetes Care. 2008;31(6):1201-6.
21. Pandey A, Usman K, Reddy H, et al. Prevalence of hand disorders in type 2 diabetes mellitus and its correlation with microvascular complications. Ann Med Health Sci Res. 2013;3(3):349-54.
22. Starkman H, Brink S. Limited joint mobility (LJM) of the hand in patients with diabetes mellitus. Diabetes Care. 1982;5:534-6.
23. Liu T, McCalmont TH, Frieden IJ, et al. The stiff skin syndrome: case series, differential diagnosis of the stiff skin phenotype, and review of the literature. Arch Dermatol. 2008;144(10):1351-9.
24. Infante JR, Rosenbloom AL, Silverstein JH, et al. Changes in frequency and severity of limited joint mobility in children with type 1 diabetes mellitus between 1976–78 and 1998. J Pediatr. 2001;138:33-7.
25. Arlan L Rosenbloom. Limited joint mobility in childhood diabetes: discovery, description, and decline. J Clin Endocrinol Metab. 2013;98:466-73.
26. Del Rosso A, Matucci Cerinic M, De Giorgio F, et al. Rheumatological manifestations in diabetes mellitus. Current Diabetes Reviews. 2006;2(4): 455-66.

27. Nagesh VS, Kalra S. Type 1 diabetes: Syndromes in resource-challenged settings. J Pak Med Assoc. 2015;65(6):681-5.
28. Rebora A, Rongioletti F. Mucinoses. In: Bolognia JL, Jorizzo JL, Rapini RP (Editors). Dermatology. London: Mosby, 2003, pp.647–58.
29. Salazar-Nievas M, Crespo-Lora V, Rubio-López J, et al. Cutaneous indurated plaque on the abdomen associated with diabetes mellitus. Aust Fam Physician. 2013;42(12):876-7.
30. Beers WH, Ince A, Moore TL. Scleredema adultorum of Buschke: a case report and review of the literature. Semin Arthritis Rheum. 2006;35(6):355-9.
31. Tran K, Boyd KP, Robinson MR, et al. Scleredema diabeticorum. Dermatol Online J. 2013;19(12):20718.
32. Gruson LM, Franks A Jr. Scleredema and diabetic sclerodactyly. Dermatol Online J. 2005;11(4):3.
33. Yaqub A, Chung L, Rieger KE, et al. Localized cutaneous fibrosing disorders. Rheum Dis Clin North Am. 2013;39(2):347-64.
34. Lin I-Chun, Chiu Hsien-Yi, Chan Jung-Yi, et al. Extensive scleredema adultorum with loss of eccrine glands. J Am Acad Dermatol. 2014;71(3):e99-101.
35. Sapadin AN, Fleischmajer R. Treatment of scleroderma. Arch Dermatol. 2002;138:99.
36. Doğramacı AÇ, Inan MU, Atik E, et al. Scleredema diabeticorum partially treated with low-dose methotrexate: a report of five cases. Balkan Med J. 2012;29(2):218-21.
37. Janiga J, Ward D H, Lim H W. UVA-1 as a treatment for scleredema. Photodermatology Photoimmunology and Photomedicine. 2004;20(4):210-1.
38. Kroff EB, de Jong EM. Scleredema diabeticorum case series: successful treatment with UV-A1. Arch Dermatol. 2008;144(7):947-8.
39. Kroft E, Berkhof N, van der Kerkhof P, et al. Ultraviolet A phototherapy for sclerotic skin diseases: a systematic review. J Am Acad Dermatol. 2008;59(6):1017-30.
40. Martín C, Requena L, Manrique K, et al. Scleredema diabeticorum in a patient with type 2 diabetes mellitus. Case Rep Endocrinol. 2011;560. 2011:560273. doi: 10.1155/2011/560273.
41. Clark C, Pentland B, Ewing D, et al. Decreased skin wrinkling in diabetes mellitus. Diabetes Care. 1984;7(3):224-7.

CHAPTER 6

Acanthosis Nigricans and Other Cutaneous Manifestations of Insulin Resistance and Metabolic Syndrome

Emilia Noemí Cohen Sabban

INTRODUCTION

Acanthosis nigricans (AN) is a distinctive cutaneous disorder, as it is the clinical marker for a variety of abnormalities. It appears in men and women, kids, teenagers and adults. A large proportion of patients are obese and diabetic; as much as 66% of teenagers who are overweight and 56–92% of children and teenagers with diabetes mellitus type 2 (DM2) develop AN. It is actually considered a marker for insulin resistance (IR) and is also associated with DM2, obesity, endocrinopathies, autoimmune diseases, drugs and even malignancies; whereby it is classified as benign or malignant AN (Table 1).

Due to the constant global increase in the prevalence of obesity and DM, AN's prevalence has also raises and nowadays it is estimated between 7–74% depending on the age, race, type of AN, the degree of obesity, concomitant endocrinopathy, etc. The different ethnicities have an influence in its prevalence; it is more common in native Americans, followed by Afro-Americans, Hispanics, and Caucasians.

Among internal malignancies, it is generally associated with adenocarcinomas mainly of gastrointestinal origin (stomach cancer) (Fig. 1). Other diseases associated with AN are autoimmune diseases like systemic lupus erythematosus, scleroderma, Sjörgen's syndrome and Hashimoto's thyroiditis.[1] Exogenous drugs that can cause AN include insulin injections, nicotinic acid, oral contraceptives, topical fusidic acid, methyltestosterone and palifermin.[2] Familiar and syndromic forms of AN have also been identified. These syndromes share clinical features like obesity, hyperinsulinemia and craniosynostosis.

TABLE 1: Acanthosis nigricans	
Prevalence	• 7% of general population • 74% of obese population
Age	All ages
Gender	Male/female
Relationship with diabetes	More frequently in diabetes type 2
Importance	Skin marker of insulin resistance

CLINICAL DESCRIPTION

Since it is clinically very characteristic, it becomes easy to diagnose in the presence of thickened bilateral, symmetrical, velvety and hyperpigmented skin plaques (Figs. 2 and 3). In the majority of cases, the disease affects localized areas of the skin, i.e. flexural posterior neck, the axilla and/or groins, but it has also been described in the folds of the upper and lower limbs, inframammary, around the belly button, on the lips, vulva, dorsum of the hands (knuckles) and the face, particularly in the case of individuals with dark skin (Figs. 4 and 5). Generalized forms appear frequently in adults with underlying malignancy (Fig. 6). Occasionally, AN lesions can affect the oral and nasal mucosa, in the larynx, and esophagus. Even the nipple areola, eyes (eyelids) and nails (leukonychia and hyperkeratosis) can be affected by this condition.

The lesions are asymptomatic, but they can occasionally itch, hurt or be smelly, due to excessive sweating and friction that favor maceration in some

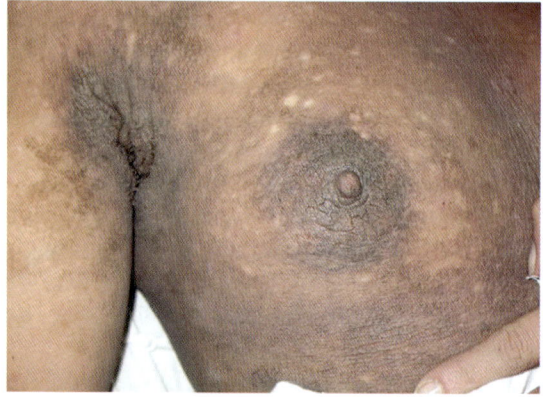

Fig. 1: Malignant acanthosis nigricans.

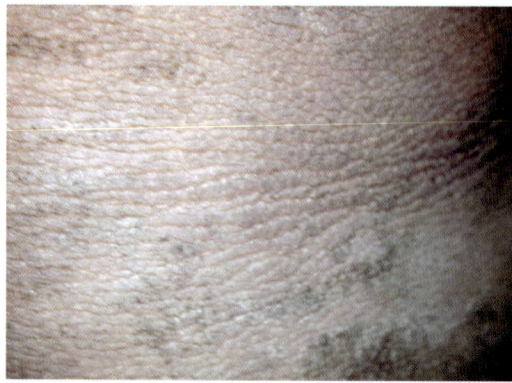

Fig. 2: Acanthosis nigricans: Plaque of velvety and hyperpigmented cutaneous thickening.

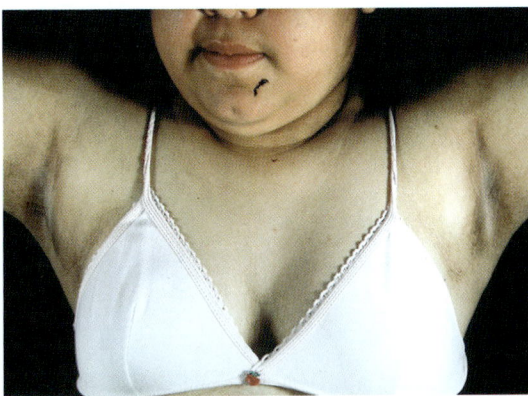

Fig. 3: Benign acanthosis nigricans located on axillary folds.

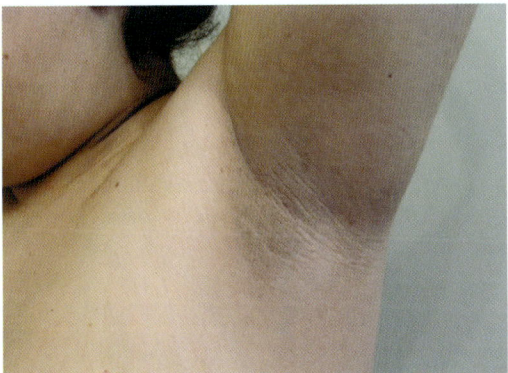

Fig. 4: Benign acanthosis nigricans located on axillary folds.

areas. Acrochordons (skin tags) share the etiopathogenesis with AN, and can be found in or around the affected areas.[3] Acanthosis nigricans in a scleredema plaque has also been described, both pathologies associated to DM.[4]

Although the mechanism by which AN arises has not been clarified completely, in its benign form there are factors involved that stimulate keratinocyte and fibroblast (FB) proliferation, like insulin and insulin-like growth factor 1 (IGF-1) thanks to its proliferative properties and differentiation. IGF-1 is expressed by keratinocytes of the stratum granulosum and dermal FBs, but not basal keratinocytes.[5]

Insulin crosses the dermo-epidermal junction (DEJ) in order to reach the keratinocytes and in small concentrations joins its classical receptor and regulates the metabolism of carbon hydrates, proteins and lipids, slightly promoting growth.

Genetic or acquired defects of the insulin receptor produce IR and compensatory pancreatic secretion of the hormone into the circulation. Insulin in high concentrations exerts powerful proliferative changes, due to direct and indirect toxic effects. The direct effect is on epidermal and dermal

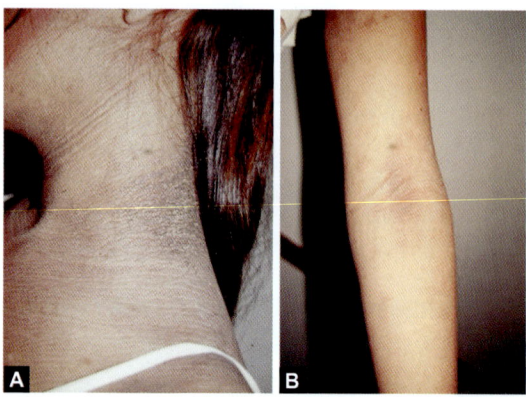

Figs. 5A and B: Acanthosis nigricans. (A) Lateral neck; (B) Upper extremity fold.

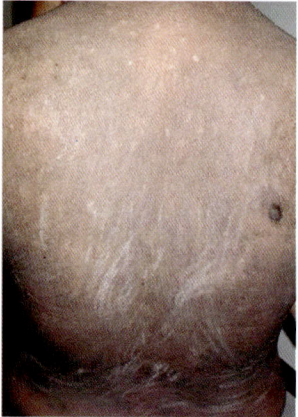

Fig. 6: Generalized acanthosis nigricans on a female patient with underlying malignancy.

cells, that along with an increase in the metabolism increase their replication and growth, which in turn becomes clinically evident through skin thickening and hyperpigmentation. The indirect effect through which hyperinsulinemia produces AN is through the increase of free IGF-1 levels in the circulation. At supraphysiological concentrations, insulin not only binds with its own receptor, but also through a high affinity binding with the IGF-1 (IGF-1R) receptor whose levels on the other side are elevated in the case of obese patients with hyperinsulinemia. IGF-1 receptor is similar in structural terms to the classic insulin receptor, but it binds 100–1,000 times with more affinity to insulin.[6]

Insulin-like growth factor 1 activity is regulated through binding proteins of the IGF [IGF binding proteins (IGFBPs)] type 1 and 2 (IGFBP-1 and IGFBP-2), which decrease in obese patients with hyperinsulinemia, increasing the plasmatic concentrations of the metabolically active "free" blood IGF, which in turn promotes growth and proliferation. It is believed that the systemic decrease of IGFBP-1 and IGFBP-2 induced by insulin could increase local levels of free IGF-1 and favor the development of hyperkeratosis and papillomatosis observed in AN.

Insulin-like growth factor binding proteins IGFBP-1 and IGFBP-2 increase the half-life of IGF-1, release IGFs to the target tissues and regulate "free" IGF-1 levels.

Other suggested mediators include tyrosine kinase receptors like the epidermal growth factor receptor (EGFR) or the fibroblast growth factor receptor (FGFR).[7]

It is believed, that in malignant AN there is a substance secreted by the tumor or in response to it, which could be the transforming growth factor alpha (TGF-α), whose structure is similar to EGF.

Benign and malignant AN lesions cannot be distinguished, but there are a couple of points to be highlighted. Benign AN has variations in its presentation depending on the race, age, etc., but without showing predilection for any gender.

Malignant AN does not have racial predilection, but its manifestation is more frequent and extensive in older patients and it also progresses quite fast. It appears sudden and dramatically, sometimes even accompanied by pruritus. The oral cavity is involved in 25–50% of the cases, specially the lips and commissures. Skin lesions become visible simultaneously in 61% of the patients and they precede in 17% of the cases or are subsequent to cancer detection.[8]

Regarding morbidity and mortality, in the benign form there are practically no complications regarding skin lesions, but we have to keep the underlying condition of IR in mind. The severity of the skin changes can be correlated with the degree of IR, which can improve with the treatment of the IR condition. On the contrary, AN associated to malignancy has a very bad prognosis, since it is associated with aggressive tumors and a short survival time after the diagnosis, which usually does not exceed 2 years.

So, in the case of a patient with malignant AN, we will usually find an association with IR or obesity. In order to assess IR, we examine insulinemia, which will most probably elevated if confirmed, being important for the detection of patients that still do not have insulin deficiency, but which could lead them to a declared DM. We perform a check-up in order to discard DM through glycosylated hemoglobin or a glucose tolerance test. In the case of older patients with extensive cutaneous or mucosa involvement, it will be necessary to get a comprehensive screening in order to rule out malignancy.

In histopathology, we can observe hyperkeratosis, acanthosis and hyperplasia of melanocytes in the epidermis, with minimal dermal variations like papillomatosis and a light perivascular lymphocytic infiltrates.[3]

Many topical and systemic drugs have been used in cases of AN, but it is mandatory to correct the underlying condition. The treatment of skin lesions is done for cosmetic reasons. A change in habits, like a low-calorie diet, an increase in physical activity and a decreased body weight can improve IR and compensatory hyperinsulinemia. The correction of the latter can revert the severity of the cutaneous injuries. The withdrawal of the drug involved or the surgical removal of the tumor can help regress the clinical picture.

Topical therapeutic agents like Vitamin D3 analogs (calcipotriol) and keratolytics like topical retinoid type, urea-based creams and salicylic acid, triple depigmentation combinations (tretinoin 0.05%, hydroquinone 4%, and fluocinolone acetonide 0.01%), and superficial peelings with trichloroacetic acid (TAA) 15% which destroys the epidermis could be beneficial.[9,10]

Systemic retinoids, isotretinoin and acitretin could be effective due to their ability to regulate keratinocytes proliferation and differentiation, but recurrence is the rule after discontinuation the drug.[11] Dermabrasion and laser (alexandrite) have also been described.

In the case of malignant AN, tumor removal is the gold standard of treatment. Cyproheptadine can inhibit the release of substances by the tumor, as well as psoralen + ultraviolet A (UVA) (PUVA) are used to decrease pruritus, if necessary.[12]

INSULIN, INSULIN-RESISTANCE AND METABOLIC SYNDROME

Insulin is a polypeptide hormone produced by pancreatic β-cells; it controls glucose levels in the blood, whereby it plays a central role in the metabolic system. When binding to its receptor, produces its own autophosphorylation and the recruitment of molecules such as insulin receptor substrates (IRS), which can also be generated through IGF-1. This implies the activation of multiple pathways which not only regulate glucose, lipids and proteins metabolism, but also control mitogenic responses through proliferation, differentiation and apoptosis control. Among these signaling cascades are PI 3-K/AKT, mammalian target of rapamycin (mTOR) and Ras/mitogen-activated protein kinase (MAPK). AKT, particularly, controls the conformation of the glucose 4 transporter (GLUT-4) at the level of the cell membrane and thus, controls the influx of glucose into the cell. The mTOR-1 complex (mTORC1) activates S6K1 kinase, which phosphorylates and inhibits the insulin substrates, and therefore decreases the uptake of glucose dependent on AKT-GLUT, the main peripheral IR mechanism.[13]

Insulin resistance consists of a biological effect whereby a fixed amount of insulin (exogenous or endogenous) is not capable to induce uptake and use of glucose as in normal individuals. This decreases the transportation of glucose to the skeletal muscle, adipose tissue and liver; and on the other side, hinders the normal compensatory response of the pancreas. This increase in the insulin secretion into the bloodstream, tries to maintain normal levels of glucose and lipid homeostasis. If hyperinsulinemia is enough to overcome IR, the regulation of glucose will stay normal; if not, DM2 happens.[14]

Effects associated to hyperinsulinemia include accelerated lipogenesis with increased production of free fatty acids and other hormonal changes, among which are low levels of sexual hormone binding globulin (SHBG), increased luteinizing hormone (LH) and follicle-stimulating hormone (FSH) levels, an increased ovarian androgen production and, thanks to its biologically active part, potential hyperandrogenism.

Insulin resistance occurs in 20% to 25% of individuals. It is a multifactorial failure that comprises genetic and acquired factors. Its detection is subject of multiple studies that link together insulinemia and fasting glucose levels. Homeostatic model assessment (HOMA) is one of the best known.[15]

$$HOMA = \frac{Insulin\ (uIU/mL) \times Glycemia\ (mg/dL)}{405}$$

The most frequent skin manifestations secondary to IR, are acrochordons and AN, present in one-third of the patients. Both are easy to recognize clinical signs of IR and noninsulin dependent DM.[16]

Acanthosis nigricans and IR are so closely related, that some consider them a clinical substitute for hyperinsulinemia in the laboratory.

Payne et al. concluded that for an instant evaluation of AN, the change in the skin's texture at the posterolateral aspect of the neck is more sensitive and specific than its hyperpigmentation and proposed for this finding the term *insulin neck* (a visibly increased texture-like lines and/or grooves and crests at the posterolateral part of the neck) (Fig. 7). Even more, the appearance of the texture avoids possible confusions with the pigmentation induced by the sun. The authors suggest that all patients with an elevated BMI should be assessed for *insulin neck* and if the texture of the neck is normal, it is less likely associated with IR.[17]

Nevertheless, for some authors even if AN and IR are closely related, obesity is a more important determinant for IR than AN; thus, AN should not be seen as an exclusive marker to predict that a child with overweight suffers from excessive insulin levels.

Other remarkable cutaneous findings are keratosis pilaris, hirsutism and signs of hyperandrogenism that include seborrhea and acne, which are accentuated in the presence of obesity. It has also been noted, that these patients have more severe infectious processes and complications in adulthood, like plantar hyperkeratosis and ulcers, among others.[18]

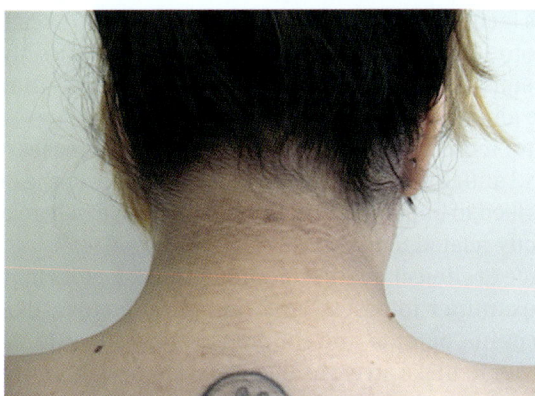

Fig. 7: Benign acanthosis nigricans located on lateral and posterior folds of the neck, in a diabetes type 2 insulin resistant female patient.

TABLE 2: Types of insulin resistance (IR).

IR type	Cause
Type A	Reduced number and dysfunction of insulin receptors
Type B	Antibodies against insulin
Type C	Postreceptor defects

Among the alterations associated to IR, we have to mention changes in the function of endothelial cells, alterations in coagulation (thrombosis and fibrinolysis) and proinflammatory phenomena.

There are different types of IR, classified into A, B and C, respectively (Table 2). Obese patients and bearers of polycystic ovary syndrome (PCOS) have type A.

The disturbance of the carbohydrate metabolism, central obesity, hypertriglyceridemia, hyperinsulinemia, cholesterol abnormalities linked to high-density lipoproteins (cHDL) and arterial hypertension (HT) are disorders related to IR that constitute a set of risk factors for DM and cardiovascular diseases, the so called metabolic syndrome (MS).

Frequently, some authors refer to IR as a synonym for MS, but IR and/or hyperinsulinemia could actually be absent in the syndrome. A patient with insulinoma (insulin-producing tumor), will clearly have hyperinsulinemia, but no higher cardiovascular risk if he/she does not have IR.

An issue still unresolved is the question of the existence of one or more causes for MS and which these would be. There are different hypotheses: fetal malnutrition and visceral obesity among others. Regardless of the mechanism definitely responsible, there is no doubt about the incidence of genetic and environmental components.

In cases of MS, hyperinsulinemia induces a lipogenic condition that promotes abdominal obesity, triglyceride production through the liver, and very low density lipoprotein release.[19] Adipose tissue, formerly considered energy storage tissue, is actually a key endocrine organ. It secretes a number of biologically active proteins named "adipokines", among which we find the tumor necrosis factor-alpha (TNF-α), interleukin-6 (IL-6), resistin, leptin and adiponectin. Some of them, e.g. resistin and adiponectin, directly and indirectly affect insulin sensitvity by modulating its signaling and that of molecules involved in the glucose and lipid metabolism.

In IR, resistin increases and serum adiponectin decreases, which have an antidiabetic and antiatherogenic action that contribute to the development of MS. Both are linked to body weight, adiponectin is inversely related to it, while resistin is directly related to it.[9]

The presence of clinical manifestations and risk factors in patients should motivate the examiner to assess environmental factors, like education at home, obese parents, parents' and children's life habits, outdoor activities and nutrition, in order to make an early diagnosis and design a treatment through changes in lifestyle, nutrition and pharmacotherapy with metformin (MET) and insulin, if necessary.[18]

INSULIN SENSITIZING AGENTS

Their goal is to reduce IR and hyperinsulinemia and improve metabolic alterations. The main agents are Metformin and thiazolidinediones (TZD), widely used in the treatment of DM2. They reduce glucose production through an increase in insulin sensitivity of the peripheral tissues, they also reduce hyperinsulinemia, weight, and body fat.

Metformin is a biguanide whose main purpose is to inhibit hepatic glucose production and increase peripheral sensitivity of the tissues to insulin; these effects have been proven in women with polycystic ovarian syndrome, where circulating insulin levels and ovarian androgens decrease. In this context, MET would act as an inhibitor for anabolic and hyperproliferative processes mediated by western civilization mTORC1 (obesity, DM, etc.).[20]

Although in the case of diabetic patients, hyperglycemia levels decrease, when administered to nondiabetics, it only decreases insulin levels without modifying glycemia. The main side effects affecting up to 50% of patients are digestive (sickness, vomit and abdominal pain). Ten to thirty percent can develop Vitamin B12 malabsorption during long-term treatments. Although not frequent, lactic acidosis is the worst complication; therefore, this drug is contraindicated in the presence of renal insufficiency. It is considered a category B drug during pregnancy. There are reports that relate MET with a decrease of the relative risk of progression of glucose intolerance (GI) status to DM, and also on its indication as protective measure against cardiovascular risks in cases of IR and insulin excess.[21]

Thiazolidinediones constitute a new class of agonist drug of the human peroxisome proliferator activated receptor gamma gene (hPPAR-γ) that after coupling with the receptor forms a complex which binds to specific genes that regulate—by stimulation or inhibition—molecules that affect the action of insulin and lipid metabolism. They exert their effects, in part, by increasing the expression and circulating levels of adiponectin (rosiglitazone). As a result, TZD improve the action of insulin and decrease IR.[22]

In those cases with hyperandrogenism, IR and AN (HAIR-AN syndrome), MET may be used in combination with oral contraceptives.[23]

REFERENCES

1. Kutlubay Z, Engin B, Bairamov O, et al. Acanthosis nigricans: a fold (intertriginous) dermatosis. Clin Dermatol. 2015;33(4):466-70.
2. Bahadursingh S, Mungalsingh C, Seemungal T, et al. Acanthosis nigricans in type 2 diabetes: prevalence, correlates and potential as a simple clinical screening tool—a cross-sectional study in the Caribbean. Diabetology & Metabolic Syndrome. 2014;6(77):2-9.
3. Ki-Heon Jeong, Seung-Joon Oh, Suk Chon, et al. Generalized acanthosis nigricans related to type B insulin resistance syndrome: a case report. Cutis. 2010;86: 299-302.
4. Lamba S, Krishtul A, Tan MH, et al. Acanthosis nigricans in a plaque of scleredema on the back of a diabetic patient: a case report. Int J Dermatol. 2005;44(1):45-7.

5. Puri N. A study of pathogenesis of acanthosis nigricans and its clinical implications. Indian J Dermatol. 2011;56(6):678-83.
6. Higgins SP, Freemark M, Prose NS. Acanthosis nigricans: a practical approach to evaluation and management. Dermatol Online J. 2008;14(9):2.
7. Deklotz CMC, Eshagh K, Krakowski AC. psoriatic Plaques "Koebnerizing" to areas of acanthosis Nigricans in an obese female clues to a common pathway? J Clin Aesthet Dermatol. 2014;7(11):40-1.
8. Piscoya Rivera A, de los Ríos Senmache R, Valdivia Retamozo J, et al. Acantosis Nigricans Maligna: Reporte de un Caso y Revisión de la Literatura. Rev Gastroenterol Perú. 2005;25:101-5.
9. Phiske MM. An approach to acanthosis nigricans. Indian Dermatology Online Journal. 2014;5(3):239-49.
10. Zayed A. Sobhi RM, Abdel Halim, DM. Using trichloroacetic acid in the treatment of acanthosis nigricans: a pilot study. J Dermatol Treat. 2014;25(3):223-5.
11. Hermanns-Lê T, Scheen A, Piérard GE. Acanthosis nigricans associated with insulin resistance: pathophysiology and management. Am J Clin Dermatol. 2004;5(3):199-203.
12. Miller JH, Rapini RP, Cruz PD Jr, et al. Acanthosis Nigricans. [cited 2014 Feb 24]. Available from: http://emedicine.medscape.com/article/1102488-overview#a0199.
13. Napolitano M, Megna M, Monfrecola G. Insulin resistance and skin diseases. Scientific World Journal. 2015;2015:479354. doi: 10.1155/2015/479354.
14. Levobitz HE. Insuline resistance: definition and consequences. Exp Clin Endocrinol Diabete 2001;109:135-48.
15. Wallace TM, Levy JC, Matthews DR. Use and abuse of HOMA modeling. Diabetes Care. 2004;27:1487-95.
16. Sadeghian G, Ziaie H, Amini M, et al. Evaluation of insulin resistance in obese women with and without acanthosis nigricans. J Dermatol. 2009;36(4):209-12.
17. Payne KS, Rader RK, Lastra G, et al. Posterolateral neck texture (insulin neck) early sign of insulin resistance. JAMA Dermatol. 2013;149(7):875-7.
18. Baselga Torres E, Torres-Pradilla M. Manifestaciones cutáneas en niños con diabetes mellitus y obesidad. Actas Dermosifiliogr. 2014;105(6):546-57.
19. Puchulu F. Sindrome metabólico en Diabetes y piel. 1era Ed. Ed. Ediciones Journal S.A. 2013: p175-81.
20. Melnik BC, Schmitz G. Metformin: an inhibitor of mTORC1 signaling. J Endocrinol Diab Obesity. 2014;2(2):1029.
21. Knowler WC, Barrett-Connor E, Fowler SE, et al. Diabetes Prevention Program Research Group. Reduction in the incidence of type 2 diabetes with lifestyle intervention or metformin. N Engl J Med. 2002;346:393-403.
22. Lebovitz HE, Banerji MA. Insulin resistance and its treatment by thiazolidinediones. Recent Prog Horm Res. 2001;56:265-94.
23. Buerger C, Richter B, Woth K, et al. Interleukin-1B interferes with epidermal homeostasis through induction of insulin esistance: implications for psoriasis pathogenesis. J Invest Dermatol. 2012;132(9):2206-14.

CHAPTER
7

Cutaneous Infections in Diabetics

PART 7A: FUNGAL INFECTIONS IN DIABETICS
Roberto Arenas, César Iván Eugenio-González

INTRODUCTION

Diabetes mellitus (DM) is a heterogeneous group of chronic and degenerative disorders characterized by serologic glucose high levels and alterations of lipid and carbohydrates metabolism. It is considered that almost 30% of patients have cutaneous manifestations and an important group has infections.[1] A susceptibility to cutaneous infections is not present when DM is under control, except for *Candida* and *Corynebacterium minutissimum* which is a causative agent of a pseudomycosis involving intertriginous zones such as gluteal groove and inframammary fold with erythematous and pigmentary macules with a fine desquamation.

Infections are more frequent and severe when an inadequate metabolic control, high glycemic levels, ketoacidosis, hypohidrosis or micro- and macroangiopathy are present. A relationship also has been found with serological hyperglycemic, hyperosmolarity and dysfunction of white blood cells.[2] It has been seen that *Candida* spp. predominate when saliva shows high concentrations of glucose. In these patients cutaneous and systemic manifestations are highly important.

CANDIDAL INFECTIONS

Infection with *Candida albicans* and *Candida glabrata* species have a high frequency and their clinical manifestations range from local mucous membrane infections to widespread systemic dissemination with multisystemic organ failure. Local manifestations are mainly oral such as oropharyngeal or thrush commonly seen in infants, elderly adults who wear dentures with false teeth and those with cellular immune deficiency; the usual symptoms are in the oral cavity, loss of taste and pain on eating and swallowing. The diagnosis is suspected when white plaques on the buccal mucosa, palate, tongue or the oropharynx with a cottony aspect are present. Diagnosis is confirmed by scraping the lesions and microscopic exam using potassium hydroxide (KOH), chlorazol black or lactophenol blue preparations observing budding yeasts with or without pseudohyphae are seen or culture of skin scrapings in Sabouraud dextrose agar can be made[3] (Figs. 1 and 2).

Vulvovaginitis, which is the most common form of mucosal candidiasis and diabetes mellitus, is a well-known condition. Clinical manifestations are primarily itching and discharge, dyspareunia, dysuria and vaginal irritation. Physical examination shows vulvar and vaginal erythema and discharge.[3]

Intertriginous candidiasis is especially present in obese patients living in tropical zones and in elderly patients with no efficient metabolic control; the warm, moist environment of the skin folds predispose for the growth of *Candida* spp. Other risk factors are obesity, hyperhidrosis, and immunodeficiency. Clinical manifestations are erythematous, macerated plaques and erosions with fine peripheral scaling and erythematous satellite papules and pustules in

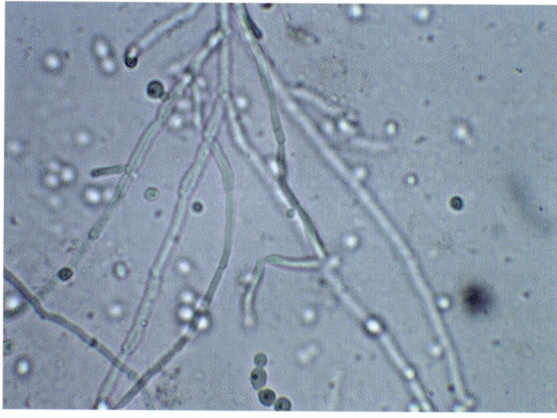

Fig. 1: Pseudohyphae and yeast in *Candida* spp. (Lactofenol blue 40x).

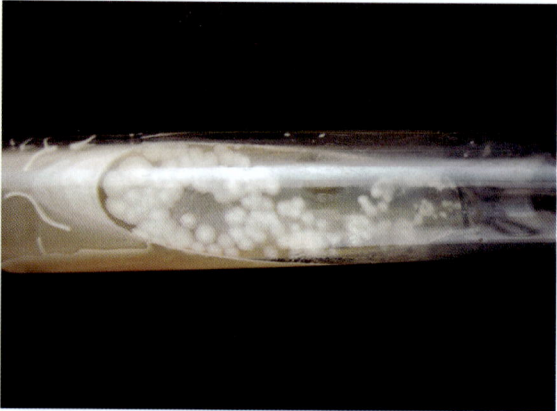

Fig. 2: *Candida* culture in Sabouraud dextrose agar.

typical locations including inguinal folds, axillae, and scrotum and intergluteal folds (Fig. 3). Many times this mucocutaneous manifestation is mandatory to evaluate the possible association with diabetes.[1]

Although *Candida* spp. are considered normal flora in the gastrointestinal and genitourinary tracts of humans, they have the propensity to invade and cause disease when an imbalance is created in the ecologic niche in which these organisms usually exists. The immune response of the host is an important determinant of the type of infection caused by these yeasts.[3]

DERMATOPHYTIC INFECTIONS

Dermatophyte infections are common worldwide, and are the prevailing causes of fungal infection of the skin, hair and nails.[4] They are as frequent as in general population, but complications in the DM context can be severe, that's why it is very important to perform a careful physical examination especially in the feet.[1] Onychomycosis is estimated to affect 12% of the United States of America populations and represents 50% of all nail disorders.[5] It is the most common fungal skin infection and it is frequently seen in the setting of other concomitant fungal diseases, the most common being tinea pedis. Infected nails become a reservoir of fungal organisms that may infect the skin and vice versa.[6] The three major clinical types of dermatophytic foot infection are: (1) Interdigital which manifests as pruritic, erythematous erosions or scales between the toes, especially between the third and fourth interdigital fold; (2) hyperkeratotic (moccasin-type) characterized by a diffuse hyperkeratotic eruption involving the soles and medial and lateral surfaces of the feet, resembling a "moccasin"; and (3) bullous (inflammatory) which presents as pruritic, sometimes painful, vesicular or bullous eruption with underlying erythema.[7] The diagnosis is confirmed with the detection of segmented hyphae in skin scrapings from an affected area with a microscopic exam with KOH preparation (Fig. 4). Isolated agents are usually *Trichophyton rubrum* in

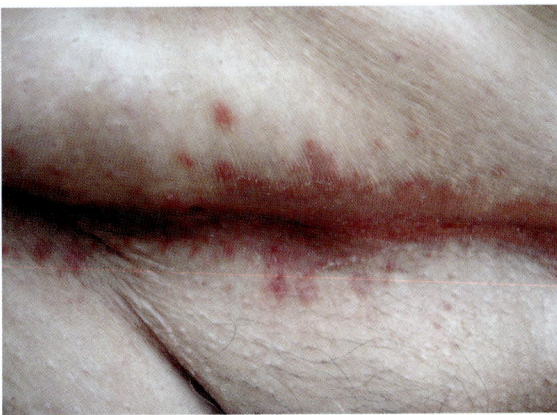

Fig. 3: Intertriginous candidiasis in an obese and diabetic woman.

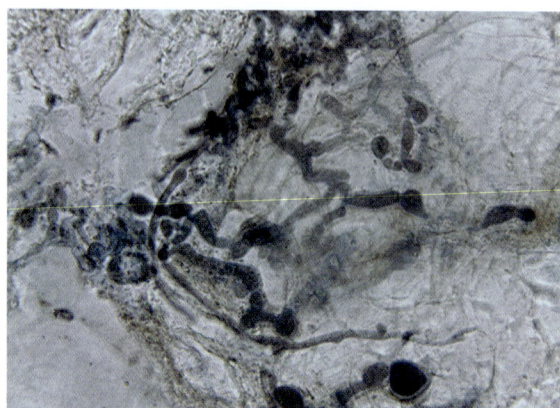

Fig. 4: Fungal hyphae under direct examination (Chlorazol black 40x).

chronic forms and *Trichophyton mentagrophytes* in acute type. Identification of the causal agent is very important in order to offer an early topical or systemic antifungal treatment.[1]

INFECTIONS CAUSED BY ZYGOMYCETES

Mucormycosis is manifested by a variety of different syndromes, particularly in immunocompromised patients and those with diabetes mellitus.[8] Clinical importance of opportunistic invasive fungal infections has significantly increased due to an increase of immunocompromised and diabetic patients who present disorders in the immune system, both at a cellular and humoral level, such as the reduction of the phagocytic activity of neutrophils and opsonization inability, particularly during ketoacidosis imbalance because hyperglycemia and metabolic acidosis reduce even further the chemotactic action of phagocytes.[9-12] The incidence of mucormycosis is difficult to estimate since it is not a reportable disease and the risk varies widely in different populations. A review of 929 cases between 1940 and 2003 noted that diabetes mellitus was the most common predisposing factor, found in 36% of cases, followed by hematologic malignancies (17%) and solid organ or hematopoietic cell transplantation (12%).[8,13] In some patients, mucormycosis was the diabetes-defining illness. Mucormycosis is characterized by infarction and necrosis of host tissues that results from invasion of the vasculature by hyphae.[14]

The most common clinical presentation of mucormycosis is rhino-orbito-cerebral infection; hyperglycemia usually with an associated metabolic acidosis is the most common underlying condition.[13] A review of 179 cases of rhino-orbito-cerebral mucormycosis found that 126 (70%) of the patients had diabetes mellitus and that most had ketoacidosis at the time of presentation.[15] Invasive fungal sinusitis caused by mucoral fungi has devastating results. It is characterized by infiltrating adjacent structures and it progresses rapidly[16] (Fig. 5).

Therefore, it frequently progresses to the rhino-orbito-cerebral form, from paranasal sinuses to the central nervous system, first for its adjacent position to the orbit and then to the cribriform plate; this form is most commonly caused by *Rhizopus oryzae*[17,18] (Fig. 6). In almost 100% of cases, the patients have facial pain and headache, but the most common symptom is periorbital edema in 41% and fever in 34% of cases.[19] The infection usually presents as acute sinusitis with fever, nasal congestion, purulent nasal discharge, headache, and sinus pain.[20] The hallmarks of spread beyond the sinuses are tissue necrosis of the palate resulting in palatal eschars, destruction of the turbinates, perinasal swelling, and erythema and cyanosis of the facial skin overlying the involved sinuses[21] (Fig. 7). A review of 208 cases of rhino-orbito-cerebral mucormycosis published in the literature between 1970 and 1993 found the following frequency of symptoms and signs: fever 44%, nasal ulceration or necrosis

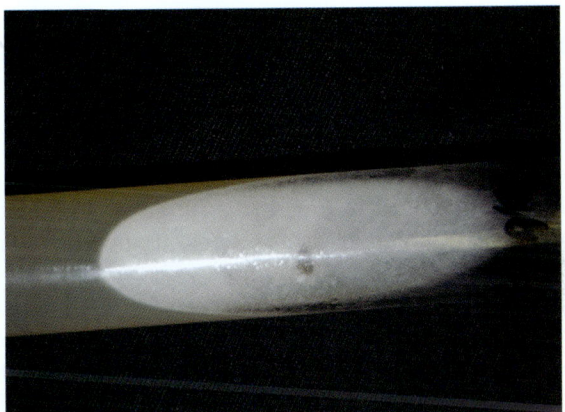

Fig. 5: Mucoral on Sabouraud dextrose agar.

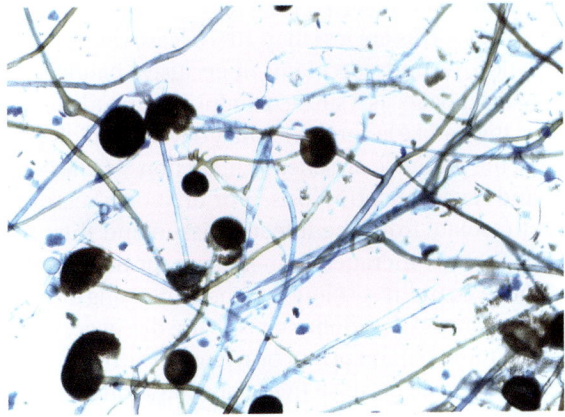

Fig. 6: Microscopic examination of *Rhizopus* spp.

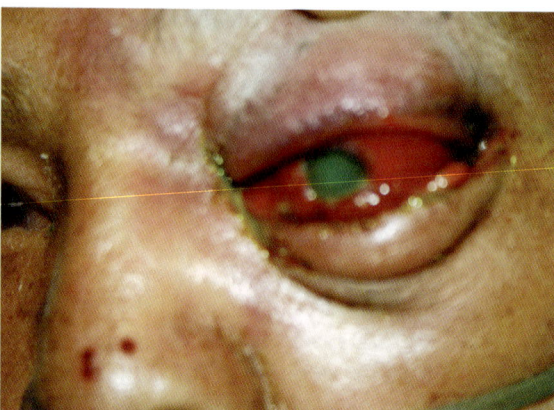

Fig. 7: Severe mucormycosis of the orbital and periorbital zone.

38%, periorbital or facial swelling 34%, decreased vision 30%, ophthalmoplegia 29%, sinusitis 26% and headache 25%.[22]

Palate conditions occur in three stages: first, erythema, followed by ulceration, and finally, a black eschar appears. Even though visualization of necrotic tissue is very suggestive of mucormycosis, it is present in 40% of cases.[17] Black necrotic tissue and black retronasal discharge are pathognomonic signs of vascular invasion which appear as a reflection of tissue necrosis and are important markers of deep tissue infection.[21]

Mucormycosis, in 1950, had a survival rate of only 16%, and most diagnoses were made postmortem.[12,17] Currently, in spite of aggressive treatment, mortality is still over 40%.[10,23] The high morbidity and mortality associated with these infections is not only the result of microorganism virulence, but also of delayed diagnosis. The stigma of intracranial disease indicates extensive disease and severe prognosis; mortality increases when the orbit is affected, and survival is rare when brain involvement is present.[24,25] The average time between diagnosis and death is 10–17 days.[26]

Primary cutaneous forms are less than 10% of cases and usually appear after traumatic inoculation, wounds, accidents or occlusive bandages but no related with DM.[27] It usually appears as a single, painful, indurated area of cellulitis that develops into an ecthyma-like lesion, which may develop rapidly progressive tissue necrosis reflecting the presence of ischemic infarction.[23] Other sites of infections are pulmonary and renal mucormycosis.[8] For unknown reasons, zygomycetes can be difficult to isolate from the infected tissue and they seldom grow in cultures[1] (Fig. 8). The first therapeutic maneuver for treatment required is an early diagnosis, followed by the resolution of the underlying disease, for example, hyperglycemia and control of acidotic states.[28] The discovery of amphotericin B marked a change in the evolution of mucormycosis. The new liposomal formulas have proved to be less toxic because their concentration increases in inflamed tissues, thus resulting in a lower systemic dose with less nephrotoxicity. Some case

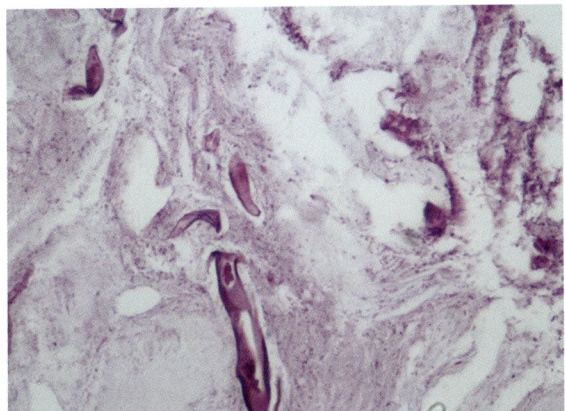

Fig. 8: Fungal structures in mucormycosis biopsy (periodic acid-Schiff 40x).

reports claim that the side effects that amphotericin B produces contributes to the morbidity of mucormycosis, so new treatments have been sought, finding success with posaconazole.[29] The most important management is extensive surgical debridement of the necrotic tissue. Evidence has shown that this treatment is essential for fungus eradication, despite the fact that some reports claim success with medical treatment exclusively. Treatment duration must be individualized and is based on the resolution of the clinical symptoms, on the stabilization of radiologic signs, and on the resolution of the underlying immunosuppression.

One of the most critical decisions in the management of rhino-orbital mucormycosis is whether the eyeball should be preserved or not. This is an important decision because the orbit is the entry port to the central nervous system. There is no standard data in the literature to guide physicians in terms of eye exenteration, and there is insufficient information concerning criteria that help make an evidence-based decision.[17] The eye exenteration is indicated in cases of fungal invasion to the orbit, particularly with inflammatory activity. We can consider that there is orbital invasion if there is vision loss, eye movement restriction, proptosis, ophthalmoplegia, conjunctival pallor, chemosis, and retinal artery occlusion.[30] We are in favor of eye exenteration; it would be performed in all the cases with ocular invasion or suspicion of rapidly progressive disease.

REFERENCES

1. Arenas R. Medical Illustrated Micologia, 5th edition. Mexico: McGraw Hill; 2014. pp. 239-80, 270-89.
2. Jelinek JE. Cutaneous manifestations of diabetes mellitus. Int J Dermatol. 1994;33:605-17.
3. Kauffman CA. Diagnosis and management of fungal urinary tract infection. Infect Dis Clin North Am. 2014;28(1):61-74.
4. Havlickova B, Czaika VA, Friedrich M. Epidemiological trends in skin mycoses worldwide. Mycoses. 2008;51 Suppl 4:2-15.

5. Borgers M, Degreef H, Cauwenbergh G. Fungal infections of the skin: infection process and antimycotic therapy. Curr Drug Targets. 2005;6(8):849-62.
6. Zeichner JA. Onychomycosis to fugal superinfection: prevention strategies and considerations. J Drugs Dermatol. 2015;14(10):32-4.
7. Goldstein AO, Smith KM, Ives TJ, et al. Mycotic infections. Effective management of conditions involving the skin, hair, and nails. Geriatrics. 2000;55(5):40-2, 45-7, 51-2.
8. Ameen M, Arenas R, Martinez-Luna E, et al. The emergence of mucormycosis as an important opportunistic fungal infection: five cases presenting to a tertiary referral center for mycology. Int J Dermatol. 2007;46:380-4.
9. Csomor J, Nikolova R, Sinkó J, et al. Mucormycosis. Orv Hetil. 2004;145:2507-13.
10. Spellberg B, Walsh T, Kontoyiannis DP, et al. Recent advances in the management of mucormycosis: from bench to bedside. Clin Infect Dis. 2009;48:1743-51.
11. Perez MI, Kohn SR. Cutaneous manifestations of diabetes mellitus J Am Acad Dermatol. 1994;30:519-31.
12. Naggie S, Perfect JR. Molds: yalohyphomycosis, phaeohyphomycosis, and zygomycosis. Clin Chest Med. 2009;30:337-53.
13. Roden MM, Zaoutis TE, Buchanan WL, et al. Epidemiology and outcome of zygomycosis: a review of 929 reported cases. Clin Infect Dis. 2005;41(5):634.
14. Petrikkos G, Skiada A, Lortholary O, et al. Epidemiology and clinical manifestations of mucormycosis. Clin Infect Dis. 2012;54 Suppl 1:S23-34.
15. McNulty JS. Rhinocerebral mucormycosis: predisposing factors. Laryngoscope. 1982;92:1140.
16. Songu M, Unlu HH, Gunhan K, et al. Orbital exenteration: A dilemma in mucormycosis presented with orbital apex syndrome. Am J Rhinol. 2008;22(1): 98-103.
17. Fisher E, Tomas A, Fisher PH, et al. Rhinocerebral mucormycosis: Use of liposomal amphotericin B. J Laryngol Otol. 1991;105:575-7.
18. Waitzman AA, Birt BD. Fungal sinusitis. J Otolaryngol. 1994;23:244-9.
19. Iwen P, Rupp ME, Hinrichs SH. Invasive mold sinusitis: 17 cases in immunocompromised patients and review of the literature. Clin Infect Dis. 1997;24:1178-84.
20. Harril WC, Stewart MG, Lee AG, et al. Chronic rhinocerebral mucormycosis. Laryngoscope. 1996;106:1292-7.
21. Rajagopalan S. Serious infections in elderly patients with diabetes mellitus. Clin Infect Dis. 2005;40:990-6.
22. Yohai RA, Bullock JD, Aziz AA, et al. Survival factors in rhino-orbital-cerebral mucormycosis. Surv Ophthalmol. 1994;39:3-22.
23. Adam RD, Hunter G, DiTomasso J, et al. Mucormycosis: emerging prominence of cutaneous infections. Clin Infect Dis. 1994;19:67-76.
24. Kauffman CA, Malani AN. Zygomycosis: an emerging fungal infection with new options for management. Curr Infect Dis Rep. 2007;9:435-40.
25. Munir M, Jones NS. Rhinocerebral mucormycosis with orbital and intracranial extension: a case report and review of optimum management. J Laryngol Otol. 2007;121:192-5.
26. Ryan M, Yeo S, Maguire A, et al. Rhinocerebral zygomycosis in childhood acute lymphoblastic leukaemia. Eur J Pediatr. 2001;160:235-8.
27. Song WK, Park HJ, Cinn YW, et al. Primary cutaneous mucormycosis in a trauma patient. J Dermatol. 1999;26(12):825-8.

28. De Pauw B, Walsh TJ, Donnelly JP, et al. Revised definitions of invasive fungal disease from the European Organization for Research and Treatment of Cancer/Invasive Fungal Infections Cooperative Group and the National Institute of Allergy and Infectious Diseases Mycoses Study Group (EORTC/MSG) Consensus Group. Clin Infect Dis. 2008;46:1813-21.
29. Van Burik J, Hare R, Solomon H, et al. Posaconazole is effective as salvage therapy in zygomycosis: a retrospective summary of 91 cases. Clin Infect Dis. 2006;42:61-5.
30. Nithyanandam S, Jacob MS, Battu RR, et al. Rhino-orbito-cerebral mucormycosis. A retrospective analysis of clinical features and treatment outcomes. Indian J Ophthalmol. 2003;51:231-6.

PART 7B: BACTERIAL INFECTIONS IN DIABETICS

Emilia Noemí Cohen Sabban

INTRODUCTION

Cutaneous infections occur in 20% to 50% of patients with poorly controlled and complicated diabetes mellitus (DM), especially type 2. Its incidence correlates with hyperglycemia, acid-base imbalances, vascular insufficiency, peripheral neuropathy, anhydrosis, decreased sebaceous secretion, trauma and impaired immune response.[1]

Bacterial and fungal infections can be the presenting feature of the disease. A recurrent candidal infection forces us to rule out an underlying diabetes.[2]

There are many reasons why patients with DM are at increased risk for skin and soft tissue bacterial infections (SSTIs). The deleterious effects of long-term DM have an impact on both specific and innate immune response. Hyperglycemia increases the nonenzymatic glycation (NEG) and the advanced glycation end-products (AGEs) output, with deleterious effects on fibroblast and endothelial cells, which are in turn key players in the wound healing process.[3]

A long-standing hyperglycemic condition in animal models has been shown to impair the skin barrier by decreasing the epidermal lipids production; by reducing the expression of antimicrobial peptides (AMPs) in the skin; and by a significant increase of serum levels of AGEs and their epidermal receptors resulting in inhibition of the defense mechanisms of the skin.[4] In the last few years, AMPs, defensins and cathelicidins have been shown to be an important step against gram-negative and gram-positive bacterial infection, including *Staphylococcus aureus*.[5]

In keratinocytes, AGEs significantly decrease human β-defensins (hBD) production through the inhibition of the signaling pathway p38MAPK.[6] In addition, keratinocytes express toll-like receptors (TLRs) and they act as a trigger of innate immune response because of their regulatory role in hBD synthesis.

Other components of the innate immunity are affected; diabetic patients have decreased neutrophil functioning (adherence, phagocytosis and cellular chemotaxis). It has been shown that intracellular bacterial killing activity of neutrophils and macrophages is impaired in vitro.[7] The NEG of antibodies leads to inconsistent humoral response, which occurs in proportion with increased glycated hemoglobin (HbA1c) levels.

The interaction between TLRs and β-defensins promotes an adaptive immune response, with recruitment of T-lymphocytes and dendritic cells to the site of invasion through intracellular signal.[8] Antigen-specific cell-mediated immunity and impaired T-lymphocytes proliferative responses to certain pathogens, such as *S. aureus*, have been described in patients with DM.[9]

The high concentration of glucose in the epidermis is an ideal environment for microbial colonization and infection.[10] Maceration and humidity stimulate bacterial colonization and growth. Other predisposing factors which play an important role are malnutrition/obesity status and the integrity of the skin barrier, since this is the first line against infections and serves as a physical defense.

Erosions, lacerations, wounds, burns and surgery can act as a port of entry by which the microbial penetration can occur.[11]

Diabetic SSTIs tend to be more severe, widespread, and recurrent. They progress rapidly and are often resistant to treatment, which in turn results in difficult wound healing and poor prognosis. Therefore, patients with DM have more associated complications and more SSTIs-related hospitalizations compared to patients without DM.[12] In a population-based study with 7-year follow-up, Benfield et al. have demonstrated that diabetes and hyperglycemia at baseline were both associated with an increased risk of infectious disease hospitalization.

Foot infections are the most important chronic complications of DM, and deserve a special consideration. *S. aureus* is the most common etiologic pathogen, although chronic infections are often polymicrobial.[13]

The diabetic foot infections are classified as mild/moderate or non-limb-threatening, and severe or limb-threatening. Based on that, if an infected foot ulcer remains untreated, the result would be necrosis, gangrene and amputation; therefore, the therapeutic approach should be based on the severity of the involvement.[14]

Normal Skin Flora and Pathogens

There are normal and pathogenic skin microflora. The former includes aerobic diphtheroids (*Corynebacterium* spp.), anaerobic diphtheroids (*Propionibacterium acnes*), coagulase-negative staphylococci (*Staphylococcus epidermidis*) and *Pseudomonas* spp.

Among the most common bacterial pathogens we can mention are *S. aureus* and group A beta-hemolytic streptococci (BHS), although *Pseudomonas aeruginosa* has also been implicated. Another pathogen is group B *Streptococcus* (*Streptococcus agalactiae*), which is responsible for the high morbimortality among neonates and pregnant women;[15] it also affects adults or elderly individuals with underlying conditions such as DM and immunocompromised patients. SSTIs are the most prevalent among the broad spectrum of its clinical manifestations including necrotizing fasciitis, toxic shock syndrome and primary bacteremia.[16] Diabetic patients are at increased risk of invasive disease with a global mortality rate of 16% based on a study of 58 diabetics, among whom the authors found that the severity of the invasion correlates with HbA1c more than 8%.[17] In our country, all the strains were penicillin and ceftriaxone sensitive.[18]

Out of all *S. aureus* infections, 90% locate in the skin and soft tissue. Thirty percent of healthy adults are carriage, with affection of the nares in the first place, followed by the skin, perineum, gastrointestinal tract and throat.

Apart from that, during the past two decades, the incidence of methicillin-resistant *S. aureus* (MRSA) has been increasing. In fact, all these pathogens tend to be more resistant to antibiotic treatment. One of the reasons is that they can form biofilms, consisting of a single or multiple bacterial species, covered by an extracellular polymeric substance. Actually, biofilm facilitates the survival and bacterial multiplication on the colonized or infected cutaneous surface; biofilm confers bacteria the possibility to evade the host immune response and, at the same time, therapeutic agents, turning them more resistant to antibiotics and more virulent. Another reason is that these bacteria count on cell surface proteins, extracellular enzymes and toxins, to become even more virulent. Among them, toxins, which are the most important, recognize two classes: endotoxins, which are lipopolysaccharides found in large amounts in the cell walls of gram-negative bacteria; and exotoxins, which produce damage through enzymatic reactions, cellular dysregulation or pore formation, with subsequent cell lysis. Some of them induce an exaggerated immune response through massive release of cytokines, in particular interleukin-1 and 17 (IL-1, IL-17) by T-cell lymphocytes.[19] One already-known toxin, and its pathogenic role, is Panton-Valentine leukocidin (PVL), which forms pores in neutrophils and has consistently been linked to suppurative cutaneous disorders such as abscesses and furunculosis.[20]

STAPHYLOCOCCUS AUREUS AND BETA-HEMOLYTIC STREPTOCOCCI

Clinical Description

Skin and soft tissue infections include a spectrum of disorders with different clinical presentation that compromise the skin and the underlying soft tissues

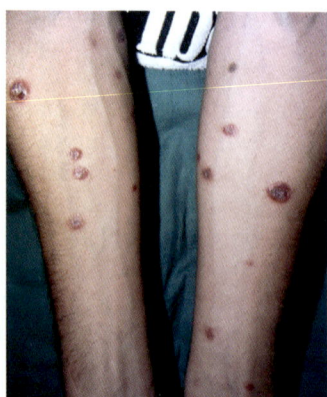

Fig. 1: Ecthyma. Multiple lesions on the upper extremities.

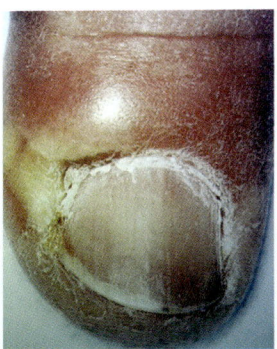

Fig. 2: Bacterial panadizo. Purulent collection.

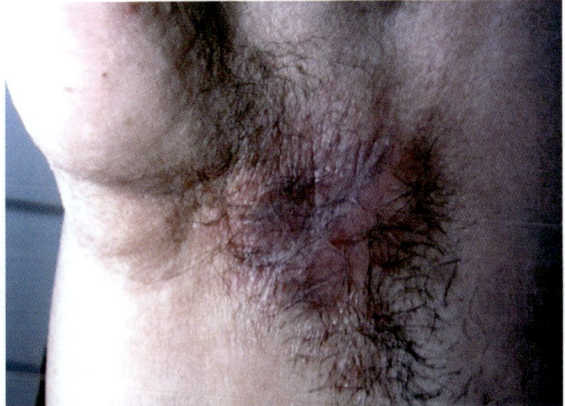

Fig. 3: Hydrosadenitis.

(Figs. 1 to 3). When the epidermal pores are involved, this may result in folliculitis and furuncles. Depending on the level of the skin that is affected, it may be erysipelas in the superficial layer while cellulitis involves the subcutaneous tissue. When the infection is still deeper, it may result in fasciitis, where the superficial fascia is involved.

There is an increased prevalence among men (60–70% of all cases) between 45 years old and 64 years old; and the lower legs are predominantly the site of involvement. They range from mild to life-threatening infections; however, around 70–75% of all cases are managed in the outpatient setting, and tend to resolve within 7–10 days. Cardinal signs and symptoms are erythema, edema, warmth, pain and/or tenderness. Based on how serious the infection is, the area involved may also develop a functional impairment (e.g. hands and legs).

In a study of 996 episodes among 841 hospitalized patients, abscesses and cellulitis/erysipelas were the most frequent, accounting for 66.7%. DM was present in 33% of the patients out of all possible comorbidities.[21]

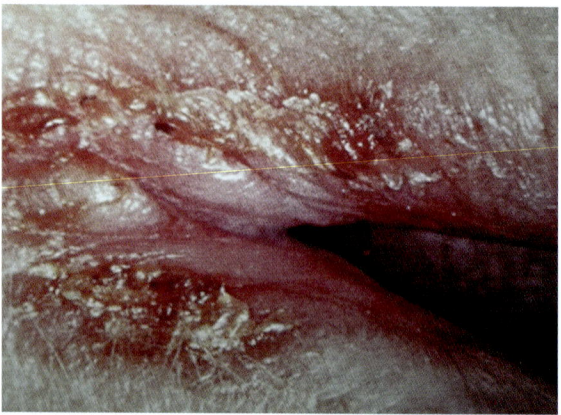

Fig. 4: Impetigo.

Impetigo

Impetigo is a common, superficial bacterial skin infection, which is most frequently encountered in children (Fig. 4).[22] There are two variants, bullous and nonbullous or crusted. The former is more frequent in children between 2 years and 5 years of age and is caused by a single organism, *S. aureus*. The production of exfoliative toxins (proteases) by this pathogen renders it virulent, causing localized blister formation at the epidermal subcorneal-granular level.[23]

Under clinical examination, it presents in the form of very small lesions measuring up to 2 cm in diameter each, initially with clear fluid, and later becoming purulent. As the blister is quite flaccid, the roof detaches easily, leading to central erosion surrounded by a collaret of scales at the periphery. It localizes predominantly in flexural areas, although it can be seen in any part of the skin. Adenopathies are not common.[11]

The nonbullous form accounts for most impetigo cases. It occurs in adults and children but rarely in those under 2 years of age. The main etiological pathogen is *S. aureus*, alone or in combination with group A BHS. Under physical examination, the lesions are very similar to that of bullous impetigo with some differences: (1) they are located on an erythematous skin of periorificial and exposed areas; (2) in their evolution, the serous or purulent content dries leading to the formation of a characteristic honey-yellowish colored crust; (3) regional adenopathy is more common and fever can be present. Self and hetero-inoculation have been described.

Erysipelas

Erysipelas is characterized by an acute onset of an erythematous and edematous plaque with ill-defined borders, which typically grows centrifugally, accompanied by local signs of inflammation and systemic manifestations (fever, chills and malaise). Lower limbs account for 80% of the cases followed by upper limbs, thorax or trunk, and head or face (Fig. 5).

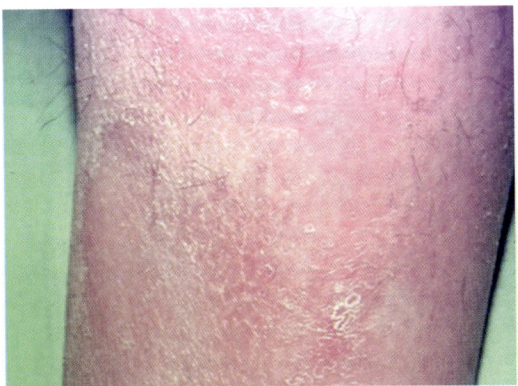

Fig. 5: Erysipelas.

Aside from DM, risk factors include lymphedema, venous insufficiency, leg ulcer, cutaneous barrier disruption such as toe web intertrigo or traumatic wounds, previous radiation therapy, any kind of localized surgery, and overweight. It is well known that women treated for breast cancer are at risk of ipsilateral erysipelas, especially if lymphedema develops.[24]

Around one-third have a positive local culture and bacteremia develops in a very low number of patients.[25]

Erysipelas has a low rate of complications like abscess formation and necrosis. In up to 30% of the cases, prophylaxis with penicillin V is recommended due to recurrence, which is the most common complication. The most frequent pathogens in adults are group A (nearly always *Streptococcus pyogenes*) and group G BHS. Whether *S. aureus* or gram-negative bacteria can cause erysipelas is still in doubt.

Furuncles

Furuncle is a deep infection of the hair follicles; therefore, it appears only in hairy areas of the body. The most common etiologic agent is *S. aureus*, which causes an abscess with purulent content and necrotic tissue affecting general extremities.

Under clinical examination it consists of an erythematous and edematous painful nodule filled with purulent fluid and devitalized tissue, which tend to be well-demarcated from the surrounded healthy skin. It may resolve with or without a scar (Fig. 6). If some adjacent follicles are involved, they form the so-called carbuncle, which has multiple openings through, the purulent content drain out from.[26] Furunculosis refers to the simultaneous or sequential presence of some furuncles. Recurrence is common and colonization by *S. aureus* strains among family members or healthcare personnel is considered an important factor for recurrence in those who are in close contact with patients, along with DM, anemia, previous hospitalization, previous antibiotic treatments, and associated dermatosis such as atopic dermatitis.[27] The virulence staphylococcal toxin PVL was correlated with chronic recurrent furunculosis.

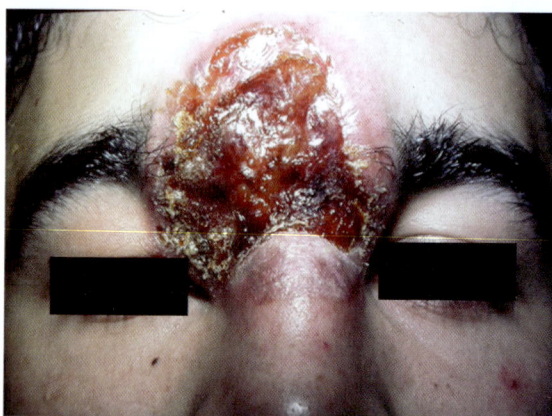

Fig. 6: Furuncle.

Necrotizing Fasciitis

Necrotizing fasciitis is a life-threatening dermatologic emergency involving the subcutaneous tissue and superficial fascia. This SSTI is more frequent in immunocompromised patients like diabetics or alcoholics, but it is also associated with small traumas, and after surgical procedures.

In diabetic patients, the infection is typically polymicrobial, caused by aerobic or anaerobic pathogens. It starts with fever and local pain-causing skin necrosis, suppurative fasciitis, vascular thrombosis, and systemic toxicity. If septicemia and systemic toxic effects occur, death in a very short period of time (2–4 days) would be the result. The most affected sites are thorax, abdominal wall, limbs, perineum and groin; the head and neck are rare localizations. Mortality rate is approximately 40% and is sometimes related to the diagnosis delayed.[28]

Diagnostic Evaluation of Skin and Soft Tissue Infections

In a skin lesion with the typical clinical signs of inflammation, we should rule out an SSTI, even more if the patient is febrile. In addition, the presence of blisters, blood extravasation, crepitus, etc. can give us good pointers to a diagnosis and which complementary exams to perform, such as ultrasound, X-ray, etc. For example, if the lesion has a fluid content similar to that of blisters or abscesses, needle aspiration is recommended. A culture swab from a purulent furuncle can reveal the etiologic agent.[29]

If we are going to swab an infected wound or a furuncle, it should be cleaned and the necrotic tissue should be previously removed. If the cultured swabs yield a positive result, we have to differentiate between a pathogenic bacteria or a simple colonization. In diabetic superficial ulcers without bone involvement, a positive swab may reveal an etiologic agent.[30]

It would be helpful to perform laboratory exams including glycemia, glycated hemoglobin and glycosuria levels, to rule out an underlying DM, as well as a complete blood count and blood culture in order to discard other internal conditions or bacteremia and systemic toxicity.

However, unfortunately in most cases, the etiology remains uncertain and the patient is treated empirically, due to lack of confirmatory microbiological cultures (blood, tissue swab or needle aspiration).[31]

Treatment

Depending on the severity of the infection, different therapeutic strategies will focus on: carriage status, topical treatment, tissue debridement, drainage of an abscess, wound care, oral or intravenous antibiotics and metabolic control.[14]

Carriage Status

The attempts to reduce the incidence of *S. aureus* infections comprise the decolonization of *Staphylococcus* carriers with mupirocin, particularly among family members or other close contacts of patients with recurrent infections.

Topical Treatment

For superficial cutaneous infections, there is good evidence that topical antibiotic treatment is very effective, with mupirocin and fusidic acid having the same efficacy.

Tissue Debridement, Drainage and Wound Care

Some purulent abscesses with necrotic tissue need incision and drainage. Applying warm sterile gauzes on the lesion surface twice a day leads to faster healing because it helps to drain the abscess.

Systemic Antibiotics

Regarding systemic treatment, bear in mind that diabetics with impaired microcirculation may interfere with antimicrobial adequate concentration in the infection focus, leading to a wrong interpretation of antibiotic treatment failure.

Almost 50% to 100% of the SSTIs are cured by antibiotics in up to 1 month's treatment (median duration of treatment 11 days). If it is a first episode of a superficial infection, the treatment of choice should cover both targets, *Staphylococcus* and *Streptococcus*. On the contrary, recurrent or chronic infections in a patient already treated with antibiotics are probably polymicrobial (Enterobacteria, coagulase-negative *Staphylococcus*, MRSA) and the therapeutic choice will include other antibiotic schedule including piperacillin-tazobactam, ceftriaxone, fluoroquinolones and the carbapenems (ertapenem, imipenem, meropenem). For *S. aureus* resistant to different antibiotics, vancomycin is the first choice, particularly for MRSA infections.[7]

In the last years, in patients with underlying diseases at high risk of morbimortality, new drugs were developed (linezolid, daptomycin, tigecycline) particularly for gram-positive cocci. Side-effects for oral antibiotic treatment were mostly gastrointestinal and mild.[21]

CORYNEBACTERIUM MINUTISSIMUM

Corynebacterium minutissimum is an etiologic agent with an increased prevalence among obese diabetic patients who have a higher susceptibility, probably due to the ability of these bacteria to ferment glucose. Some factors such as maceration, humidity and friction present in flexural areas are important.

Clinically, it consists of well-demarcated, shiny, and brown-to-red asymptomatic patches over intertriginous areas (axilla, inguinal, inframammary, inner thighs and fourth web space of the toes) (Fig. 7). They could be macerated and scaly. The most common clinical variant is the interdigital, which is very similar to tinea pedis and is sometimes misdiagnosed.[32]

The Wood lamp is very useful for diagnosis, where the bacterial porphyrin production shows a coral fluorescence, especially in the active borders of the lesions[33] (Fig. 8). If the Wood lamp yields a negative result, the confirmatory

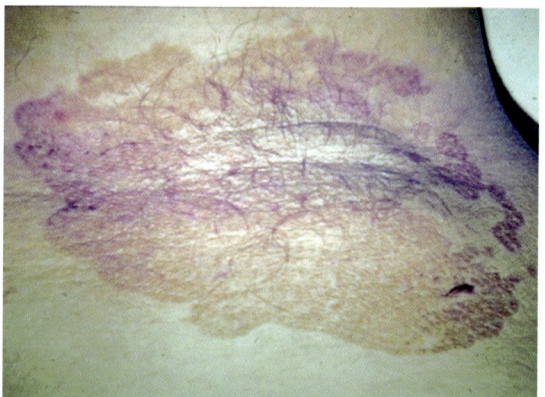

Fig. 7: Erythrasma.

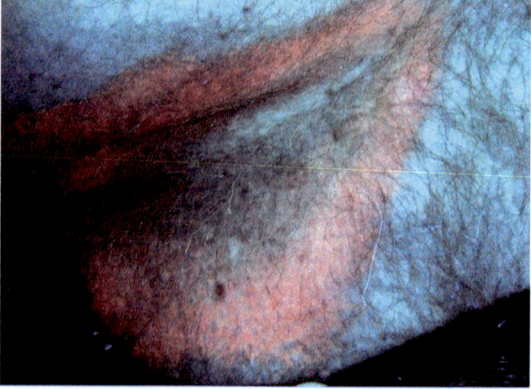

Fig. 8: Porphyrin production by the bacteria leads to a coral fluorescence observed by Wood's lamp.

diagnosis would be achieved with Gram staining, because bacterial culture erythrasma is known to be difficult for diagnosis.

The first-choice treatment is erythromycin, topical or systemic depending on the extent of cutaneous involvement, comorbidities, etc. Another option is tetracyclines.[34] Oral erythromycin at 1 g/day dose for 14 days, reaches a 100% cure rate, and is more effective compared with tetracyclines.[35]

PSEUDOMONAS AERUGINOSA

Pseudomonas aeruginosa, gram-negative bacteria, is a ubiquitous environmental microorganism, which is considered an opportunistic agent in immunocompromised individuals. It can cause onychomycosis of the toenails, ecthyma gangrenosum and a more severe infection: malignant otitis externa.[36]

Onychomycosis

Onychomycosis by *Pseudomonas* is more common in diabetics than in the general population and presents with the characteristic green discoloration. Oral antibiotics, in particular ciprofloxacin, are standard therapy.

Ecthyma Gangrenosum

Ecthyma gangrenosum is a well-recognized cutaneous manifestation of severe, invasive infection by *P. aeruginosa*, with or without bacteremia.[37] Usually, it presents in immunocompromised state, DM, hypogammaglobulinemia and other terminal conditions. It typically occurs on the extremities and gluteal and perineal regions.[38] In diabetic patients with impaired microcirculation of the lower limbs, a small lesion becomes a necrotic ulcer in a poor wound healing background. Considering the high mortality rate, early diagnosis and prompt effective treatment are mandatory.

Malignant Otitis Externa

It is a rare infection that affects older diabetic patients. In general, it is caused by *P. aeruginosa*. It is characterized by a painful purulent secretion of the external auditory duct, associated with cellulitis (Fig. 9). It progresses and invades the cartilage, into the skull base involving intracranial nerves, mainly the facial one, causing paralysis, which occurs in 50% of the cases, extending to the meninges and the brain. Clinical signs and symptoms are otorrhea associated with acute pain and hearing loss. Magnetic resonance imaging is the best procedure for diagnosis. The treatment should be initiated immediately and includes necrotic tissue debridement, drainage and oral or intravenous antibiotics for *Pseudomonas* species such as fluoroquinolones. In more severe cases, they can be combined with an antipseudomonal beta-lactam agent such as piperacillin, piperacillin-tazobactam, ceftazidime or a carbapenem. Unfortunately, it is a life-threatening condition, with high morbidity and mortality, which can reach up to 50% of the cases.[36,39]

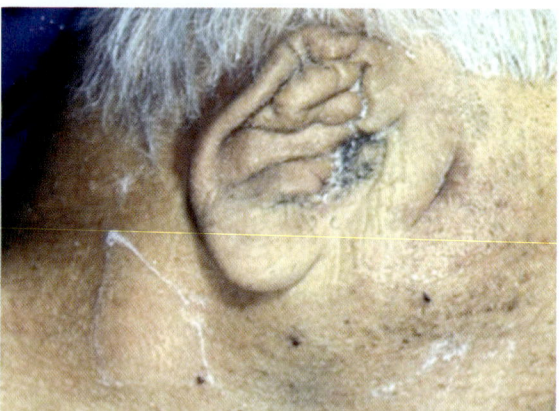

Fig. 9: Malignant otitis externa.

CONCLUSION

Glycemic control is the best preventive measure for all skin infections. In decompensated patients, these infections may be difficult to treat. If they are chronic and recurrent, the *Staphylococcus* carriage state should be suspected. Diabetic patients with SSTIs have higher rates of both SSTI-associated metabolic complications such as hypoglycemia, ketoacidosis and coma, as well as subsequent hospitalizations.

REFERENCES

1. Timshina DK, Thappa D, Agrawal A. A clinical study of dermatoses in diabetes to establish its markers. Indian J Dermatol. 2012;57(1):20-5.
2. Murphy-Chutorian B, Han G, Cohen SR. Dermatologic manifestations of diabetes mellitus: a review. Endocrinol Metab Clin North Am. 2013;42(4):869-98.
3. Gkogkolou P, Böhm M. Advanced glycation end products: Key players in skin aging? Dermatoendocrinol. 2012;4:259-70.
4. Park HY, Kim JH, Jung M, et al. A long-standing hyperglycaemic condition impairs skin barrier by accelerating skin ageing process. Exp Dermatol. 2011;20(12):969-74.
5. Hodgson K, Morris J, Bridson T, et al. Immunological mechanisms contributing to the double burden of diabetes and intracellular bacterial infections. Immunology. 2015;144(2):171-85.
6. Lan CC, Wu CS, Huang SM, et al. High-glucose environment inhibits p38MAPK signaling and reduces human β-Defensin-3 expression in keratinocytes. Mol Med. 2011;17(7-8):771-9.
7. Tong SY, Chen LF, Fowler VG Jr. Colonization, pathogenicity, host susceptibility and therapeutics for *Staphylococcus aureus*: what is the clinical relevance? Semin Immunopathol. 2012;34(2):185-200.
8. Ryu S, Song PI, Seo CH, et al. Colonization and infection of the skin by *S. aureus*: immune system evasion and the response to cationic antimicrobial peptides. Int J Mol Sci. 2014;15:8753-72.
9. Rajagopalan S. Serious infections in elderly patients with diabetes mellitus. Clin Infect Dis. 2005;40:990-6.

10. Muller LM, Gorter KJ, Hak E, et al. Increased risk of common infections in patients with type 1 and type 2 diabetes mellitus. Clin Infect Dis. 2005;41:281-8.
11. Pereira LB. Impetigo - review. An Bras Dermatol. 2014;89(2):293-9.
12. Suaya JA, Eisenberg DF, Fang C, et al. Skin and soft tissue infections and associated complications among commercially insured patients aged 0–64 years with and without diabetes in the U.S. PLoS One. 2013;8(4):e60057.
13. Benfield T, Jensen JS, Nordestgaard BG. Influence of diabetes and hyperglycaemia on infectious disease hospitalisation and outcome. Diabetologia. 2007;50: 549-54.
14. Nicolau DP, Stein GE. Therapeutic options for diabetic foot infections: a review with an emphasis on tissue penetration characteristics. J Am Podiatr Med Assoc. 2010;100(1):52-63.
15. Skoff TH, Farley MM, Petit S, et al. Increasing burden of invasive group B streptococcal disease in nonpregnant adults, 1990-2007. Clin Infect Dis. 2009;49:85-92.
16. Sendi P, Johansson L, Norrby-Teglund A. Invasive group B Streptococcal disease in non- pregnant adults: a review with emphasis on skin and soft-tissue infections. Infection. 2008;36:100-11.
17. Matsubara K, Yamamoto G. Invasive group B streptococcal infections in a tertiary care hospital between 1998 and 2007 in Japan. Int J Infect Dis. 2009;13:679-84.
18. Lopardo HA, Vidal P, Jeric P, et al. Argentinian Streptococcus Study Group. Six-month multicenter study on invasive infections due to group B streptococci in Argentina. J Clin Microbiol. 2003;41:4688-94.
19. Anaya DA, Sullivan SR, Foy H, et al. Predictors of mortality and limb loss in necrotizing soft tissue infections. Arch Surg. 2005;140:151-7.
20. Miller LS, Cho JS. Immunity against *Staphylococcus aureus* cutaneous infections. Nat Rev Immunol. 2011;11(8):505-18.
21. Raya-Cruz M, Ferullo I, Arrizabalaga-Asenjo M, et al. Skin and soft-tissue infections in hospitalized patients: epidemiology, microbiological, clinical and prognostic factors. Enferm Infec Microbiol Clin. 2014;32(3):152-9.
22. Koning S, van der Sande R, Verhagen AP, et al. Interventions for impetigo. Cochrane Database Syst Rev. 2012;1:CD003261.
23. Kevat D, Wilson D, Sinha A. A 5-year-old girl with type 2 diabetes. Lancet. 2014;383(9924):1268.
24. Bläckberg A, Trell K, Rasmussen M. Erysipelas, a large retrospective study of aetiology and clinical presentation. BMC Infect Dis. 2015;15:402-7.
25. Inghammar M, Rassmussen M, Linder A. Recurrent erysipelas - risk factors and clinical presentation. BMC Infect Dis. 2014;14:270-5.
26. Ibler KS, Kromann ChB. Recurrent furunculosis – challenges and management: a review. Clin Cosmet Investig Dermatol. 2014;7:59-64.
27. El-Gilany AH, Fathy H. Risk factors of recurrent furunculosis. Dermatol Online J. 2009;15(1):16.
28. Oguz H, Demirci M, Arslan N, et al. Necrotizing fasciitis of the head and neck: Report of two cases and literature review. Ear Nose Throat J. 2010;89(2):E7-10.
29. Hakkarainen TW, Kopari NM, Pham TN, et al. Necrotizing soft tissue infections: review and current concepts in treatment, systems of care, and outcomes. Curr Probl Surg. 2014;51(8):344-62.
30. Slater RA, Lazarovitch T, Boldur I, et al. Swab cultures accurately identify bacterial pathogens in diabetic foot wounds not involving bone. Diabet Med. 2004;21: 705-9.

31. Ray GT, Suaya JA, Baxter R. Incidence, microbiology, and patient characteristics of skin and soft-tissue infections in a U.S. population: a retrospective population-based study. BMC Infect Dis. 2013;13:252.
32. Morales-Trujillo ML, Arenas R, Arroyo S. Interdigital erythrasma: clinical, epidemiologic, and microbiologic findings. Actas Dermosifiliogr. 2008;99(6): 469-73.
33. Van Hattem S, Bootsma AH, Thio HB. Skin manifestations of diabetes. Cleve Clin J Med. 2008;75(11):772-87.
34. Holdiness MR. Management of cutaneous erythrasma. Drugs. 2002;62:1131-41.
35. Inci M, Serarslan G, Ozer B, et al. The prevalence of interdigital erythrasma in southern region of Turkey. J Eur Acad Dermatol Venereol. 2012;26(11): 1372-6.
36. Sarlangue J, Brissaud O, Labrèze C. Clinical features of *Pseudomonas aeruginosa* infections. Arch Pediatr. 2006;13 Suppl 1:S13-6.
37. Avolio M, La Spisa C, Moscariello F, et al. Aeromonas hydrophila ecthyma gangrenosum without bacteraemia in a diabetic man: the first case report in Italy. Infez Med. 2009;17(3):184-7.
38. Nakai N, Takenaka H, Kishimoto S. Ecthyma gangrenosum without pseudomonas septicemia in a kidney transplant recipient. J Dermatol. 2008;35(9):585-9.
39. Casqueiro J, Casqueiro J, Alves C. Infections in patients with diabetes mellitus: A review of pathogenesis. Indian J Endocrinol Metab. 2012;16(S1):S27-36.

CHAPTER 8

Dermatoses Most Frequently Related to Diabetes

Emilia Noemí Cohen Sabban

INTRODUCTION

These dermatoses constitute a heterogeneous group of diseases that have been associated over time with diabetes for different reasons. The coexistence of diabetes mellitus (DM) with diseases that affect the skin actually remains in the realm of speculation; and except for glucagonoma syndrome, any of them could arise in nondiabetic patients.

Although the causes for which they are associated are unknown; in some cases they share pathogenesis, others are a simple clinical observation and ultimately both pathologies could relate because one is a favorable background for the development of the other.

Some of these associations are not universally accepted yet, but in an attempt to group them and based on the findings in the last decade, we have reformulated their classification into four groups, in accordance with a possible linking mechanism with DM (Table 1).

1. *Metabolic mechanism:* Porphyria cutanea tarda (PCT), eruptive xanthomas (EX), migratory necrolytic erythema (Glucagonoma syndrome), pruritus and acrochordons or skin tags.
2. *Immunological mechanism:* Vitiligo and bullous pemphigoid (BP).

TABLE 1: Classification according to possible linking mechanisms between diabetes mellitus and different dermatoses.

Metabolic mechanism	Immunological mechanism	Unknown mechanism
Porphyria cutanea tarda	Vitiligo	Lichen planus
Eruptive xanthomas	Bullous pemphigoid	Kaposi's sarcoma
Migratory necrolytic erythema		Acquired perforating dermatoses
Pruritus		
Acrochordons or skin tags		
Psoriasis		

TABLE 2: Dermatoses related to diabetes mellitus.

Dermatosis	N = 237	%
Vitiligo	6	2.50
Psoriasis	9	3.79
Alterations of the lipid mechanism	6	2.53
Skin tags	4	1.68
Localized pruritus	4	1.68
Generalized pruritus	3	1.26

3. *Mixed mechanism (metabolic and immunological):* Psoriasis (Ps).
4. *Unknown mechanism:* Lichen planus (LP), Kaposi's sarcoma (KS) and acquired perforating dermatosis (APD).[1]

In a study that included 237 diagnosed diabetic patients that consulted consecutively the department of Internal Medicine and the skin at the Dermatology Division of the Hospital de Clínicas, Buenos Aires (UBA), Argentina. The presence of associated dermatoses was investigated (Table 2).

Among the skin diseases, the most frequent was Ps, followed in order of frequency by EX and vitiligo. Skin tags and localized pruritus showed the same incidence and generalized pruritus was the least found.[2]

METABOLIC MECHANISM

Porphyria Cutanea Tarda

Porphyria cutanea tarda is probably the most common type of porphyria, which manifests between the age of 30 years and 60 years and affects both genders equally. Its emergence is due to the specific blockage of an enzyme in the heme group synthesis pathway, called uroporphyrinogen decarboxylase (UROD) in the liver. The process, through which the decrease in the activity of this enzyme reaches a clinically manifest PCT, requires the interaction of multiple hereditary and acquired factors. In family cases, enzymatic deficiency is correlated with the mutation of the *UROD* gene and is inherited in an autosomal dominant manner. On the contrary, sporadic forms of PCT in patients genetically predisposed are more common and can be triggered due to a long list of factors: alcohol abuse, human acquired immunodeficiency virus and hepatitis C virus, estrogen therapy, oral contraceptives, chemical substances like hexachlorobenzene and other drugs. One of these drugs is chloroquine which in high doses can induce clinical PCT manifestations in latent cases, while in low doses it is used to treat this condition.

In both forms, PCT is the result of an accumulation of uroporphyrin in the skin and the liver due to the alteration in the hepatic function of the enzyme through an iron-dependent mechanism, which explains the increase of the iron parameters like serum ferritin levels.

Clinically, cutaneous and extracutaneous manifestations have been described. Skin lesions arise gradually and consist of (Figs. 1 to 5):
- *Skin fragility*: Minor injuries cause painful erosions.
- *Tense blisters:* With serous or serohematic content, which localize on healthy photoexposed skin like the dorsum of hands and which are of traumatic or actinic origin. After a couple of hours, they break, their content desiccates and forms a crust; finally, they heal and leave scars and milia. This is the most important and frequent sign of PCT.
- *Hyperpigmentation*: Progressively increases and affects exposed areas.
- *Hypertrichosis*: Although not always present, it can be an early sign and become the first manifestation.

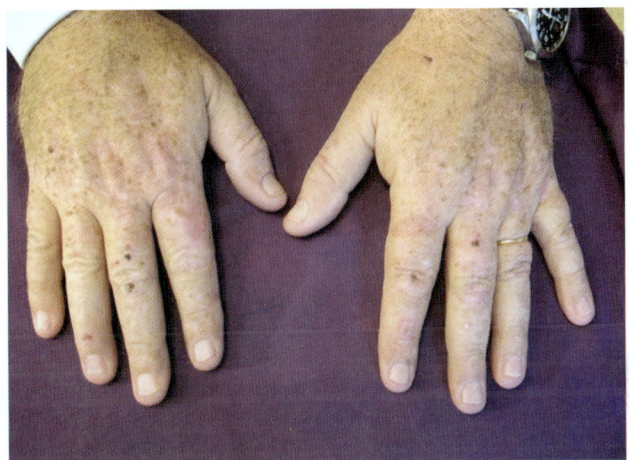

Fig. 1: Crusts formed by dried blister content, that appear on healthy skin sunexposed skin.

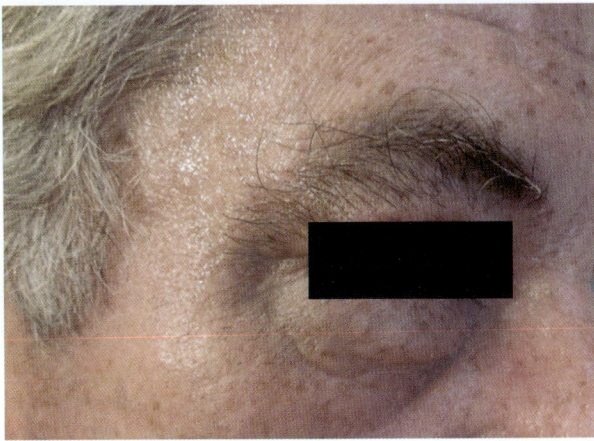

Fig. 2: Malar hypertrichosis.

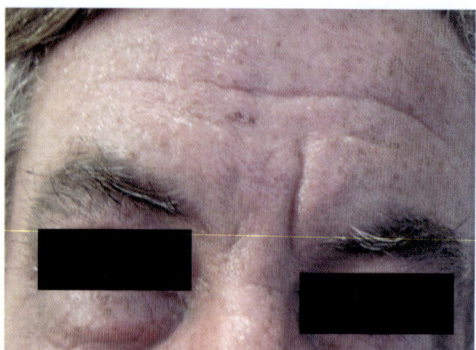

Fig. 3: Skin aging.

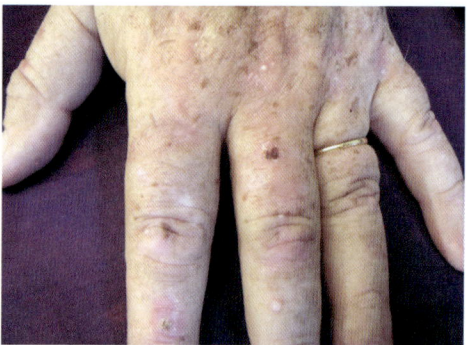

Fig. 4: Blisters with dry content covered with crusts and milia cysts.

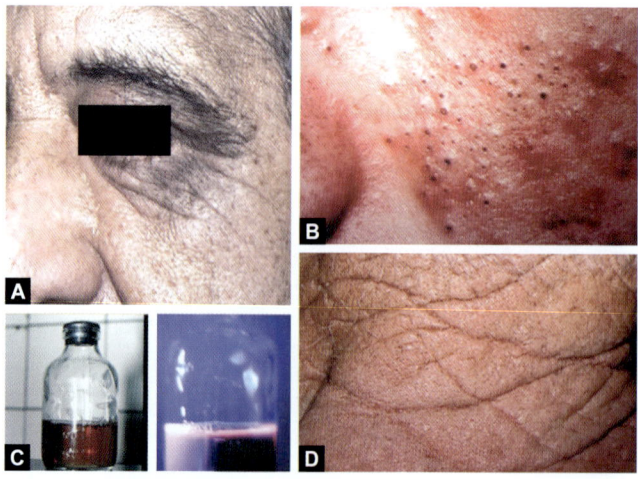

Figs. 5A to D: (A) Malar hypertrichosis and hyperpigmentation; (B) Nodular elastoidosis with cysts and comedones; (C) Dark urine from porphyric patient; through a Wood's lamp we observe the characteristic coral colored fluorescence evidencing uroporphyrins; (D) Cutis rhomboidalis.

- *Sclerodermiform changes*: They appear in photoexposed areas in patients with long-standing PCT.
- *Premature skin aging.*
- *Porphyric alopecia:* Diffuse and of sudden onset.
- *Purpuric red ectasia:* In the central facial area, its appearance is very rare.

Regarding extracutaneous manifestations, it is important to highlight those of hepatic origin, since they are present in almost 100% of the patients and predicted according to the severity levels—ocular, neurological, osteomuscular and digestive.

From the histological point of view, we can observe the presence of a subepidermic blister accompanied by a scarce inflammatory infiltrate and periodic acid-Schiff positive thickening of vessel walls. Direct immunofluorescence of skin samples obtained from photoexposed areas reveal the existence of an IgG deposit in the dermoepidermic junction and the perivascular area. In terms of blood, there is an increase of plasma iron; the diagnosis is confirmed through an increase in uroporphyrin in urine which produces the red-orange fluorescent color observed with Wood's lamp.

There is an association between DM and PCT; 25% of the patients with PCT are diabetics, more frequently men between 45 years and 75 years of age. Inversely, only around 1% of diabetics have PCT. It is believed that one of the causes of this association lies in non-enzymatic glycation (NEG) of the heme group.[3]

Eruptive Xanthomas

Eruptive xanthomas present as small yellowish papules, one or two millimeters in diameter, or nodules surrounded by an inflammatory erythematous halo, of sudden onset.[4] They are generally asymptomatic, although they can be pruritic. They localize on the buttocks, extensor areas of extremities (knees, elbows) and the torso. They can also result on pressure and touch points due to the Koebner phenomenon (Figs. 6 to 9).[5]

Xanthomas, in general, and particularly eruptive ones, are skin markers of a wide range of primary diseases (caused by a genetic disorder) like some types of familiar lipoproteinemias, or secondary to other processes among which we find DM. The reason for a higher frequency of EX in diabetics is the fact that insulin is a stimulating factor of the normal activity of lipoprotein lipase, which plays an important role in serum triglyceride metabolism and lipoproteins rich in triglycerides. In conditions of insulin deficiency like in the case of DM and thus, absence of lipoprotein lipase activity, a hyperlipidemic condition is promoted with hypertriglyceridemia and an increase in chylomicrons and very-low-density lipoproteins.[6]

The histological clue is the presence of foamy macrophages in the superficial dermis loaded with lipids with perivascular distribution and loose lipids, together with a mixed lymphocyte and neutrophil infiltrate; occasionally, giant cells of the Touton type can be observed.

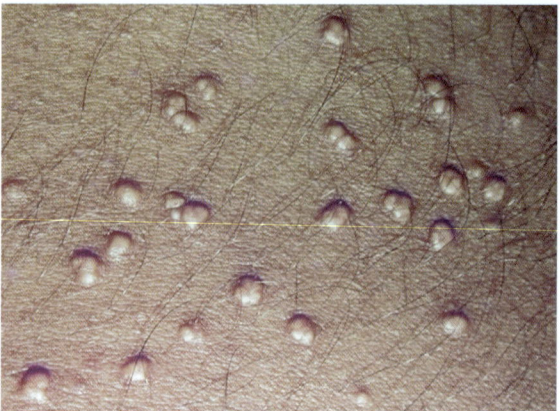

Fig. 6: Eruptive xanthomas.

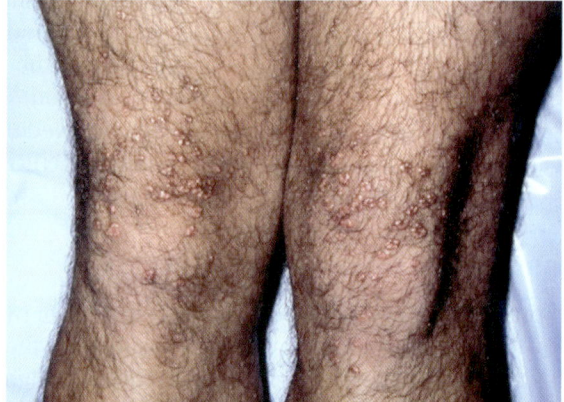

Fig. 7: Multiple eruptive xanthomas localized on both knees.

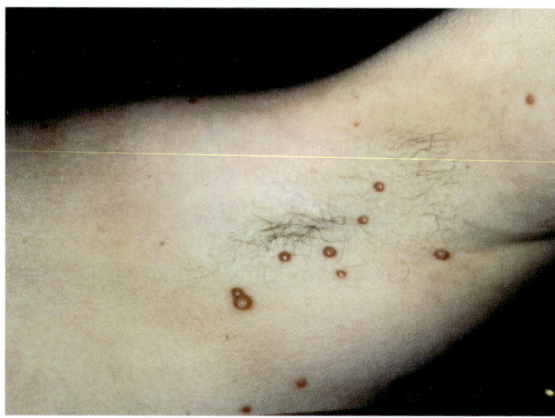

Fig. 8: Eruptive xanthomas surrounded by erythematous halo on underarm.

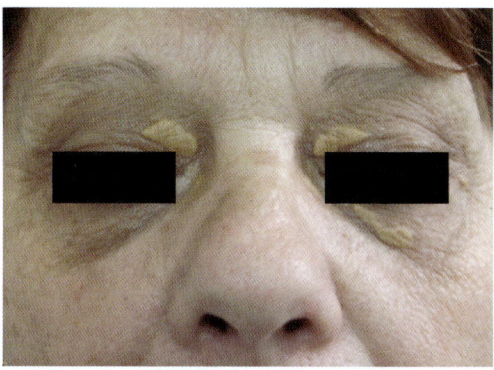

Fig. 9: Xanthelasmas associated to hypertriglyceridemia in a diabetic patient.

Xanthomas manifest in patients with a poorly controlled disease, with hyperglycemia, hypertriglyceridemia and glucosuria. The tendency to the rapid resolution (weeks) of EX through metabolic control is what allows us to consider them for the monitoring of the internal metabolism. For this same reason, those patients with sudden EX without any other diagnosis at the moment, should be assessed in order to discard an underlying metabolic disease. The treatment has to focus on the standardization of carbohydrates and lipids, adjusting insulin and statins for dyslipidemia.

Although the incidence of EX is estimated at less than 0.1% of diabetic patients, its association is well established.

Migratory Necrolytic Erythema

A glucagonoma is a rare pancreatic endocrine tumor that originates from pancreatic alpha cells and its clinical manifestations constitute the so-called glucagonoma syndrome, defined by the presence of:
- Glucagon hypersecretion due to a tumor of pancreatic alpha cells (VN: 59–177 pg/mL).
- Moderate to severe DM, or an abnormal glucose tolerance in 76–94% of patients with glucagonoma. Elevated serum levels of glucagon trigger the occurrence of DM at the expense of glycogen stored in muscular and adipose tissue.[7]
- Weight loss, anemia, diarrhea with steatorrhea and abdominal pain.
- Cutaneomucous manifestations characterized by:
  - Migratory necrolytic erythema (MNE), characteristic lesion, but not pathognomonic. Can be pruritic and painful. MNE is the presentation sign in 50–70% of the cases and can precede the diagnosis of glucagonoma in 1-6 years, so that its presence should be an alert sign. It appears between the fourth and sixth decade of life, without distinction of gender.[8]
  - Red and painful atrophic tongue (glossitis).
  - Angular cheilitis.
  - Blepharitis.

- High incidence, approximately 10–30% of thromboembolic phenomena (deep venous thrombosis, pulmonary embolism), which can cause death in 50% of the cases.
- Neuropsychiatric Symptoms have also been described in 20% of patients with glucagonoma, like dementia, psychosis, paranoid hallucinations, ataxia and hyperreflexia.

Glucagon itself could be responsible for most signs and symptoms observed in the syndrome. Although until today, the pathogenesis of MNE is uncertain, there are several hypotheses which include glucagon excess; plasmatic zinc deficiency, essential fatty acids and amino acids, release of inflammatory mediators induced by glucagon and generalized malabsorption.

Clinically, consist in erythematous annular or figurative plaques, with vesicle blisters and pustules tending to coalesce. They show central regression and centrifugal growth forming large geographic areas with circled but well-defined limits. Lesions with liquid content lose their roof leaving erosions that develop into crusts, then flake and finally leave residual hyperpigmentation. They localize preferably in intertriginous, periorificial areas (perinasal, perioral, perineal, perianal); they can also appear on buttocks and extremities. Their characteristic evolutional pattern includes spontaneous remissions within weeks and exacerbations with emergence of new lesions following a cyclic chronicle course.[9]

The diagnosis of glucagonoma is based on a clinical recognition of the cutaneous eruption and DM, and an associated serum glucagon increase. To confirm, computed tomography and magnetic resonance imaging are very useful as well as selective angiography (celiac and hepatic); although invasive, they are considered the gold standard because glucagonoma is a hypervascularized tumor.[10]

From a histological point of view, confluent parakeratosis, spongiosis and necrolysis of the upper layers of the epidermis can be observed, with vacuolated pale keratinocytes and mononuclear dermal perivascular infiltrates. These findings are also present in cases of pellagra, acral necrolytic erythema or zinc deficiency. Immunohistochemistry can be positive for glucagon, synaptophysin and chromogranin.

Surgical removal of the primary tumor will be followed by the resolution of skin lesions. Prognosis and survival depend on the tumor stage, where almost 50% of the cases are already in a metastasic phase at the moment of the diagnosis. The most frequent sites of metastasis are the liver, lymph nodes, peripancreatic areas, bones, adrenal gland, kidney and lungs.

Metastasis, in general, is difficult to resect surgically apart from the fact that glucagonoma is resistant to chemotherapy; since it is a slow growing tumor and has a 5-year survival rate in 70% of the cases.

In these cases, long-acting somatostatin analogs like octreotide and lanreotide have been successfully used as palliative treatments. These molecules are powerful inhibitors of tumoral glucagon secretion, significantly reducing their concentrations and actions; although there is no consensus regarding its efficacy to control metastasic tumoral growth.[11]

The relationship between DM and glucagonoma differs with other described associations. In this case, DM is an example of secondary disease to another pathological process. It is important to highlight the preponderant role of the dermatologist who, in the face of characteristical mucocutaneous lesions, can suspect of an underlying tumoral process in an early stage of the disease.[12]

Pruritus

Pruritus (from the Latin word *pruritus,* meaning itch) is the need to scratch and a relevant symptom of many dermatologic, systemic, neurological and psychogenic diseases (Figs. 10 to 13). It is not pathognomonic, but very common in cases of DM. 14–24% of patients with generalized pruritus, without apparent cutaneous cause, have a systemic origin and DM is one of them.

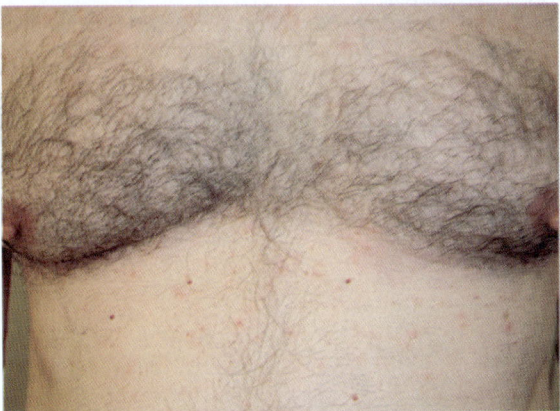

Fig. 10: Multiple pruritic lesions in a diabetic patient to whom other causes of pruritus have been ruled out.

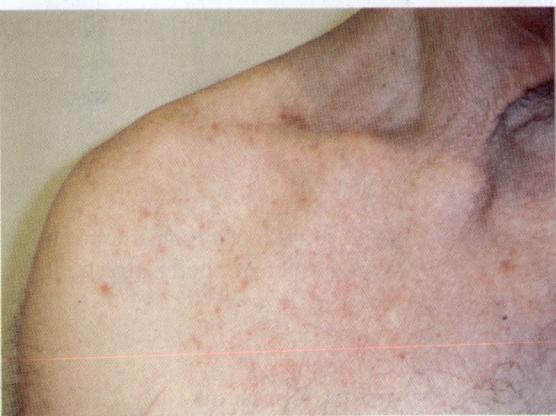

Fig. 11: Rash in a diabetic patient to whom other causes of pruritus have been ruled out.

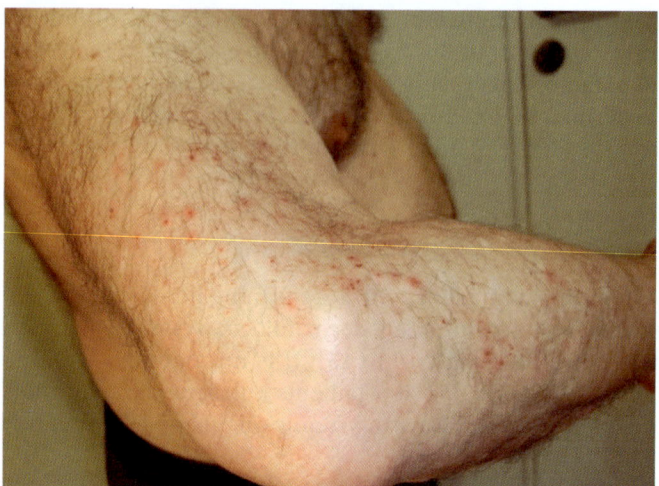

Fig. 12: Pruritus. Lesions on upper extremity.

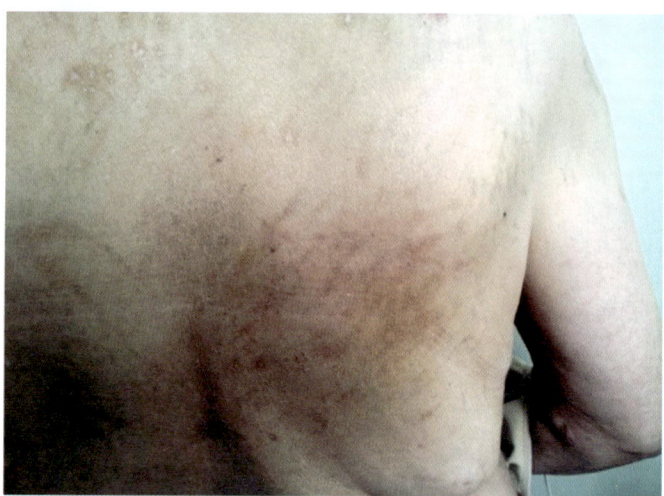

Fig. 13: Pruritus on the back with scratching signs.

It is so uncomfortable that it has a direct impact on the patients' life quality. From 385 patients with DM type 2 and extended pruritus, almost half of them suffer from sleep disorders due to pruritus.[13]

Pruritus can be acute or chronic, which lasts more than 6 weeks and is refractory to conventional treatments.

In DM, generalized pruritus represents only 2.7% of the cases. In a prospective study by Polat et al.[14] where they investigated the causes for generalized pruritus, from 41 healthy control patients and 55 patients with pruritus, they found 12 patients to have an underlying systemic disease like DM (hypothyroidism, leukemia, hepatitis C and B, etc.), where pruritus turned out to be the symptom of presentation in 8 of them.

In the case of diabetic patients, pruritus has more frequently a localized presentation, and topographically the most common are anal/genital, scalp and lower limbs.

Almost 20% of diabetic women suffer from pruritus in genital and anal regions. It is advised to always discard a fungal infection of the *Candida* type (*Candida albicans, Candida glabrata*), that is correlated with a state of hyperglycemia and in turn proofs a bad metabolic control. Due to its resistance to treatment, it requires more than one dose of fluconazol 150 mg/week and sometimes a complementary treatment with suppositories of boric acid during 14 days.[15]

Localized pruritus on the scalp is intimately related with peaks of hyperglycemia and improves clearly with DM control.

In the limbs, especially the lower limbs, it is linked to neuropathy. Autonomic neuropathy causes sudomotor alterations with the resultant hypo/anhidrosis that clinically leads to xerosis.

Concomitantly, the skin of the diabetic patient has an altered cutaneous barrier and this causes dry skin. Xerosis with pruritus is one of the most frequent cutaneous manifestations of DM; it can be observed in 25% of diabetics. When there are also microcirculation alterations of the lower limbs, distal areas are the ones with major itching; that in turn, can be affected by the coexistence of tinea pedis (Athlete's foot), contributing to exacerbation of pruritus.

In these cases, the treatment consists mostly of general measures, as for example:
- Avoid hot water baths.
- Use soft moisturizing soaps.
- Apply every day after the bath, body emollients, in order to improve xerosis, reduce pruritus and peeling, and improve the cutaneous barrier.

Sensory peripheral neuropathy that affects small not myelinated nervous fibers or group C fibers present on the skin, peripheral nerves and organs, also manifests with pruritus.[16] One type of pruritus of unknown origin is the one on the body trunk [truncal pruritus of unknown origin (TPUO)], which is considered by some a manifestation of diabetic polyneuropathy. In a large scale study that included 2,656 diabetic patients, the interrelation between pruritus and diabetic neuropathy was evaluated, comparing genders, duration of the DM, HbA1c, reflex of the Achilles tendon and abnormal leg sensation in 499 diabetic control patients. TPUO prevalence turned out significantly higher in diabetic patients in comparison with control patients (11.3% vs 2.9%), while the prevalence of other types of pruritus was not different in the studied groups. In the case of diabetics with TPUO, the finding of diabetic neuropathy was confirmed (arreflexia of the Achilles tendon, lack of sensibility in the feet, etc.).[17]

Anti-pruritus therapy is directed toward a variety of targets that include central and peripheral symptom mechanisms, among which the epidermal barrier, the immune system and the nervous system are included. Topic or systemic indications of specific substances can influence the neuroreceptors of the sensory nervous fibers of the skin and suppress pruritus.

Topical agents like capsaicin and calcineurin inhibitors (tacrolimus and pimecrolimus) should be considered along with emollients.

Among systemic treatments we include antihistamines, antiepileptic drugs, antidepressants, antagonists of opioid receptors, thalidomide, ondansetron, phototherapy with ultraviolet (UV) B, cyclosporine, and others. While antihistamines, cyclosporine and phototherapy with UVB act on skin pruritus elicitation; anticonvulsants, opioid antagonists and antidepressants block the signal processing in the central nervous system.

There is no doubt that the approach has to be multidisciplinary including general measures, treatment of the underlying cause (candidiasis) and topical and systemic medication, depending on the case.

The interrelation between pruritus and systemic diseases, among which we find DM, is very close.

In the case of a patient with pruritus, we cannot discard the possibility of an underlying DM. Pruritus relates to DM basically due to a metabolic mechanism; the higher hyperglycemia and increase in HbA1c, the more pruritus.

Acrochordons or Skin Tags

Skin tags are pedunculated exophytic proliferations of small size that vary between 1 mm and 6 mm in diameter. They have skin color or are hyperpigmented; their surface can be flat or irregular and they settle preferably on the neck, eyelids and folds (axillary, inframammary and inguinal). A slight predilection for the female gender can be observed between the fourth and fifth decade of life and its prevalence increases with age. They are considered as multiple, when they add up eight or more (Figs. 14A to D). There are reports on the interrelation between skin tags and hypertension, DM and other metabolic alterations of glucose/insulin (glucose intolerance–IGT, insulin resistance–IR) and family history of DM. They are also associated with colon polyps, abnormal hepatic enzymes and obesity. For some authors, there could be a correlation with high leptin serum levels, but nevertheless, others failed in finding such correlation.[18] Shah et al. proved the correlation between an atherogenic profile and the increase in total cholesterol, triglycerides, low-density lipoprotein cholesterol, low levels of high-density lipoprotein cholesterol and the presence of acrochordons, and also the increase of systolic and diastolic pressure.[19]

The association with DM can be observed in approximately 66–75% of patients with skin tags and more than 80% present carbohydrates metabolic alterations, specially if they are multiple, bilateral and large. As it happens with acanthosis nigricans (AN), this relation seems to be associated to the proliferative effect that hyperinsulinemia has on keratinocytes and fibroblasts.[20]

Dermatoses Most Frequently Related to Diabetes

In is not necessary to start treatment, but in case the patient needs one, common methods like cleavage with scissors, electrocoagulation or cryotherapy are useful therapeutic tools.[21]

IMMUNOLOGICAL MECHANISM

Vitiligo

It is an acquired pigmentary disorder of unknown etiology. There is an evident association between vitiligo and autoimmune diseases like hypothyroidism, DM type 1 (DM1) and the so-called autoimmune polyglandular syndrome (APS). This syndrome is characterized by the coexistence of glandular insufficiency of at least two endocrine glands, due to an autoimmune mechanism. Although type 2 APS is more common (adrenal failure, autoimmune thyroid disease or DM1), vitiligo is more frequent in cases of APS type 1.

Its pathogenesis, although uncertain, is considered multifactorial. Among multiple mechanisms that have been described, genetic predisposition,

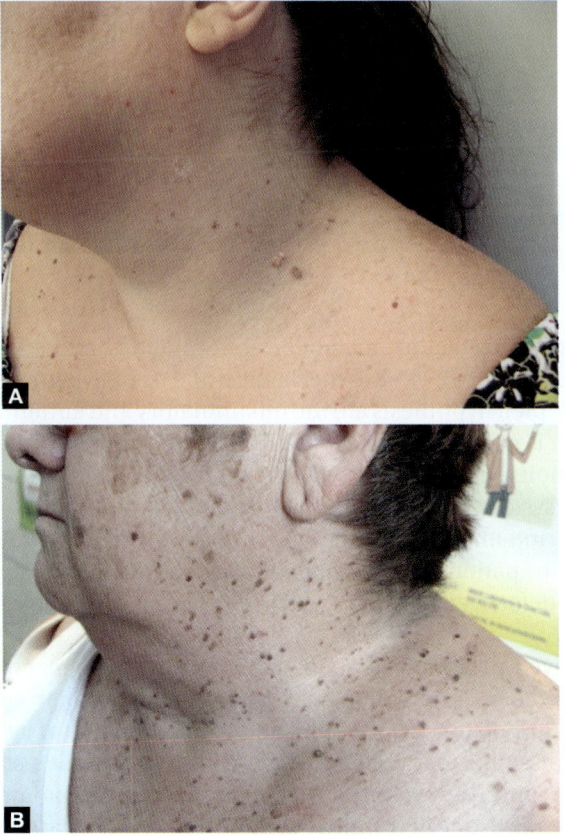

Figs. 14A and B

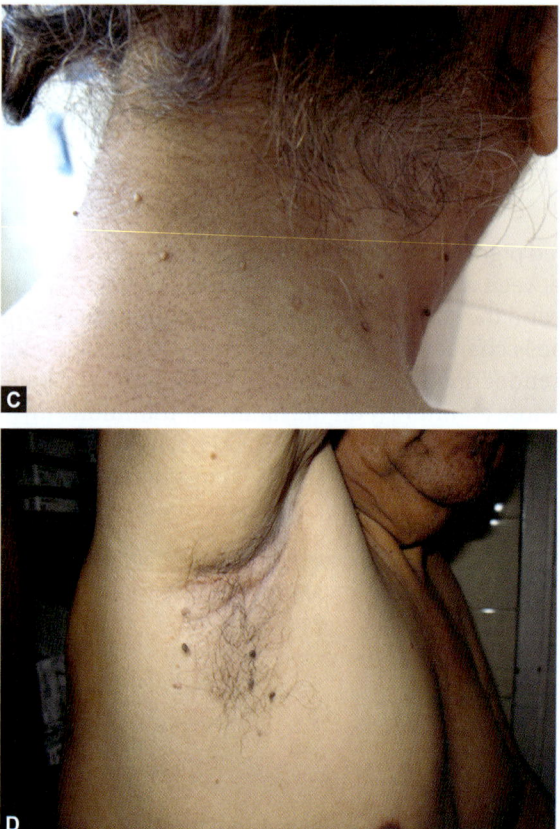

Figs. 14A to D: Skin tags or acrochordons.

microenvironmental factors, metabolic abnormalities, altered inflammatory and immune responses as well as mechanical and oxidative stress are included. The most accepted hypothesis are the inflammatory and autoimmune factors and the result is cellular destruction through a specific cytotoxic melanocyte immune response on predisposed skin due to a defect in the melanocyte adhesiveness system.[22] Wagner et al. highlighted the role of adhesion molecules like E-cadherina and sustain that there is an intrinsic primary defect of melanocytes in patients with vitiligo, in which under stressful conditions and due to a defective adhesion system, cohesion loss of those molecules is induced.[23]

One to seven percent of diabetic patients have vitiligo, compared with 0.2–1% of the general population, with a peak incidence between the ages of 10 and 30. In 30% of the cases, we can find familiar history of vitiligo.[24]

The loss of epidermal melanocytes—cells that produce skin pigment–originates the clinical appearance of hypochromic or asymptomatic achromic macules with well-defined limits, symmetrical and bilateral, that settle preferably in periorificial (eyes, nose, mouth, ears, belly button, genitals) and acral areas, compromising the hair in the area involved (Figs. 15A to C). The lack of melanin in the skin makes it more sensitive to sun burns. Between 10% and 30% of patients diagnosed with vitiligo also have ophthalmological alterations.

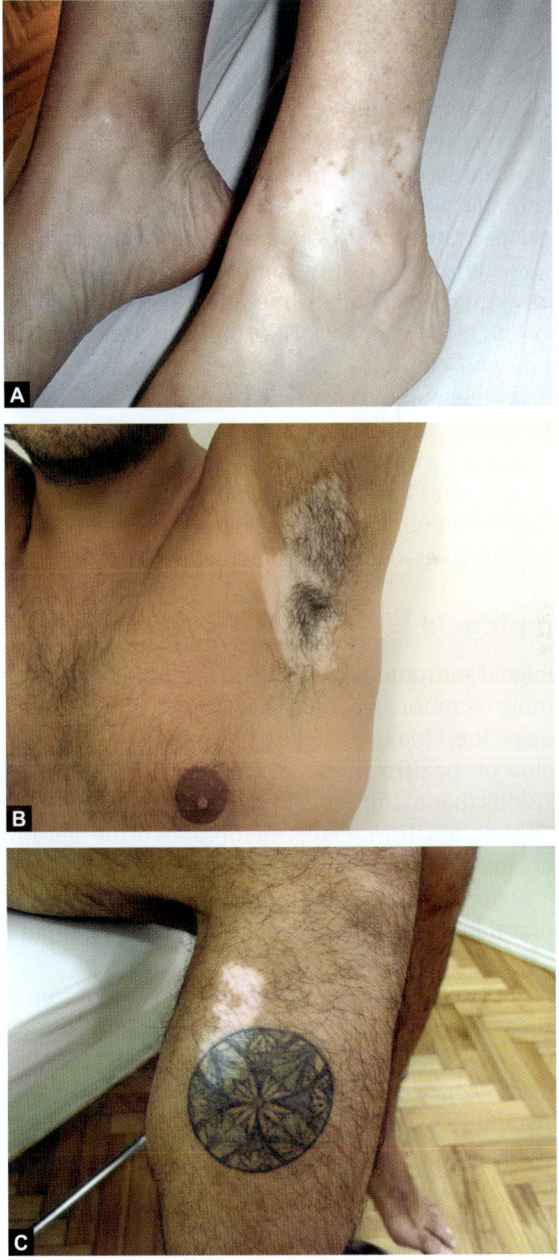

Figs. 15A to C: Vitiligo.

The finding of serum antimelanin antibodies explains the association of vitiligo with other organ-specific autoimmune diseases like, for example, Grave's disease, pernicious anemia, suprarenal insufficiency, idiopathic hypoparathyroidism, which can manifest clinically or maintain a subclinical state. In the case of a patient with vitiligo, it is important to discard thyroid disorders and/or DM.

Few cases resolve spontaneously, on the contrary, most of them are persistent. There are different recognized trigger factors like stress and diverse types of trauma, like insect bites or cuts which determine the appearance of the isomorphic Koebner phenomenon. Vitiligo treatment is unsatisfying. In the case of localized vitiligo, we prefer topical corticosteroids, calcineurin inhibitors, vitamin D analogs (calcipotriol), etc; while for generalized vitiligo the treatment with systemic corticosteroids, narrowband UVB, psoralens + UVA (PUVA), azathioprine constitute additional options. There are also laser treatments and surgical procedures. Ultimately, the combination of treatments like calcipotriol and PUVA, clobetasol and oral immunosuppressants are more effective than monotherapy. The application of wide spectrum sunscreen is mandatory. Cover makeup is a cosmetic solution.

Regarding the relationship between vitiligo and DM1, it has been proven recently that patients with vitiligo and DM1 have a seric increase of the tumor necrosis factor-α (TNF-α), interleukin (IL)-1beta and IL-6 compared with vitiligo patients alone, specially the latter to which is given a role in the development of vitiligo associated with diabetes.[25]

Bullous Pemphigoid

Bullous pemphigoid is an autoimmune disease that affects the skin and mucous membranes, more common in people over 60 and with a slight predominance for the female sex. It is characterized by the appearance of big, tense blisters that can develop on healthy or erythematous skin, urticarial plaques and eczema-like lesions that mainly affect lower limbs and groins, the abdomen, the trunk and underarms. The mucous membranes of the digestive, respiratory and genital tract may be involved. It is asymptomatic or more frequently itchy and in the case of the latter, of variable intensity. Depending on the amount of anatomical areas that are affected–one or more–it is classified into localized and generalized (Figs. 16 to 18).

Among comorbidities, the most reported are hypertension, DM and neurological diseases (seizures, depression, Parkinson's disease); being the cardiovascular diseases a dubious association. For this reason and in spite of the existence of enough evidence that systemic corticosteroids are the first-line choice, corticosteroid savers have been incorporated into the BP therapeutic scheme.[26]

Its pathogenesis is autoimmune and caused by antibodies directed against proteins of the hemidesmosomes [structure that joins keratinocytes of the epidermal basal layer with the basement membrane zone (BMZ)]. This antigen (Ag) is divided into two fractions, bullous pemphigoid antigen (BPAG)

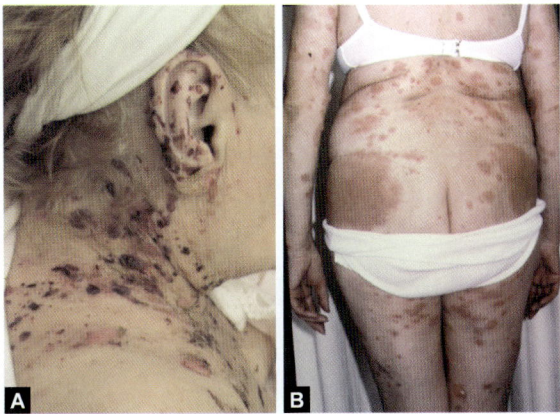

Figs. 16A and B: Bullous pemphigoid. (A) Eroded blisters on lower limbs; (B) Tense blister.

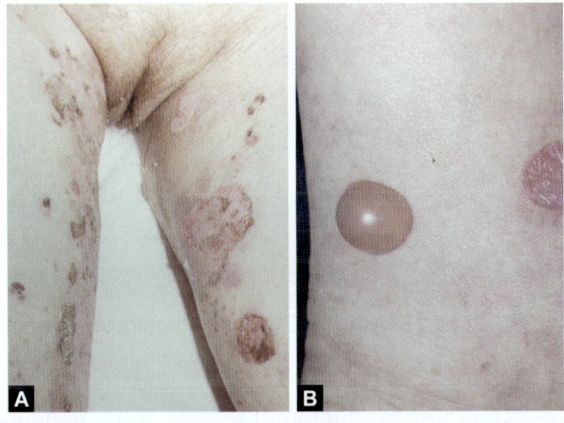

Figs. 17A and B: Bullous pemphigoid. Different evolutionary stages, some tense blisters, other already eroded and some with dry content and covered with crusts.

1 and BPAG2 (part of collagen XVII), one of greater molecular weight and another of lower molecular weight; 230 kD and 180 kD, respectively. Formed autoantibodies, which are pathogenic, join antigen fractions originating the detachment in the dermoepidermal junction, at the level of the lamina lucida of the BMZ and, in consequence, form blisters.[27]

The diagnosis is confirmed through histopathology, where subepidermal blisters with an inflammatory infiltrate, predominantly eosinophils, must be present; and direct immunofluorescence of perilesional skin samples where we found a linear deposit of immunoglobulin G (IgG) and/or C3 and C4 along the BMZ. Serological studies detect circulating IgG autoantibodies attached to the epidermal side of the blister by salt split technique, or detected antibodies against BP180 by enzyme-linked immunosorbent assay (ELISA) or Western

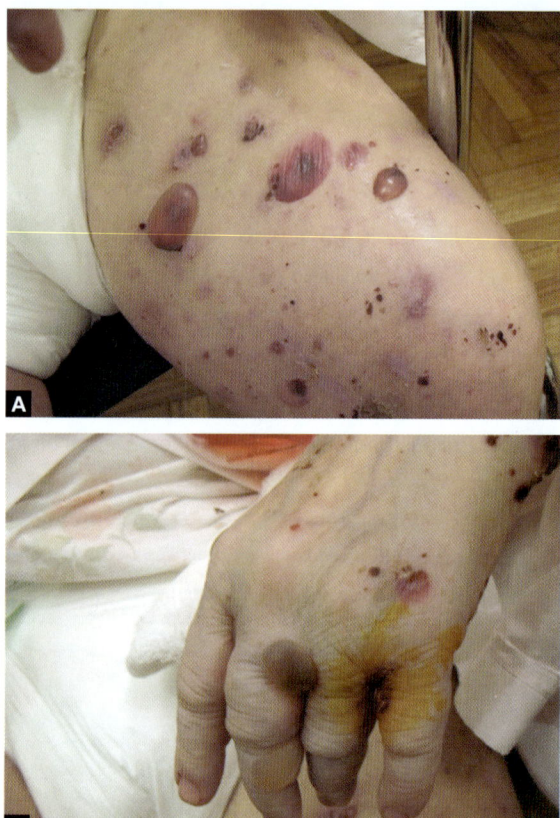

Figs. 18A and B: Bullous pemphigoid.

blot. These circulating IgG can be found in 70% of the patients and have a diagnostic but not prognostic value because they do not correlate with disease activity.

From an immunological point of view, DM and BP can be associated; according to the different reports, such combination has an incidence of 20–41%. There are two factors that contribute to blister formation in diabetic patients; on one side, they have less resistance to blister induction through trauma, and on the other side, nonenzymatic glycation of structural proteins of BMZ would make them more antigenic.

With regards to treatment and based on the extension and severity of BP, one will choose between powerful topical corticosteroids, which have shown to be very effective and safer than those administered orally. The systemic adverse effects are so few that for some authors this would be the first-line drug.[28] Systemic corticosteroids are the most validated drugs for the treatment of generalized BP, but doses exceeding 0.5 mg/kg/day produce multiple adverse effects, including a decrease in survival. The effectiveness of the combination with immunosuppressants like azathioprine, methotrexate, mycophenolate mofetil, cyclophosphamide, cyclosporine as corticosteroid-sparing agents or tetracyclines and nicotinamide, or plasmapheresis; are not yet totally clarified. But nevertheless, complications related to long-term use of corticosteroids could be avoided, which are dose dependent, such as DM/glucose intolerance, hypertension, infection and septicemia risk, psychiatric disorders and osteoporosis.[29]

Unfortunately, DM has an unfavorable impact on skin diseases. The patient needs to be hospitalized under strict glycemia monitoring if the treatment chosen is systemic corticosteroids. Generally, the attack dose is higher than the one for nondiabetic patients, and on the contrary, the response is lower and slower. Factors of worse prognosis are advanced age, stroke and DM at the time of the diagnosis, associated with mortality; with infections and cardiac diseases being the most frequent causes of death.[30]

MIXED METABOLIC IMMUNOLOGICAL MECHANISM

Psoriasis

Psoriasis is a chronic inflammatory skin disease, at present considered systemic and immunologically mediated, that affects 2–5% of the population. Clinically, it is characterized by papules and plaques of erythematous color, covered by whitish flakes. During the last decade, various reports demonstrated that psoriatic patients have a high-risk of developing cardiovascular and metabolic diseases like DM, obesity, IR and metabolic syndrome, which would be linked by a common pathogenic mechanism.

Numerous factors are responsible for the connection between Ps and these metabolic alterations, where excess adipose tissue and secreted adipokines play an important role. An example is adiponectin, an anti-inflammatory adipokine, whose plasmatic levels are reduced in all of these pathologies. This adipocytokine has metabolic and immunological actions. Among the first, it participates in the metabolism of glucose and lipids and in the appearance of IR, and immunologically in the release of cytokines and differentiation of T lymphocytes, actively participating in the pathophysiology of Ps and its connection with the mentioned metabolic alterations previously.

Tumor necrosis factor-α, one of the main actors in Ps physiopathology, is another example of the interrelation between this skin disease and IR. TNF-α induces defects in the insulin signaling pathway, acting on adipocytes and muscle cells and suppressing adiponectin secretion of adipocytes.[31]

Even controlling all these factors, psoriatic patients have a greater risk of mortality, especially young people, particularly those with serious illness. Systemic inflammation in Ps generates the elevation of C-reactive protein, homocysteine and proinflammatory cytokines: TNF-α, IL-6, IL-17, IL-20, IL-22 and IL-23 that contribute to the global morbidity and mortality of these patients.

Psoriatic patients have also a higher risk of DM, especially type 2, based on the chronic inflammatory state that would cause them to be more resistant to insulin compared to healthy individuals. At the same time, IR itself is able to influence homeostasis of keratinocytes and thus, participate in the pathogenesis of Ps.[32]

On the skin, the most common form is vulgar Ps which consists of systemic, bilateral erythematous scaly plaques in extension areas such as elbows and knees, the scalp and lumbosacral region. Other clinical varieties are ungueal Ps and the one that affects joints (arthropathic Ps), inverse Ps (intertriginous areas), palmoplantar Ps and generalized Ps, which if it compromises more than 80% of the body surface, is called erythrodermic form and is a reason for hospitalization, because the loss of proteins (albumin) and electrolytes leads the patient to hemodynamic decompensation[33] (Figs. 19A to D).

In the case of minor trauma, like described in the isomorphic Koebner phenomenon, a new Ps lesion appears on the affected site.

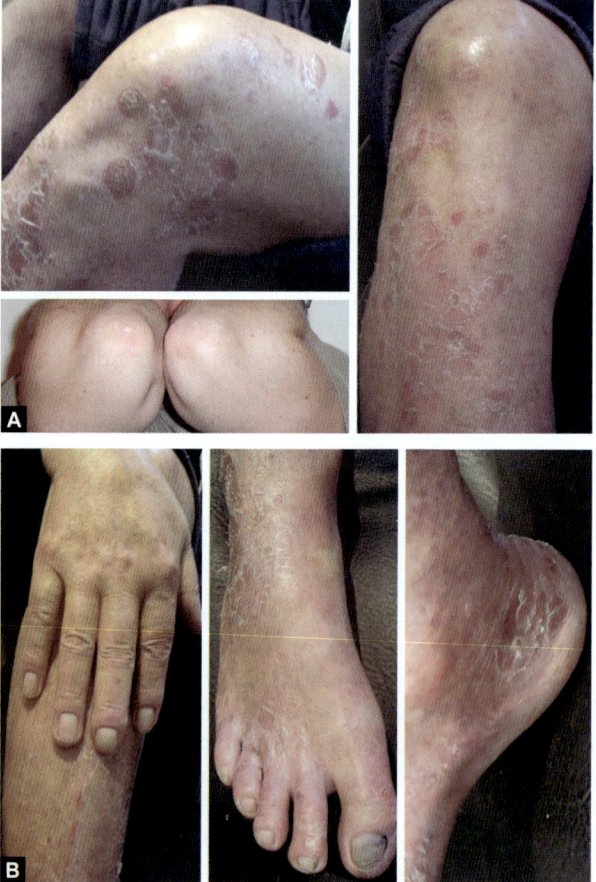

Figs. 19A and B

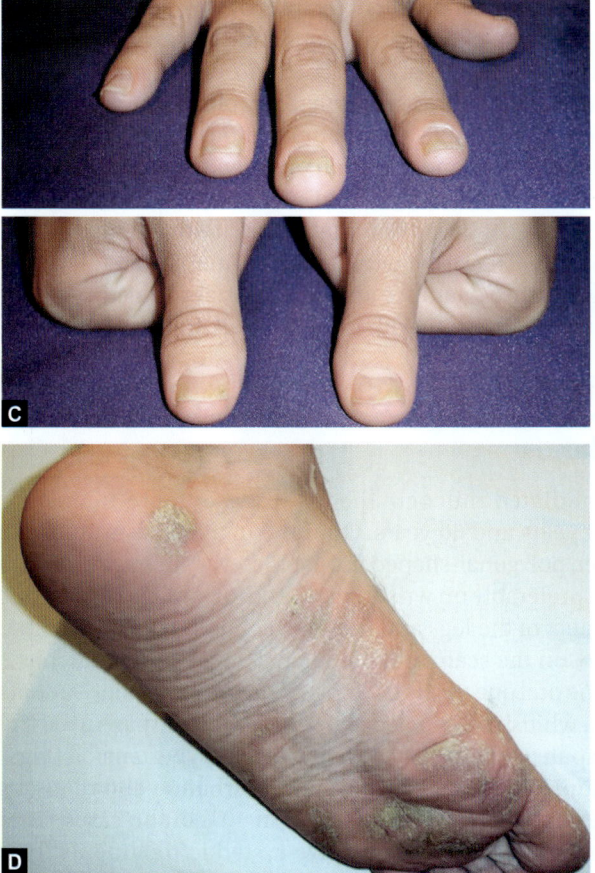

Figs. 19A to D: Psoriasis.

There are factors that can exacerbate Ps, like stress, obesity, alcohol and some drugs like systemic corticosteroids, lithium and chloroquine, nonsteroidal anti-inflammatory drugs and beta blockers.

Although most cases get better with UV radiation, there is a small percentage of patients that present photosensitivity.

As an accompanying symptom, pruritus is not constant and varies in intensity because it is more severe in acute flares, in scalp Ps and anogenital area.[34]

With regards to physiopathology, the fundamental disorder is centered on cell kinetics; keratinocytes cellular cycle which usually lasts 28 days is shortened to four. Histologically, there are epidermal alterations: hyperkeratosis and parakeratosis, polymorphonuclear microabscesses in the stratum corneum, agranulosis and regular acanthosis. In the dermis, a mononuclear inflammatory infiltrate and elongated, dilated and congested superficial capillaries can be observed.[35]

The treatment exceeds the objectives of this book, but it is important to highlight that those patients with moderate to severe Ps have to be treated with celerity and effectively; apart from putting emphasis on correcting cardiovascular risk factors and particularly obesity and smoking.

In the association of Ps with comorbidities, there could be genetic links. Environmental factors and common underlying inflammatory pathways play a role too. As for the coexistence of DM and Ps, its frequency varies between 2.5% and 25%. It is believed that there is greater incidence of DM in psoriatic patients; 25–29% of these patients have abnormal glycemic levels with evidence of abnormal glucose tolerance and 24% refer family history of DM. About 50% have DM prior to Ps, while with the other half, the opposite happens.

UNKNOWN MECHANISM

Lichen Planus

Immune-mediated mucocutaneous disease, more frequently in women between 30 years and 60 years. On the skin, it consists of the appearance of bright, violet, polygonal-shaped flat papules, very itchy, with a size of 1–10 mm. They locate preferably on wrists and the flexor surface of forearms and thighs, anterior aspect of the legs and trunk, even though it can be disseminated as, for example, on the scalp and the ungual areas. In the mucous membranes, especially the oral one that is the most frequently affected, it adopts a pattern of fern leaf of a whitish color or it can be erosive and be part of the triad described by Dr Grinspan: oral erosive LP, diabetes and hypertension (Figs. 20A to H).

It is chronic and shows periods of exacerbation and remission. Although the disease can involve spontaneously in 40% of the cases, intense pruritus motivates the initiation of aggressive systemic treatments. First-line drugs are topical or systemic corticosteroids according to the localization and/or extension of the disease, associated or not to antihistamines.[36]

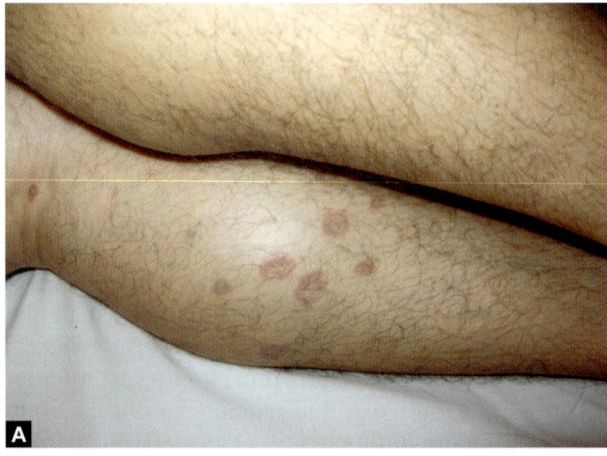

Fig. 20A

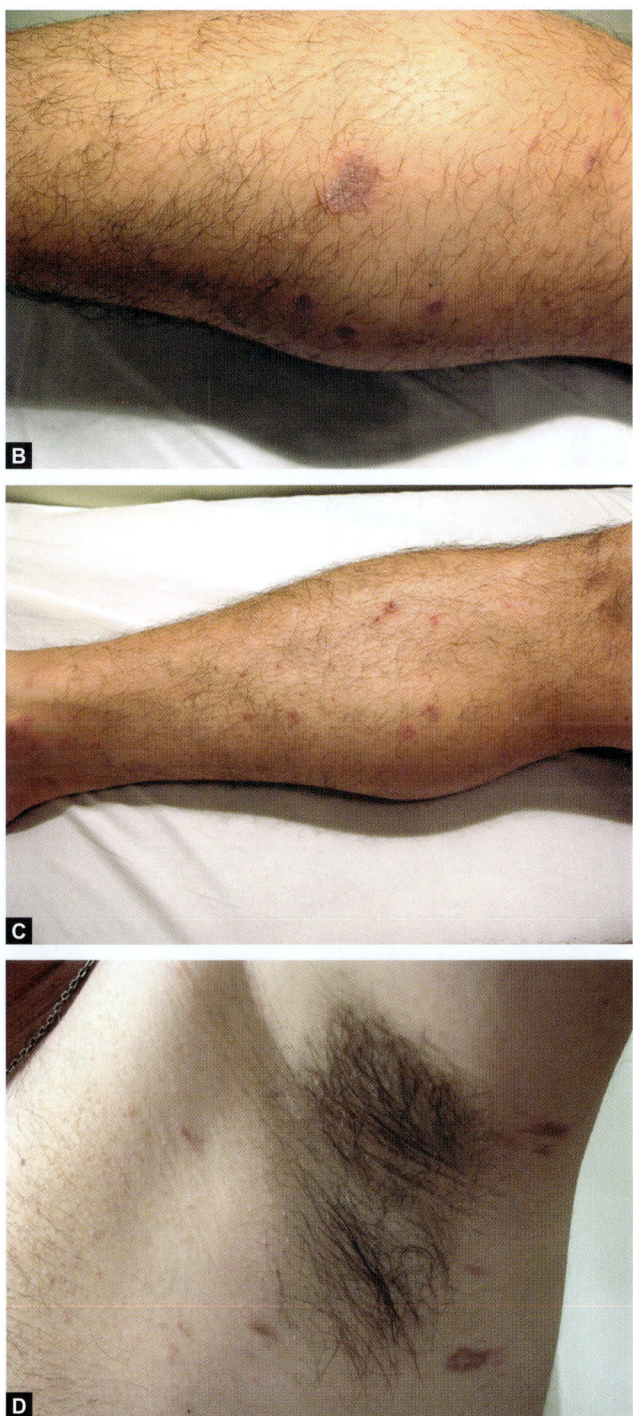

Figs. 20B to D

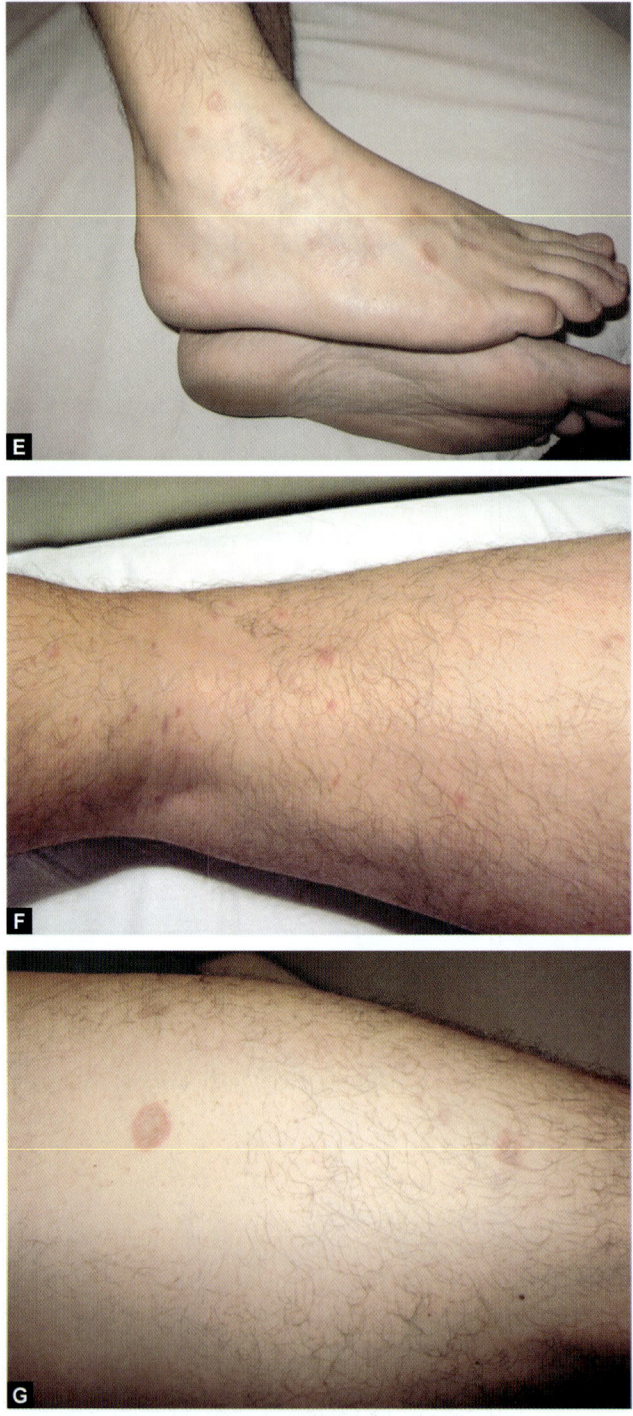

Figs. 20E to G

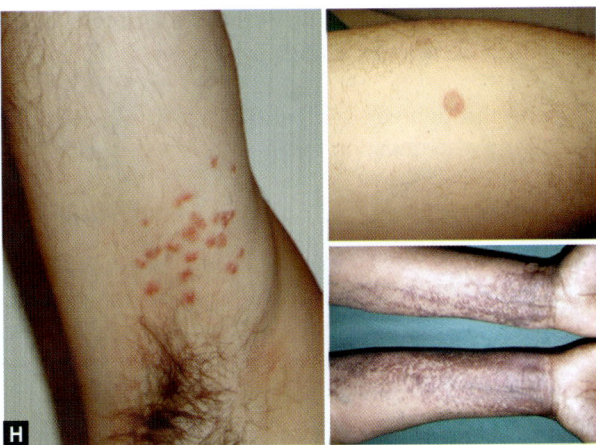

Figs. 20A to H: Lichen planus.

Although its etiopathogenesis is not totally clear, basal keratinocytes express altered antigens on the surface, generating an immune response of lymphocytes, particularly, CD8-positive lymphocytes, which reach the skin through the blood stream. Adhesion molecules (E-selectin) and other mediators of Th1 response released by these activated lymphocytes, like TNF-α, interferon-gamma, induce the release of chemokines related to the skin and endothelial intercellular adhesion molecules.

These autoantigen are presented by the antigen presenting cells, as for example Langerhans (CL) to T-lymphocytes and stimulate their epidermotropism, damaging keratinocytes. This cytotoxic process is mediated by diverse cytokines, TNF-α, IL-6, IL-10 and IL-4, which explains the association of LP with some components of metabolic syndrome such as dyslipidemia.[37]

From the histological point of view, it is an example of mixed dermo-epidermic papules. Hyperkeratosis, focal hypergranulosis, irregular acanthosis and hydropic degeneration of the base membrane can be observed. In the dermis, we observe a band or lichenoid distribution of the mononuclear infiltrate (along the dermoepidermal junction) and the presence of free pigment or free pigment or within the macrophages (melanophages).

This disease has been described in association with different systemic conditions such as hypertension, DM, hepatitis C, primary biliary cirrhosis, etc. There are also reports on the relationship between chronic inflammatory conditions, like LP and metabolic syndrome (dyslipidemia, IR and obesity), and cardiovascular risk factors (hypertension, atherosclerosis, myocardial infarction, etc.), especially in patients with oral LP.

The relationship between DM and LP, particularly oral LP, has been subject of many investigations. The incidence of LP in diabetic patients reaches 1.6%, instead, in a population of Iranian patients with LP, 20% where diabetics and 17.5% had an abnormal glucose tolerance test; which had been documented years ago with similar results by Seyhan et al.[38]

With regards to oral LP, particularly its erosive form, the coexistence was with insulin dependent diabetics with glycemia levels above 240 mg/mL and smokers.[39]

The mechanism through which LP and DM are linked is unknown. Even more, there are many who question this hypothesis.

Kaposi's Sarcoma

Classic KS, described in 1872 by Moritz Kaposi, is a very rare neoplasm, characterized by mixed proliferation of fibroblast like cells and vascular origin cells. It has a higher prevalence between Jewish men (4.7:1) of the Mediterranean and East Europe that have passed the sixth decade of life.

Until 1994, the etiology of KS was unknown, when it started to be linked to human herpes virus-8 (HHV-8), whose deoxyribonucleic acid was identified practically in 100% of the samples. A high index of antibodies against HHV-8 was found, with differences between South America, the Mediterranean region and Africa, for example; and at the same time, within the same population, among Amerindians and the rest. Despite this, actually it is believed that HHV-8 is necessary, but not enough to cause KS and other factors such as immunosuppression play a very important role.[40]

From the clinical point of view, it starts with one or multiple red-violaceous, oval or lanceolate macules with well-defined limits (Figs. 21A and B). During their evolution, the size increases and confluences in big plaques, nodules and tumors commonly asymptomatic. Generally, they localize on the lower third of the legs and can be accompanied by lymphedema. They can stay in that location or extend to other regions like the trunk or the face. They also involve mucous membranes, especially oral mucosa, lymph nodes and internal organs, such as the digestive tract and lungs; however, their dissemination and multicentricity can be observed in a low percentage of patients. Histologically, it consists of a proliferation of vascular lights lined by atypical endothelial cells, with few mitoses and a certain polymorphism, extravasated erythrocytes and macrophages loaded with hemosiderin, along with a discrete dermal mononuclear infiltrate.[41]

The disease tends to be indolent and of good prognosis, with an average survival time of 8–13 years. Some cases of spontaneous regression have been described, which apparently respond to intralesional thrombosis or to an immunological reaction of the host. Treatments for KS such as radiotherapy, surgery and chemotherapy are associated to more severe adverse effects, especially in diabetic patients. Local treatment, although it does not prevent the emergence of new lesions in other cutaneous sites or internal disease, it avoids systemic treatment toxicity.[42]

The association between KS and latent or manifest DM is controversial. For some authors, both pathologies appear together with a higher frequency than expected. The incidence of DM in patients with classic KS varies between 15% and 25%. There has not been found any connection with other forms of KS.

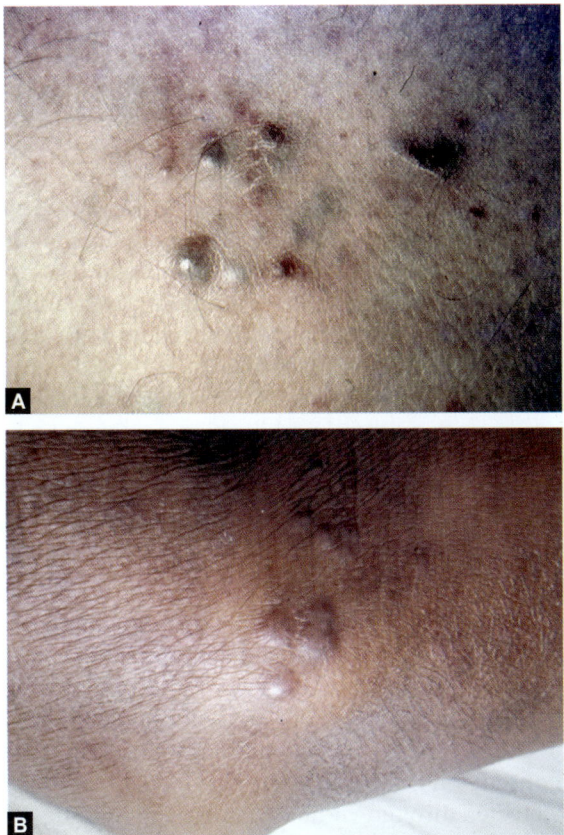

Figs. 21A and B: Kaposi's sarcoma.

Acquired Perforating Dermatosis

Acquired perforating dermatoses in adult age appear in patients with renal failure or DM type 1 and 2 with nephropathy and renal insufficiency that require hemodialysis.

They constitute a group of disorders, whose common denominator is the transepidermal elimination of one or more dermal components. Four classic forms of perforating dermatosis have been described: Elastosis perforans serpiginosa (EPS), generally associated to Down's and Ehlers-Danlos syndrome; perforating folliculitis (PF) secondary to local trauma; Kyrle disease and acquired perforating collagenosis (APC), which appears during childhood in hereditary form or in acquired form in adulthood. Because the pathogenesis involves an active role of the epidermis and not merely a perforation of the epidermis, the authors prefer the term transepidermal elimination disease rather than perforating dermatosis. On the other side, upper dermis would contribute to inflammation which would stimulate the epidermis toward hyperplasia, especially around the eliminated material. Once inside the epidermis, it is obvious to think that all that content formed by collagen, elastic fibers, nuclear debris and polymorphonuclear leukocytes will be eliminated transepidermically toward the surface together with normal maturation of the keratinocytes.

The relation between APD and DM is widely described in the literature and it is estimated that its incidence is between 5% and 10% in patients with hemodialysis.[43]

Even though its etiopathogenesis is unknown, microtrauma due to pruritus and chronic scratching, diabetic microangiopathy, increase of the transforming growth factor beta, degradation of the extracellular matrix due to metalloproteinases, acquired collagen or elastic fiber abnormalities and the deposit of substances that cannot be removed through dialysis (increase in Vitamin A), are the most known theories.

With small differences, all share the clinical aspect which consists of cupuliform papules with a central umbilication containing a hyperkeratotic plug or pruriginous nodules, whose size is between 2 mm and 10 mm (Figs. 22A to D). Sometimes, in response to trauma, they show a linear distribution (Koebner phenomenon). They locate preferably on extremities, the trunk and dorsum of hands and less frequently in the face (exposed areas).[44]

From a histological point of view, some authors propose to classify them according to the follicle involvement and the eliminated content. In most cases, there is an epidermal invagination containing corneal material and cellular detritus, accompanied by mixed infiltrate of lymphocytes and polymorphonuclear neutrophils. If the trichrome staining turns out positive, and that of the elastic fibers negative, findings indicate that the diagnosis is APC. On the contrary, in case of EPS, the eliminated material are thickened elastic fibers, detected through Verhoeff-van Gieson staining. If both staining procedures turn out negative, there is cellular detritus but no fibers, we are facing EK. In PF, dilated follicles contain necrotic material and corneal plugs with perforations of the follicular epithelium. There can also be collagen fibers in the eliminated material.

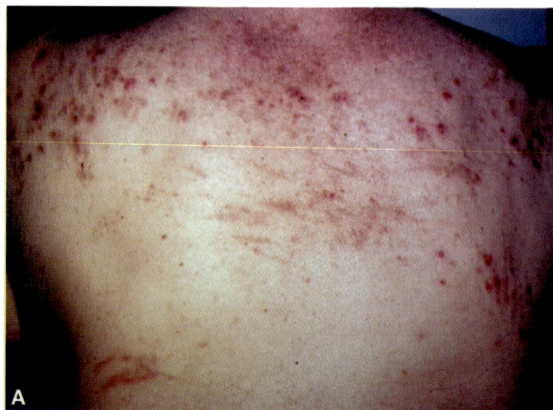

Fig. 22A

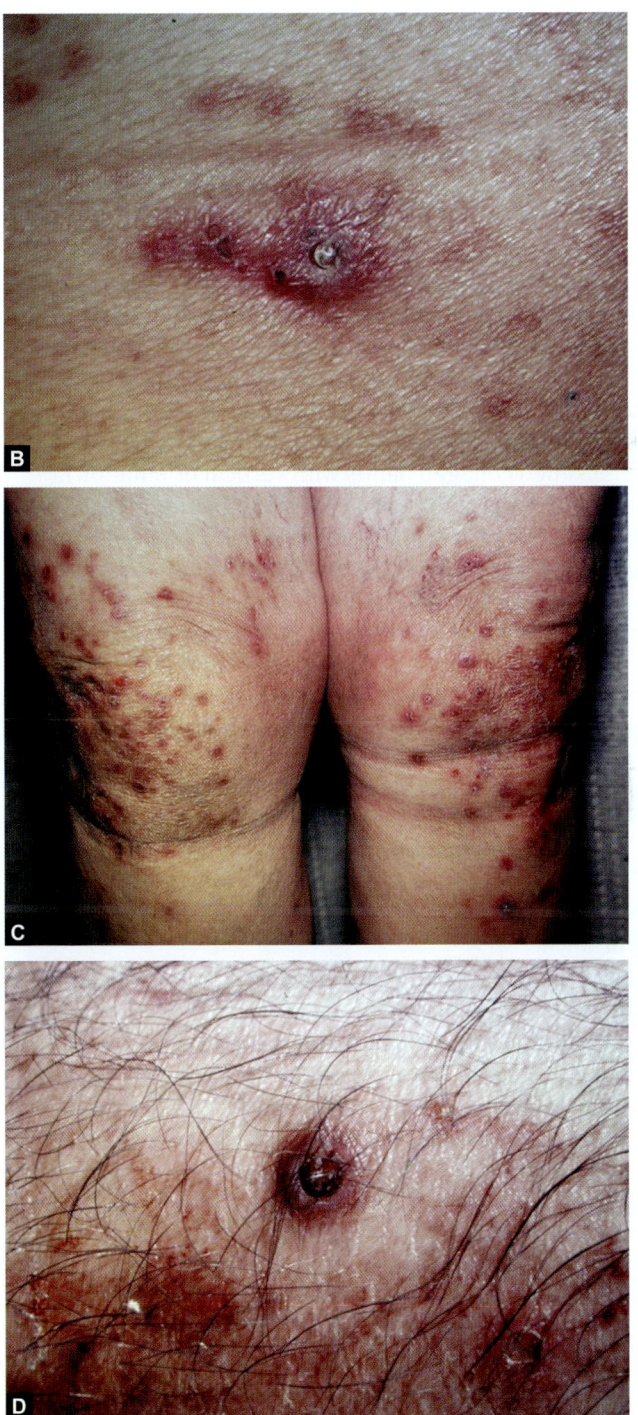

Figs. 22A to D: Acquired perforating dermatosis.

Ultrastructurally, the transepidermal elimination process reveals reduplication and discontinuation in the BMZ (basal lamina), direct contact between the dermal content and basal cells, widening of the intracellular space due to edema between keratinocytes (spongiosis) and degenerative changes of the latter.

Sometimes, clinical-histological criteria overlap and in biopsies performed in the same patient, it is not easy to differentiate between these dermatoses, therefore, it has been proposed that, in diabetic or renal failure patients, these findings represent different stages or different types of lesions of the same pathological process.[45]

In recent years, the field of dermatoscopy has added a diagnostic tool. White shiny areas are described in the middle of the lesion which correspond to a dilated infundibulum filled with keratin and cellular detritus, surrounded by a greyish structureless area which corresponds to the combination of epidermal (acanthosis, hypergranulosis, hyperpigmented basal keratinocytes) and dermal changes (thickened collagen bands with vertical orientation).[46]

Treatment is aimed to the relief of pruritus and controlling the disease or underlying diseases. Topical corticosteroids with oral antihistamines constitute the first therapeutic step. But nevertheless, other options like PUVA, narrowband UVB, topical and systemic retinoids and systemic corticosteroids, etc., are necessary, according to the extension and overall status of the patient.

Finally, acquired perforating skin diseases or transepidermal elimination diseases in adults are associated with diabetic patients and especially those with nephropathy in the stage of chronic renal insufficiency. This relation could be due to microangiopathy and other mechanisms like oxidative stress, nonenzymatic glycation, etc.[47]

CONCLUSION

Knowing the long list of skin diseases, associated most frequently to DM, has triple importance:
- From the diagnostic point of view, it allows to suspect and make an early diagnosis of an unknown DM.
- Regarding the prognosis, these skin diseases in diabetic patients evolve more awkwardly than in the general population.
- Ultimately, and linked to the anterior concept, the treatment should be more aggressive and longer.

REFERENCES

1. Cohen Sabban E, Cabo H. Dermatoses most frequently related to diabetes. J Clin Dermatol. 1999;2:15-22.
2. Cohen Sabban E. Enfermedades que se asocian con frecuencia a la Diabetes. In: Cabo H (Ed). Manifestaciones Cutáneas de la Diabetes Mellitus. Argentina, Buenos Aires: Ed A. Macchi 1996;139-63.
3. Muñoz-Santos C, Guilabert A, Moreno N, et al. The association between porphyria cutanea tarda and diabetes mellitus: analysis of a long-term follow-up cohort. BJD. 2011;165:486-91.

4. Nayak KR, Daly RG. Eruptive xanthomas associated with hypertriglyceridemia and new-onset diabetes mellitus. N Engl J Med. 2004;350:1235.
5. Wani AM, Hussain WM, Fatani MI, et al. Eruptive xanthomas with Koebner phenomenon, type 1 diabetes mellitus, hypertriglyceridaemia and hypertension in a 41-year-old man. BMJ Case Rep. 2009;2009. http://dx.doi.org/10.1136/bcr.05.2009.1871.
6. Kala J, Mostow EN. Images in clinical medicine. Eruptive xanthoma. N Engl J Med. 2012;366:835.
7. Guerrero Vázquez R, Oliva Rodríguez R, Cuenca Cuenca JI, et al. Malignant glucagonoma: an uncommon cause of new onset diabetes. Endocrinol Nutr. 2011;58:199-201.
8. Eldor R, Glaser B, Fraenkel M, et al. Glucagonoma and the glucagonoma syndrome cumulative experience with an elusive endocrine tumour. Clin Endocrinol (Oxf). 2011;74:593-8.
9. Halvorson SAC, Gilbert E, Hopkins RS, et al. Putting the pieces together: necrolytic migratory erythema and the glucagonoma syndrome. J Gen Intern Med. 2013;28(11):1525-9.
10. Granero Castro P, Miyar de León A, Granero Trancón J, et al. Glucagonoma syndrome: a case report. J Med Case Rep. 2011;5:402.
11. Lobo I, Carvalho A, Amaral C, et al. Glucagonoma syndrome and necrolytic migratory erythema. Int J Dermatol 2010; 49:24-29.
12. Wei-Fu LV, Jian-Kui Han, Xin Liu, et al. Imaging features of glucagonoma syndrome: a case report and review of the literatura. Oncol Lett. 2015;4:1579-82.
13. Ko MJ, Chiu HC, Jee SH, et al. Postprandial blood glucose is associated with generalized pruritus in patients with type 2 diabetes. Eur J Dermatol. 2013;23(5):688-93.
14. Polat M, Oztas P, Ilhan MN, et al. Generalized pruritus: a prospective study concerning etiology. Am J Clin Dermatol. 2008;9:39-44.
15. Atabek ME, Akyürek N, Eklioglu BS. Frequency of vaginal candida colonization and relationship between metabolic parameters in children with type 1 diabetes mellitus. J Pediatr Adolesc Gynecol. 2013;26(5):257-60.
16. Misery L, Bodere C, Genestet S. Small-fibre neuropathies and skin: news and perspectives for dermatologists. Eur J Dermatol. 2014;24(2):147-53.
17. Yamaoka H, Sasaki H, Yamasaki H, et al. Truncal pruritus of unknown origin may be a symptom of diabetic polyneuropathy. Diabetes Care. 2010;33(1):150-5.
18. Sadaf Idris, Sunitha S. Assessment of BMI, serum leptin levels and lipid profile in patients with skin tags. J Clin Diagn Res. 2014;8(9):CC01-3.
19. Shah R, Jindal A, Patel N. Acrochordons as a cutaneous sign of metabolic syndrome: a case-control study. Ann Med Health Sci Res. 2014;4(2):202-5.
20. Barbato MT, Criado PR, Silva AK, et al. Association of acanthosis nigricans and skin tags with insulin resistance. An Bras Dermatol. 2012;87(1):97-104.
21. Higgins JC, Maher MH, Douglas MS. Diagnosing common benign skin tumors. Am Fam Physician. 2015;92(7):601-7.
22. Picardo M, Bastonini E. A new view of vitiligo: looking at normal-appearing skin. J Invest Dermatol. 2015;135(7):1713-4.
23. Wagner RY, Luciani F, Cario-André M, et al. Altered E-Cadherin levels and distribution in melanocytes precede clinical manifestations of vitiligo. J Invest Dermatol. 2015;135(7):1810-9.
24. Sheth VM, Guo Y, Qureshi AA. Comorbidities associated with vitiligo: a ten-year retrospective study. Dermatology. 2013;227(4):311-5.
25. Farhan J, Al-Shobaili HA, Zafar U, et al. Interleukin-6: a possible inflammatory link between vitiligo and type 1 diabetes. Br J Biomed Sci. 2014;71(4):151-7.

26. Kibsgaard L, Bay B, Deleuran M, et al. A retrospective consecutive case-series study on the effect of systemic treatment, length of admission time, and co-morbidities in 98 bullous pemphigoid patients admitted to a tertiary centre. Acta Derm Venereol. 2015;95(3):307-11.
27. Furue M, Kadono T. Bullous pemphigoid: what's ahead? J Dermatol. 2016;43(3):237-40.
28. Sobocinski V, Duvert-Lehembre S, Bubenheim M, et al. Assessment of adherence to topical corticosteroids in bullous pemphigoid patients. Br J Dermatol. 2015; doi: 10.1111/bjd.14285.
29. Sakanoue M, Kawai K, Kanekura T. Bullous pemphigoid associated with type 1 diabetes mellitus responsive to mycophenolate mofetil. J Dermatol. 2012;39(10):884-5.
30. Lee JH, Kim SC. Mortality of patients with bullous pemphigoid in Korea. J Am Acad Dermatol. 2014;71:676-83.
31. Napolitano M, Megna M, Monfrecola G. Insulin Resistance and Skin Diseases. The Scientific World Journal Volume 2015, Article ID 479354, 11 pages.
32. Gyldenløve M, Storgaard H, Holst JJ, et al. Patients with psoriasis are insulin resistant. J Am Acad Dermatol. 2015;72(4):599-605.
33. Gottlieb AB, Dann F. Comorbidities in patients with psoriasis. Am J Med. 2009;122: 1-9.
34. Farley E, Menter A. Psoriasis: comorbidities and associations. G Ital Dermatol Venereol. 2011;146:9-15.
35. Cabo H, Cohen Sabban E. Psoriasis y Diabetes. Texto para libro con formato de Disco Compacto 2002. Autores: E Chouela; A Bessone; N Poggio.
36. Krupaa RJ, Sankari SL, Masthan KM, et al. Oral lichen planus: An overview. J Pharm Bioallied Sci. 2015;7(Suppl 1):S158-61.
37. Baykal L, Arıca DA, Yaylı S, et al. Prevalence of metabolic syndrome in patients with mucosal lichen planus: a case-control study. Am J Clin Dermatol. 2015;16(5):439-45.
38. Seyhan M, Ozcan H, Sahin I, et al. High prevalence of glucose metabolism disturbance in patients with lichen planus. Diabetes Res Clin Pract. 2007;77(2):198-202.
39. Atefi N, Majedi M, Peyghambari S, et al. Prevalence of diabetes mellitus and impaired fasting blood glucose in patients with lichen planus. Med J Islam Repub Iran. 2012;26(1):22-6.
40. Mohanna S, Maco V, Bravo F, et al. Epidemiology and clinical characteristics of classic Kaposi's sarcoma, seroprevalence, and variants of human herpesvirus 8 in South America: a critical review of an old disease. Int J Infect Dis. 2005;9:239-50.
41. Errihani H, Berrada N, Raissouni S, et al. Classic Kaposi's sarcoma in Morocco: clinico-epidemiological study at the National Institute of Oncology. BMC Dermatol. 2011;11:15.
42. Vassallo C, Carugno A, Derlino F, et al. Intralesional vinblastine injections for treatment of classic Kaposi sarcoma in diabetic patients. Cutis. 2015;95(5):E28-34.
43. Lynde CB, Pratt MD. Acquired perforating dermatosis: association with diabetes and renal failure. CMAJ. 2009;615.
44. Saray, D Seçkin, B Bilezikçi. Acquired perforating dermatosis: clinicopathological features in twenty-two cases. JEADV. 2006;20:679-88.
45. Schreml S, Hafner C, Eder F, et al. Kyrle disease and acquired perforating collagenosis secondary to chronic renal failure and diabetes mellitus. Case Rep Dermatol. 2011;3:209-11.
46. Ramirez-Fort MK, Khan F, Rosendahl CO, et al. Acquired perforating dermatosis: a clinical and dermatoscopic correlation. Dermatol Online J. 2013;19(7):18958.
47. Akoglu G, Emre S, Sungu N, et al. Clinicopathological features of 25 patients with acquired perforating dermatosis. Eur J Dermatol. 2013;23(6):864-71.

CHAPTER

9

Cutaneous Manifestations Induced by Antidiabetic Treatment

Emilia Noemí Cohen Sabban, Marina Luz Margossian

INTRODUCTION

The worldwide incidence of diabetes mellitus (DM), increases continuously, so the modern therapeutic strategy is to use earlier intensive regimens of insulin with the goal of achieving better control of blood glucose levels and reduce the long-term risks associated with the disease.[1]

The cutaneous manifestations induced by antidiabetic treatment, which according to the general classification belong to group 4, are divided according to the therapy instituted by insulin and non-insulin (Table 1).[2]

INSULIN THERAPY

Insulin therapy is associated with significant adverse effects on the skin, which may interfere with absorption kinetics and cause variations above and below blood glucose levels.[1] Fortunately, these complications have been declining since the advent of the new generations of insulin.[3] However, we should mention them:
- Administration failures: intraepidermal injection.
- Idiosyncrasy.
- Insulin allergy.
- Lipodystrophies.

Other complications such as keloids, keratotic papules, purpura, infectious abscesses and circumscribed pigmentation may appear from the injection of insulin (Fig. 1).

Insulin Allergy

Impurities in the preparation, presence of animal-origin (bovine, porcine), insulin molecule in itself, preservatives or additives can cause allergic reactions to insulin.[4] They can be localized or generalized. Local allergic

TABLE 1: Skin manifestations induced by the pharmacological treatment of diabetes mellitus.[27]

Type of drug	Incidence	Skin manifestation	Pathogenesis	Treatment
Non-insulin Sulfonylureas	1–5% 1–5% 1–5% 10–30%	• Maculopapular rash • Photoallergy • Phototoxicity • Flushing (Chlorpropamide) • Acute vasomotor	• Unknown • Mediated by cells • Toxic • Opioids IV	Change treatment Suspend drug
DPP-4 inhibitors	Infrequent	• Pemphigoid blister	• Alteration of immune response • Antigenic modification in ZMB	Suspend drug
GLP-1 analogs	Infrequent	• Urticaria • Pruritus • Allergic reaction at injection site	IgE-mediated reaction	Rotate application site
SGLT-2 inhibitors	Infrequent	Hyperhidrosis, stomatitis and herpes zoster	Not known	Suspend drug
Insulin Animal origin	10–50%	• Lipoatrophy • Erythema • Papules and pruriginous nodules (urticarial reaction)	• IgE cell mediation; IgG • Changes in tertiary structure	Rotate the IHR
Human recombinant	Rare <3%	Lipoatrophy	Lipolytic components of insulin and immune complexes	Highly purified IHR injection in the periphery

(DPP-4: Dipeptidyl-peptidase 4; IV: Intravenous; GLP-1: Glucagon-like peptide; IgE: Immunoglobulin E; IgG: Immunoglobulin G; IHR: Recombinant human insulin; SGLT-2: Sodium-glucose cotransporter-2; BMZ: Basement membrane zone).

reactions to insulin clinically manifest with erythema, papules and nodules with pruritus and induration. These reactions are usually transient and resolve spontaneously within weeks. The reaction localized at the site of immediate application reaches maximum intensity in 15–30 minutes and usually disappears within the first hour. Under clinical examination, the presence of erythema, which may evolve into urticarial wheals and is probably mediated by immunoglobulin E (IgE), is observed.[4] The immediate localized form may

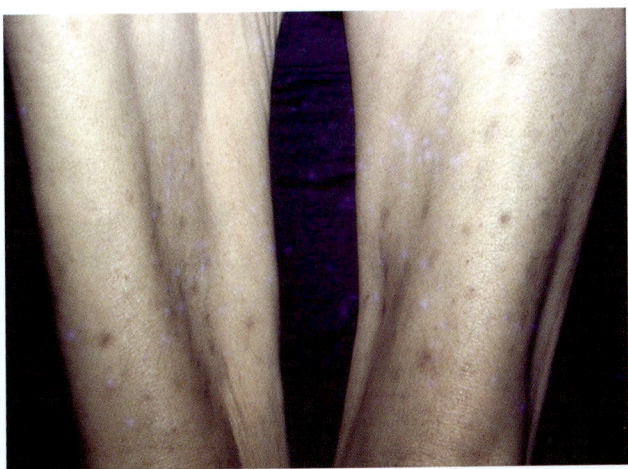

Fig. 1: Residual hyperpigmented lesions at insulin injection sites.

progress to a generalized form similar to an accelerated urticarial reaction or, less frequently, to an Arthus reaction.[1,4] The delayed hypersensitivity reaction is the most common, it appears around 2 weeks after the initiation of insulin therapy, and its clinical manifestation is a pruriginous nodule at the application site, 4–24 hours after injection. The biphasic or dual reaction is extremely rare and consists of a delayed local reaction and general malaise similar to serum sickness. They are considered to be immune-mediated reactions of Arthus type.[4] Sometimes adding dexamethasone to insulin injection, desensitization to insulin, or changing the delivery system is helpful for better treatment of these reactions.[1]

Lipodystrophies

They are one of the complications of subcutaneous insulin injection and include lipoatrophy and lipohypertrophy, which can coexist in the same patient. They are more common in obese children and women. They can be caused by lipolytic components of the preparation or by an inflammatory process mediated by immune complexes. Other theories refer to cryotrauma of refrigerated insulin, mechanical trauma due to injection angle, surface contamination with alcohol or local hyperproduction of tumor necrosis factor alpha (TNF-α) by macrophages induced by insulin injection. Insulin deposits have also been implicated and that is why some authors suggest its replacement with rapid-acting insulin. Since the introduction of highly purified recombinant human insulin, lipoatrophy is quite unusual. Lipoatrophy occurs clinically as a depressed and circumscribed area of skin at the site of application, 6–24 months after therapy initiation. Histologically, there is a decrease or absence of subcutaneous fat without inflammatory signs (Fig. 2). Repeated use of the injection at the same site increases the risk of lipoatrophy; over time, patients learn that these areas are relatively nonpainful and continue to use them.

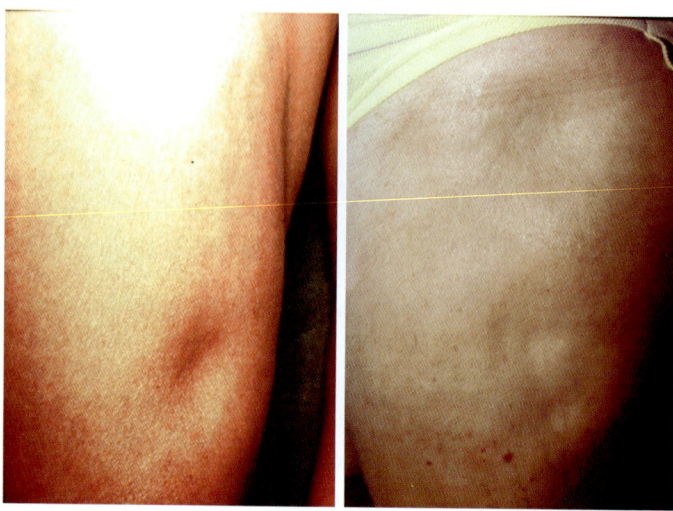

Fig. 2: Lipoatrophy by insulin injections.

However, insulin absorption in the lipoatrophic areas is erratic and frequently leads to the difficulty of achieving optimal blood glucose control.[5]

With the increasing use of rapidly absorbed modified insulin analogues, the frequency of lipoatrophy has declined in recent years. The probability of its appearance can be reduced through the regular rotation of the injection site, but once developed, practical benefits can be obtained due to the insulin injection near the injured area.[1,6]

Lipohypertrophy is the most common cutaneous complication of insulin therapy, regardless of its origin or mode of administration (Fig. 3).[7] Clinically, it resembles a lipoma, such as a soft consistency tumor in the dermis, in the injection site (Figs. 4 and 5). It is considered a local response to the anabolic action of insulin over fat metabolism. It may be accompanied by hypoalgesia. Histologically, an increase of local adipocytes is observed, that gathered in groups, separated from each other by fibrous tracts.

New insulins have also reduced their prevalence considerably, as with lipoatrophy, although their adverse effects on DM control are similar due to worsening of insulin absorption into the systemic circulation.[1]

The introduction of new therapies and new delivery systems would seem to reduce skin problems associated with long-term insulin use, and although many of the cutaneous manifestations are decreasing with the use of new insulins, they may still influence glycemic control and increase the risk of hypoglycemia, as well as cause some cosmetic impact.

The treatment of choice for the immediate localized allergic reaction is to rotate to a more purified insulin. Other options include antihistamines, the addition of corticosteroids to insulin, discontinuing insulin and desensitization, or changes in the delivery system.

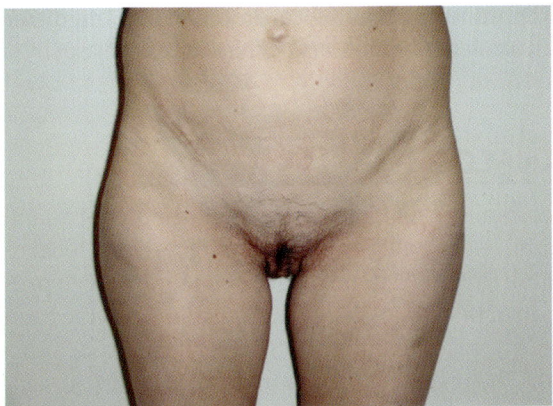

Fig. 3: Lipohypertrophy.

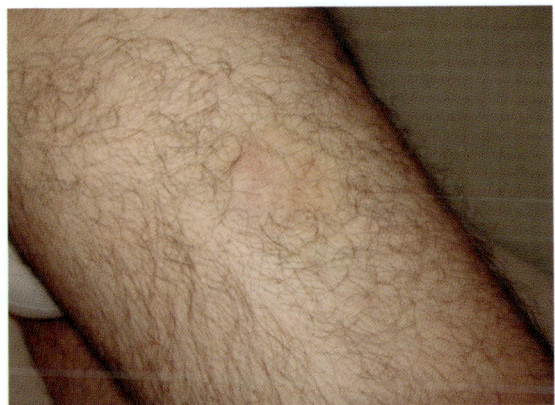

Fig. 4: Lipohypertrophy.

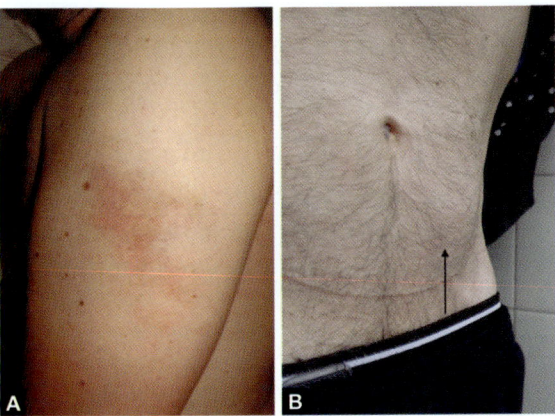

Figs. 5A and B: (A) Lipohypertrophy of recent appearance. (B) Older lipohypertrophy.

The most important immunological problem is IgE-mediated anaphylaxis, which can be controlled by temporary decrease of the dose or by desensitization to insulin.

INSULIN ANALOGUES

They are not common, but some cases of IgE-mediated anaphylaxis, a case of vitiligo (insulin lispro), allergy (insulin glargine), and local reactions at the site of application (insulin detemir) have been reported. At present and since the introduction of insulin analogs (altered amino acid sequence compared to natural insulin), cases of lipoatrophy have decreased, although there are reported cases.[8] The respective exposure to analogs lispro, aspartic, glargine and detemir prior to the development of lipoatrophy, varied considerably between 4 weeks and 2 years.[9] The treatment will depend on the reaction area and it includes desensitization, changes in insulin type, rotation of the injection site, changes in the delivery system (continuous subcutaneous infusion of insulin [CSII] through a portable pump) or a combination of the above.[4]

NON-INSULIN THERAPY

Non-insulin Hypoglycemic Agents

Just like insulin, there are first-generation oral hypoglycemic agents that have been followed by newer ones, with the aim of reduce adverse events. They can produce skin reactions described below.

First-generation Sulfonylureas (Chlorpropamide, Tolbutamide)

Between 1% and 5% of patients taking first-generation sulfonylureas develop skin reactions within the first 2 months of treatment. The most frequent form of manifestation consists of a maculopapular exanthema that disappears with the discontinuation of the drug (Fig. 6).

Between 10% and 30% of patients taking chlorpropamide develop alcohol-induced flushing, acute vasomotor syndrome manifested by erythema and heat, nauseas, vomiting, headaches, tachycardia and, occasionally, dyspnea beginning 15 minutes after alcohol consumption. The symptoms usually go away after an hour. This pattern of reaction appears to be of autosomal dominant inheritance.

Both phototoxic and photoallergic photosensitivity reactions may occur.

Other skin reactions including urticaria, pruritus, fixed erythema, erythema multiformi, erythema nodosum, Lyell's syndrome and toxic epidermal necrolysis have also been observed.

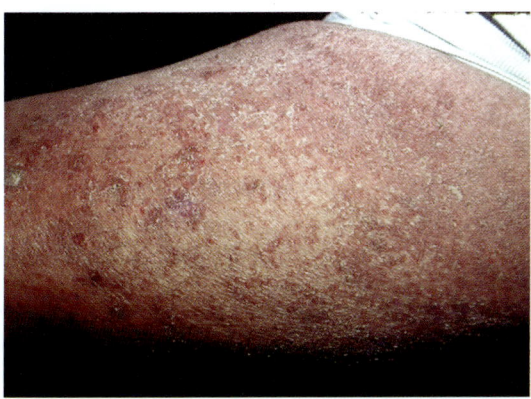

Fig. 6: Maculopapular exanthema.

Second-generation Sulfonylureas (Glipizide, Glimepiride)

Second-generation sulfonylureas also produce skin reactions. Of those associated with glipizide, photosensitivity, urticaria and pruritus were mentioned, which are less frequent with glimepiride.

Biguanides

Metformin is a biguanide with hypoglycemic effect and it is considered first-line oral treatment for patients with DM2. Its main action is to inhibit the hepatic production of glucose and increase peripheral tissue sensitivity to insulin. Cutaneous adverse events include psoriasiform drug reactions, leukocytoclastic vasculitis, and erythema multiforme. Erythema, rash, pruritus, and urticaria have also been reported.

Alpha Glycosidase Inhibitor (Acarbose)

Acarbose inhibits the absorption of glucose at the intestinal level. It rarely causes adverse effects since it is minimally absorbed in the digestive tract. There are reports of generalized erythema multiforme induced by the drug and generalized acute exanthematous pustulosis.

Thiazolidinediones (Rosiglitazone and Pioglitazone)

Rosiglitazone and pioglitazone interfere with receptor activation for advanced glycation end products (RAGE) using a soluble form. Specifically, these drugs improve the action of insulin and, therefore, the control of glycemia and decrease insulin resistance by mechanisms not completely clarified. They reduce levels of free fatty acids of insulin-resistant patients and change the distribution of body fat.[9] The treatment of insulin-resistant type 2 diabetic patients with thiazolidinediones not only improves the control of blood glucose and diminish insulin resistance, but also improves many abnormalities that are part of the insulin resistance syndrome, such as dyslipidemia, hypertension, glucose intolerance, hypercoagulability, obesity, hyperinsulinemia and mild inflammation, all cardiovascular risk factors.[10,11] It is known that through the peroxisome proliferator-activated receptor (PPARγ), which is expressed in endothelial cells, endothelial function is modified and vascular complications of DM are prevented or decreased.[12] PPARγ are transcription factors belonging to the superfamily of nuclear receptors and as such regulate the expression of numerous genes that affect glycemic control, lipid metabolism, vascular tone, and inflammation.[11]

In a randomized, open-label, parallel-group study, thiazolidinediones were compared with sulfonylureas, the authors found that glycosylated hemoglobin (HbA1c) was decreased at 6 months, but only thiazolidinediones had modulation effects on circulating RAGE levels.[13] Edema has been reported as a cutaneous side effect of rosiglitazone and pioglitazone.

Incretins

It is called the "incretin effect" to release insulin after glucose administration and is equivalent to 60% of the total release of insulin after ingestion. Faced with the observation that this phenomenon is diminished in DM2, a new pharmacological target appears to counteract this deficit.

Incretins are a group of hormones produced in the gut in response to food intake. There are two main ones and they are generated at the duodenal level: (1) Glucose-dependent insulinotropic peptide (GIP) and (2) glucagon-like peptide (GLP-1). When these nutrients are ingested, these peptides are secreted which cause increased glucose-dependent pancreatic secretion of insulin, suppress the secretion of postprandial glucagon and slow down gastric emptying.

Incretins in turn are divided into two pharmacological subgroups to treat DM2:[14,15]

1. *Inhibitors of dipeptidyl-peptidase 4 (DPP-4)* are those that inhibit the enzyme that degrades H1 called DPP-4, therefore, increasing their endogenous levels, prolonging their half-life, and generating an antihyperglycemic effect. As monotherapy, they do not produce hypoglycemia because they act in a dependent glucose form, that is to say, they do not act with glycemias inferiors to 77 mg/dL. This subgroup includes sitagliptin, saxagliptin, vildagliptin, alogliptin, linagliptin, and teneligliptin. They are indicated orally, alone or in combination with other drugs. Among its general adverse effects, we can mention headache, nasopharyngitis, urinary tract infections, and hypoglycemia (in a combined therapeutic regimen). At the cutaneous level, blister and blistering diseases produced by all but tenegliptin are described as follows:
    - Hypersensitivity reactions (sitagliptin, saxagliptin, teneligliptin)
    - Skin rash (sitagliptin, linagliptin, teneligliptin)
    - Angioedema (sitagliptin, linagliptin)
    - Steven-Johnson's syndrome (sitagliptin)

- Anaphylaxis (sitagliptin)
- Facial edema (saxagliptin)
- Eczemas (tenegliptin)
- Pruritus (tenegliptin)
- Hyperhidrosis by vildagliptin when associated with sulfonylureas.

Several cases of bullous pemphigoid (BP) (Fig. 7) associated with DPP-4 inhibitors, and more specifically vildagliptin and sitagliptin, have recently been reported in relation to blistering diseases. Bullous pemphigoid is the most common autoimmune blistering disease in which antibodies are produced against components of the basement membrane zone (hemidesmosomes) of the skin. In the cases described, although in most cases gliptin was associated with metformin, there are no cases of BP reported in patients treated with metformin alone. On the other hand, the association between DM and BP is well-known (*see* Chapter 8), but the participation of the drug was clear when despite oral or topical treatment with corticosteroids such as clobetasol, with which a transient remission was achieved after 3 months, the final remission was only obtained by gliptin discontinuation. The exact mechanism is still unknown but it is believed that gliptins could modify the immune response in genetically predisposed patients or alter the antigens of the epidermal basement membrane. However, prospective, confirmatory studies are needed to see if the effect of these drugs could trigger a subclinical disease, or its acceleration, in the group of elderly diabetic patients with pruritic dermatosis.

Cases of skin disorders associated with gliptines were published by pharmacovigilance of the European Medicines Agency until August 2014 in the European Economic Area (Tables 2 and 3).[16-23]

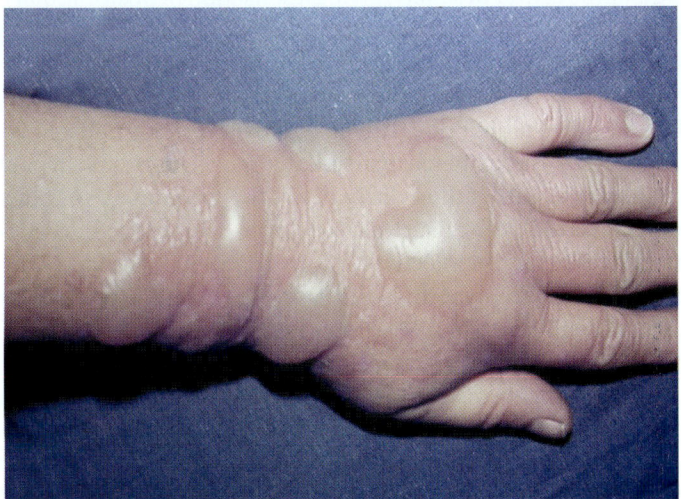

Fig. 7: Bullous pemphigoid produced by incretins.

TABLE 2: Cases of blistering diseases associated with gliptines according to reaction [high-level terms (HLT) of the MedDRA Terminology Classification].[21]

	Vildagliptin	Sitagliptin	Saxagliptin	Linagliptin
Blistering diseases	121	70	6	6

TABLE 3: Description of the different blistering diseases associated with gliptines according to reaction [preferred terms (PT) of the MedDRA Terminology Classification].[21]

Injury	Vildagliptin	Sitagliptin	Saxagliptin	Linagliptin
Blister	40	23	3	4
Blistering dermatitis	32	8	1	1
Pemphigoid blister	72	28	2	1
Pemphigus	8	2	–	–
Erythema multiforme	1	6	–	–
Toxic epidermal necrolysis	2	–	–	–
Stevens Johnson syndrome	–	4	–	–

2. *Glucagon-like peptide-1 agonists* maintain an H1-mimetic effect.[14,15] These drugs are molecularly analogous to the GLP-1 peptide, binding to its receptor with an affinity similar to incretins. They act as the native peptide, but are not degraded by the enzyme DPP-4. Within its pharmacological effects we can mention the stimulation of insulin secretion by the pancreatic β-cell and the inhibition of glucagon secretion. Unlike DPP-4 inhibitors, they slow down gastric emptying and act on the hypothalamic center of satiety, giving a sensation of postprandial fullness, decreased appetite and consequently, weight loss. They are administered subcutaneously and according to their formulation, the dose can be daily or weekly. Of this subgroup, we can mention exenatide, liraglutide, lixisenatide and albiglutide. Adverse effects include nausea, vomiting, diarrhea, dyspepsia, asthenia, pancreatitis, renal failure, and hypoglycemia (in association with sulfonylureas). Of the cutaneous manifestations observed we highlight pruritus, urticaria, anaphylactic reaction and allergic reaction at the injection site. In addition, postmarketing reports of exenatide include hyperhidrosis, alopecia, maculopapular exanthema and angioneurotic edema, whereas with lixisenatide there were cases of reaction to the excipient metacresol. Injection site reactions were reported in 3.9% of patients receiving the drug over a 24-week period, versus 1.4% of the placebo group. As the intensity of these was mild, no treatment was required. Allergic reactions were observed in 0.4% of patients versus 0.1% of the placebo group, they were mild in intensity and included anaphylactic reaction, angioedema, and urticaria.[14-16]

Sodium-glucose Cotransporter 2 Inhibitors (SGLT-2)

Sodium-glucose cotransporter 2 (SGLT-2) is a protein that is expressed at the level of the proximal renal tubule and acts as a cotransporter of sodium, glucose, low affinity and high capacity reabsorbing more than 90% of the filtered glucose. Inhibitors of this transporter inhibit glucose reabsorption, generating glucosuria, a β-cell non-dependent mechanism. There are two drugs approved so far: (1) dapagliflozin and (2) canagliflozin. Glycosuria approximately 70 g/day, generates transient increase of natriuresis and excretion of uric acid, in addition to helping in weight loss. It also promotes an improvement in blood pressure.

The adverse effects of these drugs are: genitourinary infections, symptoms of volume depletion (dizziness, hypotension and dehydration), increased creatinine and hypoglycemia. Some skin adverse events include hyperhidrosis, stomatitis and herpes zoster, but they are very rare. In the genital area, erythema, itching and balanoposthitis and vaginitis can be seen.[24-26]

REFERENCES

1. Richardson T, Kerr D. Skin-related complications of insulin therapy: epidemiology and emerging management strategies. Am J Clin Dermatol. 2003;4:661-7.
2. Perez MI, Kohn SR. Cutaneous manifestations of diabetes mellitus. J Am Acad Dermatol. 1994;30:519-31.
3. Piérard-Franchimont C, Hermanns-Lê T, Scheen AJ, Piérard GE. Cutaneous complications of insulin therapy. A drug-induced condition on the decline. Rev Med Liege. 2005;60:564-5.
4. Van Hattem S, Bootsma A, Bing Thio H. Skin manifestations of diabetes. Cleve Clin J Med. 2008;75:772-87.
5. Del Olmo MI, Campos V, Abellán P, Merino-Torres JF, Piñón F. A case of lipoatrophy with insulin detemir. Diabetes Res Clin Pract. 2008;80:20-1.
6. Saraceno EF. Manifestaciones Cutáneas del tratamiento Antidiabético. In: Cabo H (Ed). Manifestaciones Cutáneas de la Diabetes Mellitus. Argentina, Buenos Aires: Ed A. Macchi; 1996 pp. 165-78.
7. Radermecker RP, Piérard GE, Scheen AJ. Lipodystrophy reactions to insulin: effects of continuous insulin infusion and new insulin analogs. Am J Clin Dermatol. 2007;8:21-8.
8. Babiker A, Datta V. Lipoatrophy with insulin analogues in type I diabetes. Arch Dis Child. 2011;96:101-2.
9. Holstein A, Stege H, Kovacs P. Lipoatrophy associated with the use of insulin analogues: a new case associated with the use of insulin glargine and review of the literature. Expert Opin Drug Saf. 2010;9:225-31.
10. Lebovitz HE, Banerji MA. Insulin resistance and its treatment by thiazolidindiones. Recent Prog Horm Res. 2001;56:265-94.
11. Martens FM, Visseren FL, Lemay J, de Koning EJ, Rabelink TJ. Metabolic and additional vascular effects of thiazolidindiones. Drugs. 2002;62:1463-80.
12. Caballero AE, Saouaf R, Lim SC, et al. The effects of troglitazone, an insulin-sensitizing agent, on the endothelial function in early and late type 2 diabetes: a placebo-controlled randomized clinical trial. Metabolism. 2003;52:173-80.

13. Tan KC, Chow WS, Tso AW, et al. Thiazolidinedione increases serum soluble receptor for advanced glycation end-products in type 2 diabetes. Diabetologia. 2007;50:1819-25.
14. Ruiz M, Lombardo F. Nuevos fármacos: incretinas. In: Ruiz M (Ed). Diabetes Mellitus, Cuarta edición. Akadia; 2011. pp. 273-86.
15. Meier J, Gethmann A, Nauck M, et al. The glucagon-like-peptide-1 metabolite GLP-1 amide reduces postprandial glycemia independently of gastric emptying and insulin secretions in humans. Am J Phisiol Endocrinol Metab. 2006;290:e1118-23.
16. European Medicines Agency. (2017). [online] Available from http://www.ema.europa.eu [Accessed February 2017].
17. Bastuji Garin S, Joly P, Lemordant P, et al. Risk factors for bullous pemphigoid in the elderly: a prospective case-control study. J Invest Dermatol. 2011;131(3):637-43.
18. Béné J, Jacobsoone A, Coupe P, et al. Bullous pemphigoid induced by vildagliptin: a report of three cases. Fundam Clin Pharmacol. 2014;29(1):112-4.
19. Murrel DF, Daniel BS, Joly P, et al. Definitions an outcome measures for bullous pemphigoid: recommendations by an international panel of experts. J Am Acad Dermatol. 2012;66:479-85.
20. Sundaram M, Adikrishnan S, Murugan S. Co-existence or rheumatoid arthritis, vitíligo and bullous pemphigoid as multiple autoinmune síndrome. Indian J Dermatol. 2014;59(3):306-7.
21. Unidad de fármacovigilancia del País Vasco. Inhibidores de la dipeptidil peptidasa 4 (gliptinas) y penfigoide ampollar. Boletín n°38, septiembre 2014.
22. Attaway A, Mersfelder T, Vaishnav S, et al. Bullous pemphigoid associated with dipeptidyl peptidase IV inhibitors. A case report and review of literature. J Dermatol Case Rep. 2014;8(1):24-8.
23. Skandalis K, Spirova M, Gaitanis G, et al. Drug-induced bullous pemphigoid in diabetes mellitus patients receiving dipeptidyl peptidase–IV inhibitors plus metformin. J Eur Acad Dermatol Venereol. 2012;26(2):249-53.
24. Taharani AA, Barnett AH, Bailey CJ. SGLT inhibitors in management of diabetes. Lancet Diabetes Endocrinol. 2013;1:140-51.
25. Leiter L. Symposium of Safety and Adverse Effects. The role of SGLT2 inhibitors in the treatment of type 2 diabetes. 74th Congress American Diabetes Association. San Francisco, California. 2014.
26. De Fronzo RA, Davidson J, Del Prato S. The role of the kidneys in glucose homeostasis: a new path towards normalizing glycaemia. Diabetes Obes Metab. 2012;141(1):5-14.
27. Miracle López S, Barreda Becerril F. Manifestaciones cutáneas de la diabetes mellitus, una manera clínica de identificar la enfermedad. Rev Endocrinol Nutr. 2005;13(2):75-87.

CHAPTER

10

Cutaneous Manifestations due to Vasculopathy, Neuropathy and Diabetic Foot Syndrome

Emilia Noemí Cohen Sabban

INTRODUCTION

Diabetes mellitus (DM), undoubtedly, is one of the most important health problems worldwide. Its complications are responsible for the great morbidity and mortality of the disease, which in turn has a great socioeconomic impact. Alterations related to vasculopathy and diabetic neuropathy appear more frequently in the 2nd decade of life, as they result from chronic hyperglycemia and its metabolic complications.

Although the vascular and neuropathic manifestations of DM have decreased in the last decades, their prevalence follows an epidemic behavior, due to the increase of sedentarism, bad dietary habits, and the parallel increase of the obesity.[1] Unfortunately, major microvascular complications of DM (retinopathy, nephropathy, and peripheral vascular disease) remain the long-term cause of blindness, kidney failure and amputations.[2]

CUTANEOUS MANIFESTATIONS DUE TO DIABETIC VASCULOPATHY (FIGS. 1 TO 19)

Diabetes mellitus is a group of metabolic diseases in which glucose is not used properly, resulting in a chronic hyperglycemia state, which regulates vascular inflammation, alters the expression of cytokines and growth factors, and promotes activation of platelets and macrophages; favoring the development and progression of vascular complications.[3]

Vascular involvement occurs through several pathogenic mechanisms that manifest in the skin, such as activation of protein kinase C, stimulation of the polyol pathway with excess formation of sorbitol, generation of reactive oxygen species by oxidative stress and increased formation of advanced glycation end products (AGEs). When AGEs bind with their cell membrane surface receptor (RAGE), they trigger a cascade through the activation of nuclear factor-kappa B (NF-κB) and nicotinamide adenine dinucleotide phosphate (NADPH) oxidases, which ultimately increase levels of inflammation and oxidative stress. The accumulation of these products is possibly responsible for the structural

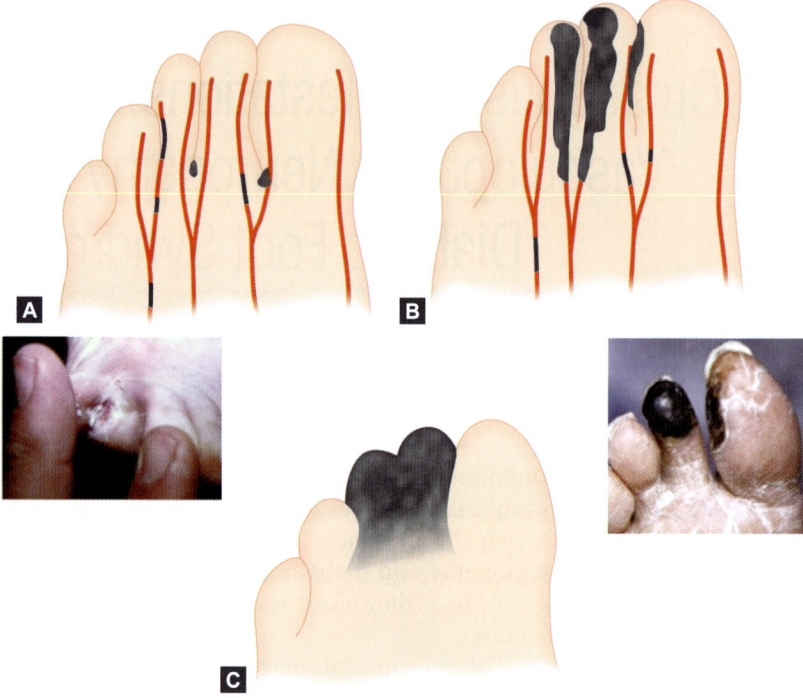

Figs. 1A to C: Outline of the irrigation of the foot. (A) An infection increases the metabolic demand. As in the presence of vasculopathy, the vessel does not dilate because it is more rigid, accelerates the flow to compensate. Small occlusions are generated due to their terminal type behavior, compromise the tissue life; (B) At the beginning, it takes the outer face of one finger (2nd finger) and the inner side of the other finger (3rd finger); and (C) Severe compromise.

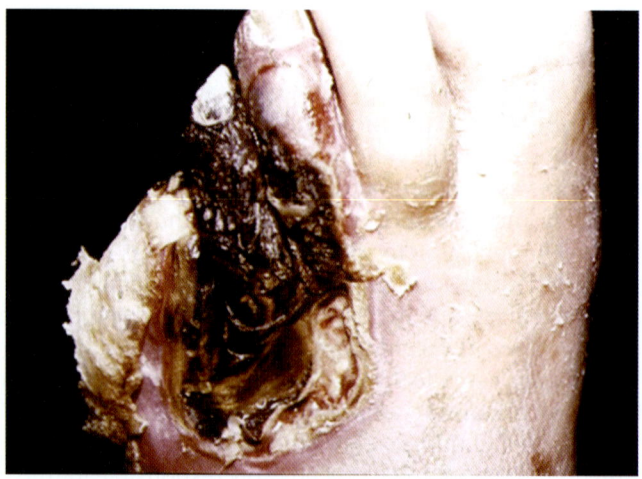

Fig. 2: Tissue necrosis, anterior aspect of the foot.

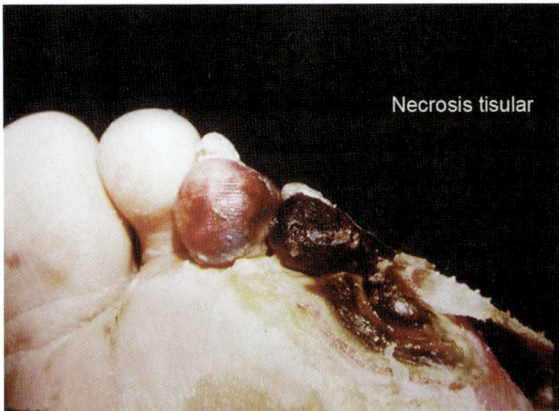

Fig. 3: Tissue necrosis plantar aspect of the foot.

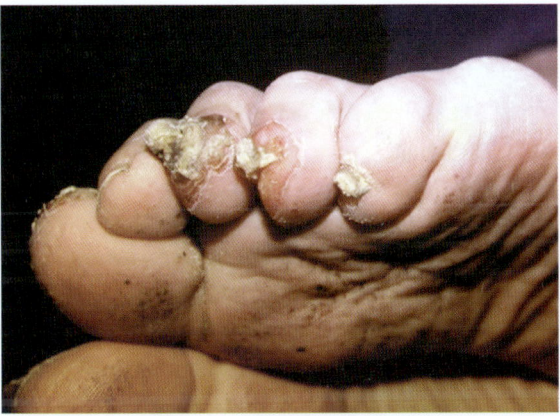

Fig. 4: Ungual dystrophy.

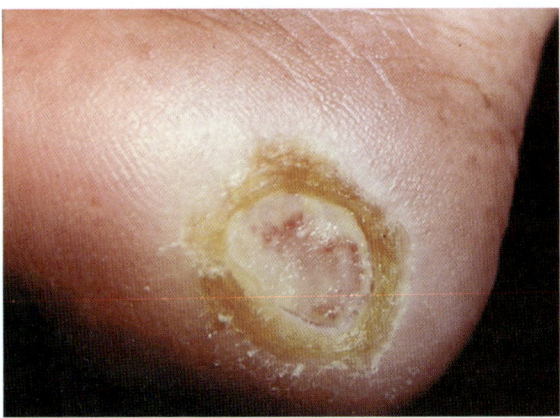

Fig. 5: Mixed, vascular and neuropathic ulcer.

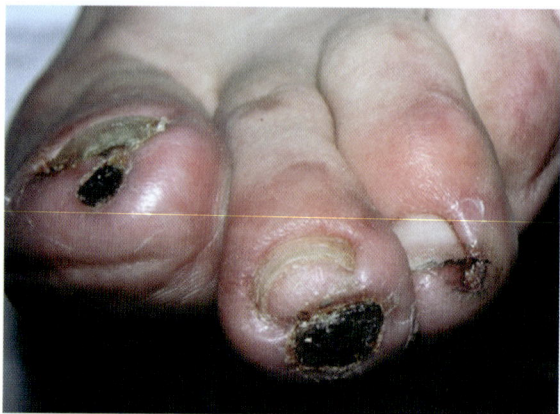

Fig. 6: Areas of cutaneous necrosis, erythema and swelling of the toes.

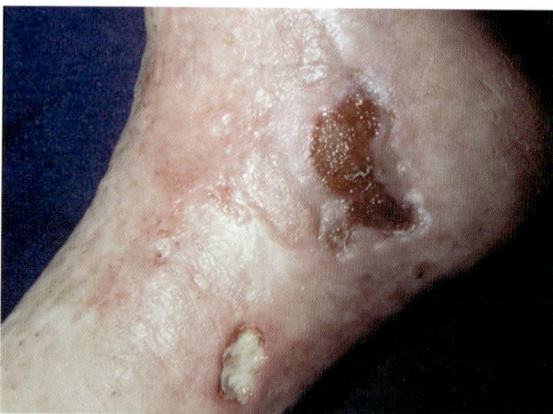

Fig. 7: Vascular ulcers.

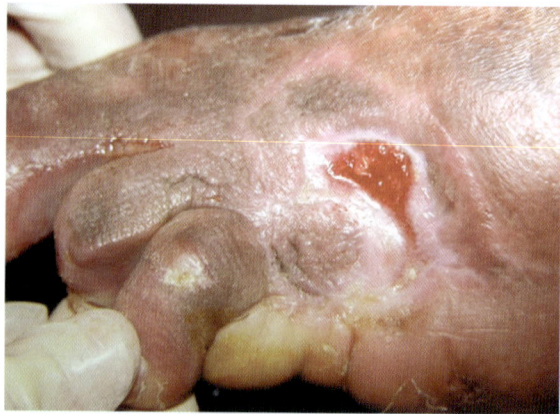

Fig. 8: Vascular foot, arterial ulcer and amputation of the distal phalange of the 2nd toe.

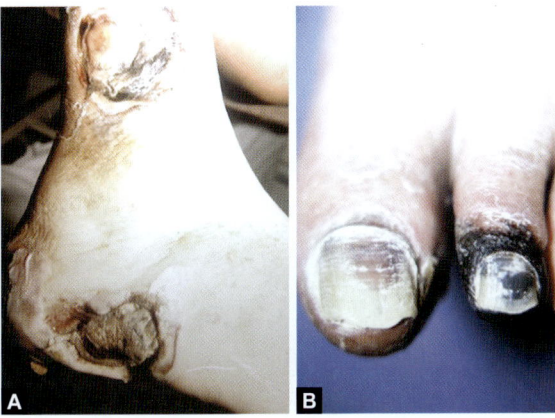

Figs. 9A and B: (A) Vascular ulcers with necrotic tissue; and (B) Necrosis and gangrene of first and second toe.

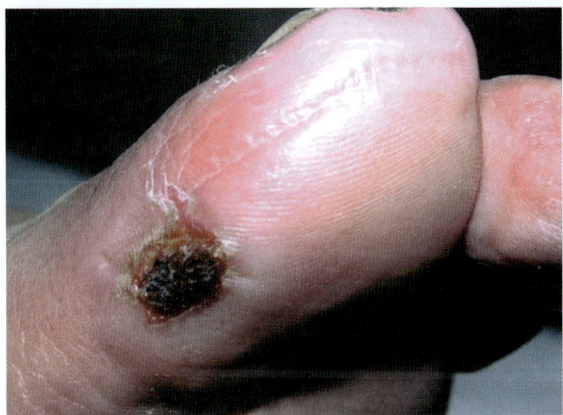

Fig. 10: Ulcer covered with necrotic tissue.

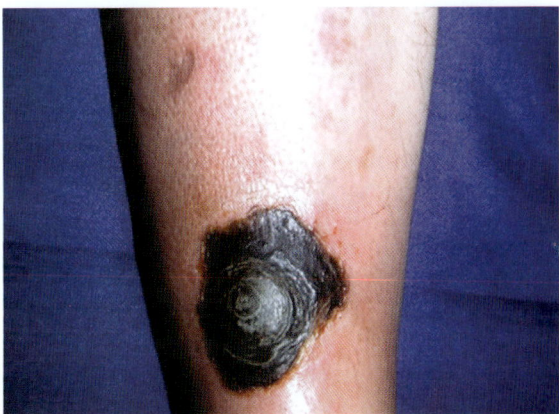

Fig. 11: Anterior leg necrosis, shiny erythematous skin and hair loss.

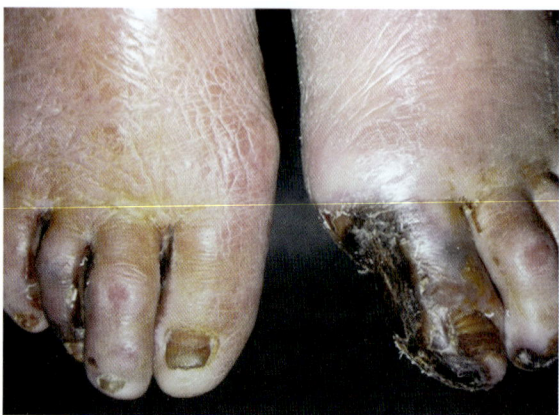

Fig. 12: Gangrene, shiny and atrophic skin, loss of hair and ungual dystrophy.

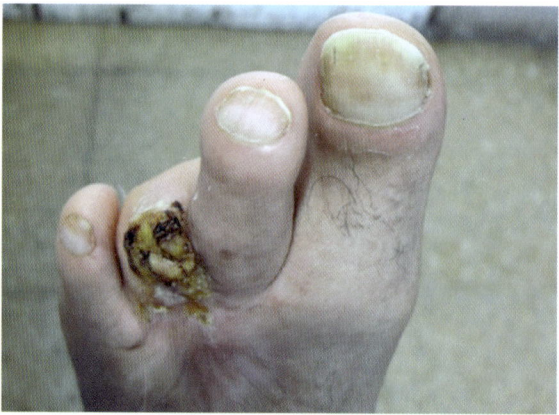

Fig. 13: Osteomyelitis and amputation of 4th toe.

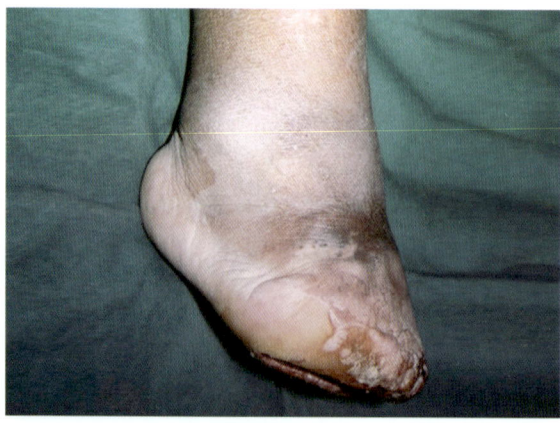

Fig. 14: Amputation.

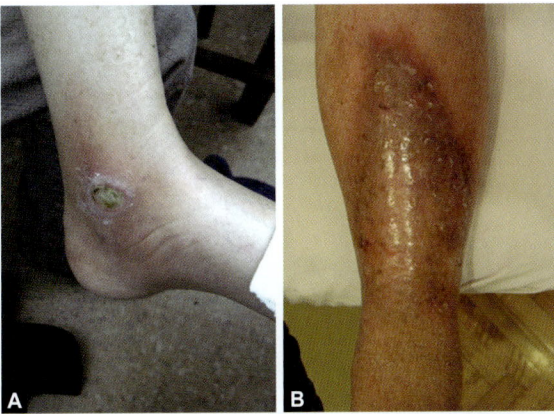

Figs. 15A and B: Vasculopathy. (A) Arterial ulcer in internal malleolus; and (B) Ocre dermatitis, advanced stage of the disease.

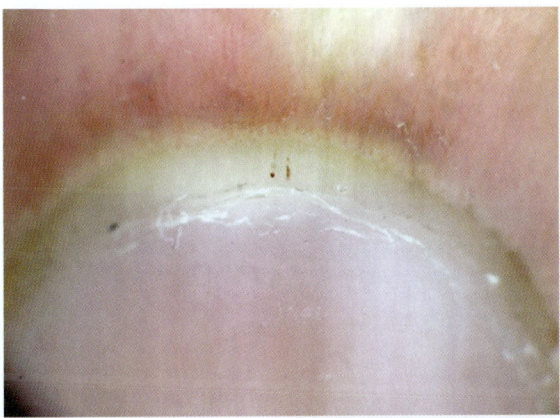

Fig. 16: Capillaroscopy: periungual erythema, tortuous and dilated capillaries and minimal microhemorrhages.

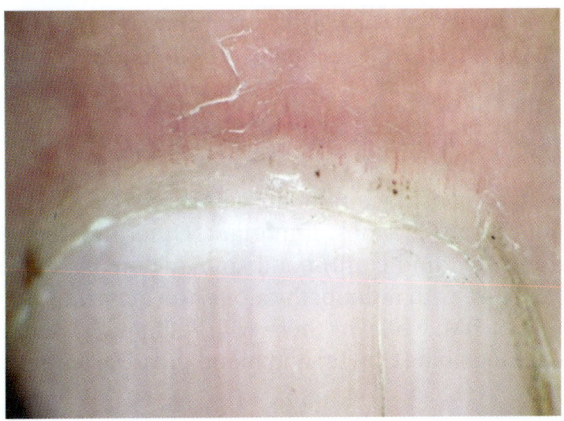

Fig. 17: Capillaroscopy: microhemorrhages, tortuous vessels and periungual erythema.

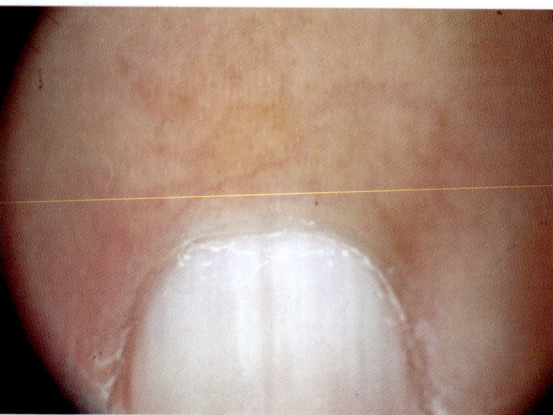

Fig. 18: Capillaroscopy: loss of capillaries (avascular area). Patient with diabetes mellitus type 1 of 50 years of evolution, with retinopathy, neuropathy and nephropathy in chronic renal failure.

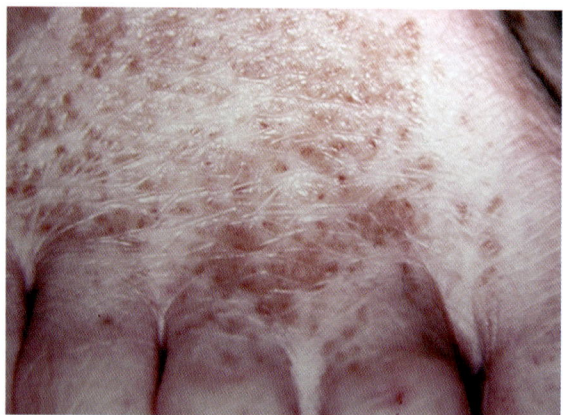

Fig. 19: Pigmentary purpura.

and functional modifications of the macromolecules as well as non-enzymatic glycation (NEG) of collagen in the vascular wall, which gives the vessel greater stiffness.[4,5]

Among the different risk factors for diabetic vasculopathy, glycemic control and duration of DM are the most important. Other modifiable risk factors such as hypertension, lipid control and smoking are also involved. It was observed that in those with retinopathy alone, the most important risk factor was the duration of DM; while for those with retinopathy and nephropathy, both glycated hemoglobin (HbA1c) and blood pressure levels were the most important.[6]

Vasculopathy affects small vessels, medium vessels and large vessels. Diabetic macroangiopathy is similar to atherosclerotic disease, affects medium- and large arterial vessels (cerebral, coronary, and lower limbs) and is seen in patients with long-standing DM. If it compromises the coronary territory, it will lead to the appearance of ischemic heart disease; while strokes are the result of altered cerebral circulation; if it affects the peripheral circulation, especially that of the lower limbs, will manifest as peripheral vascular disease (PVD).[7]

Diabetics have a higher incidence of PVD, especially in young people, and the tibial arteries are the most affected. Vascular compromise results in a decrease in the elasticity and endothelial vasomotor function of the peripheral arteries. This means that, in view of an increase in the metabolic demand generated by minimal infections (intertrigo) or cutaneous microtrauma, in the presence of microangiopathy, the vessels cannot vasodilate to increase blood flow, so they try to compensate, with acceleration. This, in turn, causes the formation of microthrombi which, if they occlude the vascular lumen, would result in ischemia, necrosis, gangrene and finally amputation. It is considered that, in the diabetic population, the presence of PVD is the main risk factor for amputation.[8]

From the clinical point of view, it is manifested by intermittent claudication, cold feet, pain at night and at rest, absence or decrease of pulses, pallor to limb elevation, delayed venous filling, subcutaneous fat atrophy, loss of hair on the feet, nail dystrophy (thickened nails), ulcer, gangrene and amputations.[9]

Diabetic microangiopathy, on the other hand, affects small-caliber vessels and is most frequently observed in insulin-dependent youngsters. Because the skin has a thermoregulatory function, there is usually an excess of capillaries; due to their loss, such as occurs in diabetic patients, a failure in microvascular perfusion is generated. The inadequate perfusion of the small vessels is the most important cause of the inability to heal small wounds that will eventually result in the subsequent formation of ulcers, which is the most relevant clinical manifestation of microangiopathy, forming part of the so-called diabetic foot syndrome.

The easy access to cutaneous capillaries makes capillaroscopy a useful tool to evaluate diabetic microangiopathy. In diabetics, the observation of the proximal periungual fold reveals the presence of periungual erythema and telangiectasia's. With the dermatoscope in early stages and with little metabolic control, the capillaries appear tortuous and dilated homogeneously, in particular the venous or afferent branch. In a patient who has suffered several years of illness and with control, only tortuosity remains, but there are no dilated capillaries. When microangiopathy is already severe, microhemorrhages and areas of the microcirculation can be seen without irrigation.[10] The more microvascular complications, the more avascular areas will be seen in capillaroscopy. We also found correlation between HbA1c levels and the number of microhemorrhages. Avascular areas were significantly more frequent in patients with microvascular complications of type 1 diabetes (retinopathy or microalbuminuria).[11]

Histopathologically, structural changes in the microvasculature include proliferation and hypertrophy of endothelial cells and thickening due to the deposition of a periodic acid-Schiff (PAS) positive material in the basement membrane of the arterioles, capillaries and venules. There may also be obliteration of vascular lumen.[11]

However, since these changes considered diagnostic have not always been demonstrated in the skin of diabetic patients, and they have also been observed in normal skin and in diseases other than DM, the concept of functional microangiopathy is born, which is characterized by two alterations: (1) increased blood viscosity and slow blood flow and (2) capillary hypertension. "Functional microangiopathy" manifests clinically in red-faced or rubeosis faciei, periungual telangiectasia, erysipelas-like erythema and pigmentary purpura, in addition to diabetic dermopathy (see Chapter 4: Cutaneous Markers of Diabetes Mellitus).

Rubeosis is a frequent finding of DM and is the prototype of functional microangiopathy. It is directly related to the degree of engorgement and, therefore, dilation of the superficial venous plexus of the dermis. Another possible mechanism could be the increased affinity of oxygen-glycosylated hemoglobin. Clinically, there is a reddish coloration on the face and neck, with no increase in temperature.[12] Decompensated young women are the most affected. In a study of diabetic patients, it was found that the prevalence of this manifestation reached 7% of insulin-dependent patients.[13]

Erysipelas-like erythema is characterized by a well-defined redness of the skin of the lower limbs or the dorsum of the feet, without clinical or laboratory signs of infection (fever, erythrocyte sedimentation or leukocytosis), which occurs in elderly diabetic patients. It correlates with an underlying bone alteration in the radiological study (bone destruction) and predicts incipient gangrene.

Pigmentary purpura results from extravasation of red blood cells from the superficial venous plexus by abnormal capillary permeability. The skin acquires a patchy ocher color (salt and pepper type), which is seen in the lower limbs and the dorsum of the feet of elderly patients with edema due to cardiac decompensation. This finding usually manifests in conjunction with diabetic dermopathy, in which some lesions are usually seen to evolve into atrophy.[14]

CUTANEOUS MANIFESTATIONS DUE TO DIABETIC NEUROPATHY (FIGS. 20 TO 29)

Up to 50% of patients with DM present some variant of neuropathy. The most common form is mixed distal motor/sensory polyneuropathy (DPN), which has been defined under international consensus as "the presence of signs and/or symptoms of peripheral nerve dysfunction in people with DM after excluding other causes".[15] Apparently, it is the sustained hyperglycemia and the metabolic disorders that it causes, such as the accumulation of AGEs and their binding to RAGE, which would determine the damage of the peripheral nerves. Increased levels of RAGE expression in diabetic neuropathy were also

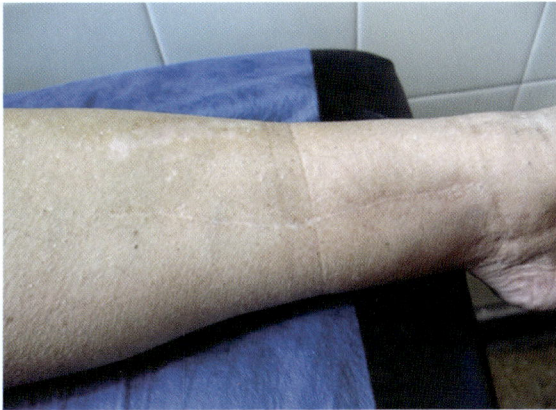

Fig. 20: Xerosis.

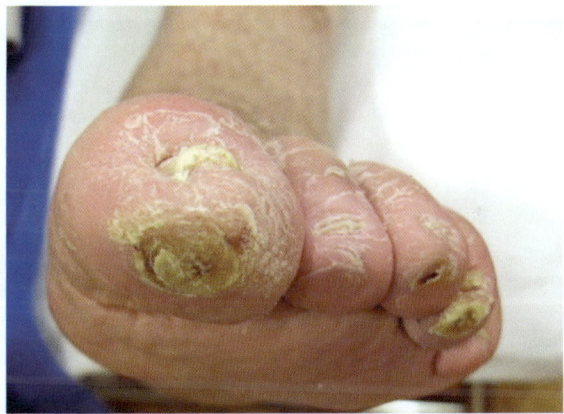

Fig. 21: Neuropathic foot, extreme dryness of the skin and neuropathic ulceration on the hallux and 4th toe.

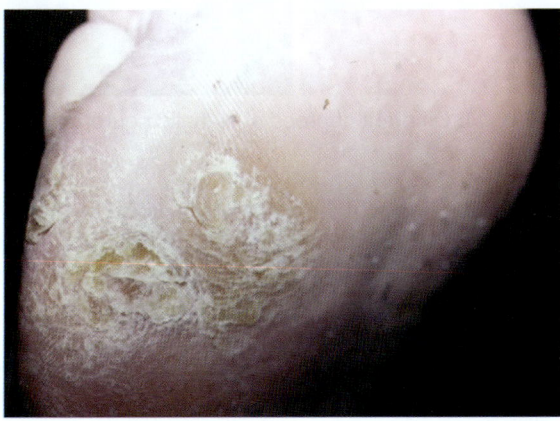

Fig. 22: Callus formation in new weight bearing points under continuous pressure.

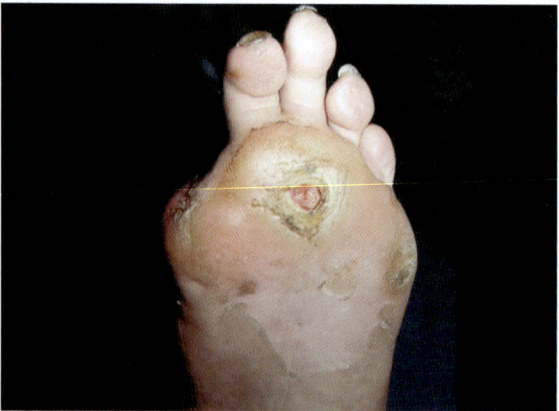

Fig. 23: Mal perforans.

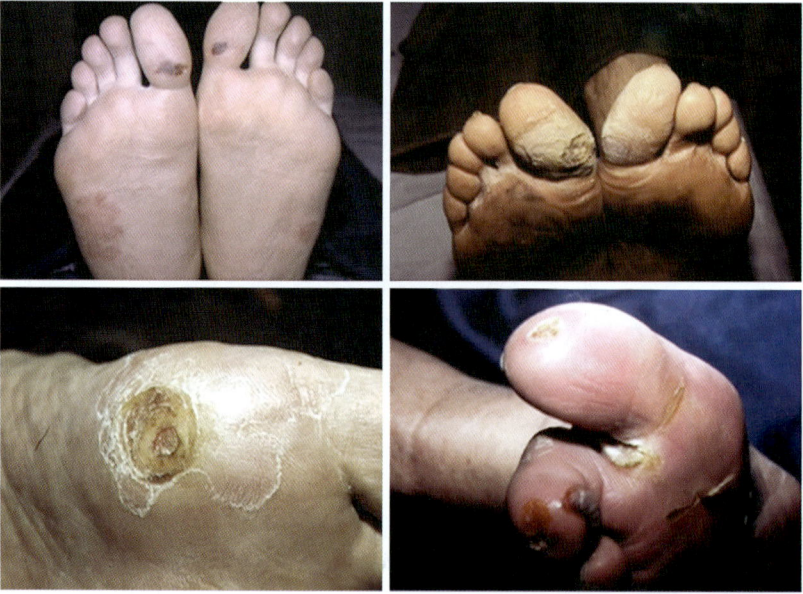

Fig. 24: Different degrees of diabetic neuropathy.

correlated with dyslipidemia, which is currently believed, which would have an implication in the progression of diabetic neuropathy. The situation would be further complicated by the ischemia of the vasa nervorum. The quantification of intraepidermal nerve fiber density (IENFD) by performing skin biopsies in diabetic patients showed that it is very reduced since early stages even when nerve conduction is still normal. The longer the duration of DM and the greater neuropathic deficits, the lower the density of the nerve fibers.[4] As in the optical microscopy of the vessels, there is a thickening of the basement membrane of

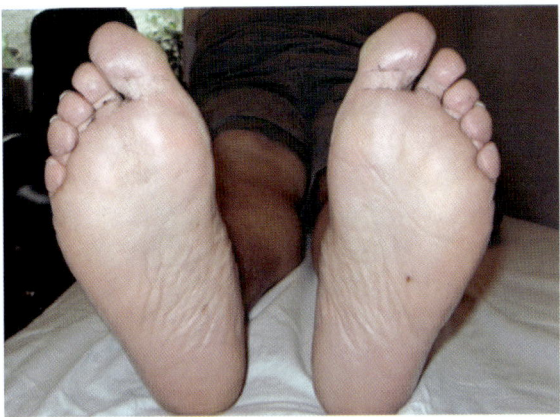

Fig. 25: Widening and loss of normal foot architecture.

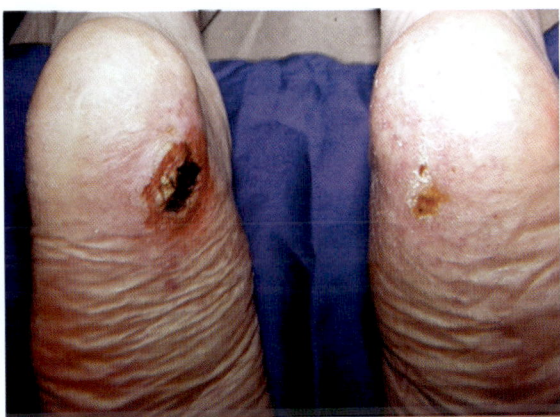

Fig. 26: Neuropathic foot, plantar erythema, mal perforans and dry skin.

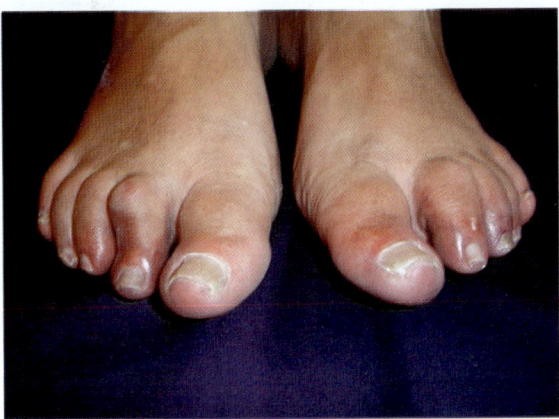

Fig. 27: Widening of the feet and claw toes.

Cutaneous Manifestations of Diabetes

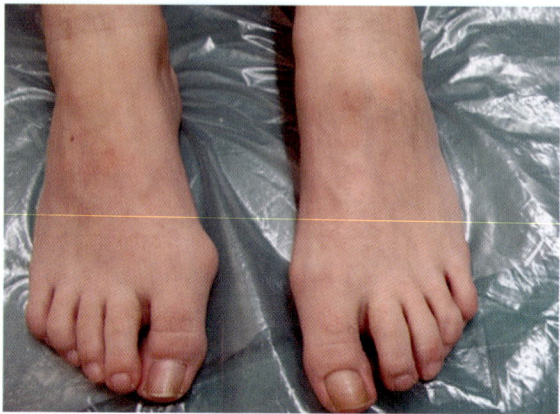

Fig. 28: Diabetic foot.

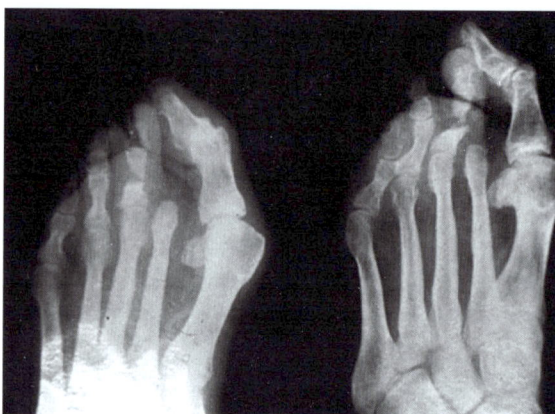

Fig. 29: Radiological signs of diabetic foot. Charcot neuroarthropathy is a complication of diabetic neuropathy, with fragmentation or destruction of the joints and bones.

the vascular wall, which has been demonstrated by electron microscopy. There is a thickening of the basal membrane of the vasa nervorum.

Diabetic neuropathy affects the autonomic sphere as well as the motor and sensory.

Autonomic Neuropathy

It is a very common and problematic complication of DM, which can affect various organs and systems throughout the body. Generally, it coexists with other types of neuropathy and with other complications of DM, although it may appear in isolation. In early stages, it is asymptomatic or manifests with less specific symptoms.[16] It consists of the peripheral and non-central lesion of the sympathetic nerves. Autonomic neuropathy manifests clinically with

erectile dysfunction, altered esophageal motility, loss of skin integrity and abnormal vascular reflexes. Within the early manifestations there are two that are very important:
1. *Alterations in the microcirculation especially of the foot:* The disruption of the cutaneous capillary blood flow and the regulation of the arteriovenous shunts depends on the sympathetic innervation. Neuropathy conditions a permanent opening of the arteriovenous shunts, thus, a system of regulation of blood flow is lost.[17]
2. The innervation of the sweat glands with alteration of the sudomotor function.

The resulting neurovascular dysfunction coupled with impaired sweating are responsible for heat intolerance, heat sensation, burning or pruritus, along with hyperhidrosis of the upper half of the body and anhidrosis in lower limbs. The loss of sweating leads to extreme xerosis (dryness) of the skin due to lack of hydration of the horny layer, with the consequent appearance of cracks that constitute an important portal of entry for different microorganisms. These changes, finally, favor the development of ulcers, gangrene and amputation.[18]

Motor Neuropathy

It is associated with hypotrophy or atrophy and weakness of the interosseous muscles that determine the loss of the normal architecture and functionality of the foot. The bone changes determine the impairment of the stabilizing function of the interphalangeal and metatarsophalangeal joints; widening of the foot and appearance of new points under pressure, especially at the level of the first and fifth metatarsal heads accompanied by the dynamic contracture of the extensors and long flexors, leading to an alteration of the phalanges resulting in the so-called "claw toes or hammer toes". There is a displacement of the plantar pads and the protrusion of the metatrsal heads occurs that are directly supported on the skin, accompanied by radiological signs of osteolysis. All these changes, added to the friction exerted by inadequate footwear, either because it is too tight or because it leaves part of the exposed foot (toes, heels), explains the appearance of skin fissures, neuropathic ulcer and subsequent infections.[19]

Sensory Neuropathy

It is characterized by degeneration and progressive loss of peripheral nerve fibers. Examination of the lower limbs may result in loss of sensation to pain, pressure, thermal and vibration as the fibers of small and large size are affected, and absence of reflexes. Clinical features are paresthesias, hyperesthesia, hypoesthesia, radicular pain, loss of deep tendon reflexes, tingling, numbness, etc. As a consequence of these alterations, diabetic patients do not perceive microtrauma, the presence of a foreign body in the footwear or major insults in their feet, with the consequent formation of blisters, calluses, callosities on pressure points and ulcers such as mal perforans.

Mal perforans is a round shaped ulcer, that begins with a thickening in weight bearing points, and then evolving to a painless ulcer surrounded by hyperkeratosis, associated with loss of pain and thermal sensation and absence of Achilles reflexes, which can become infected and form deep abscesses or osteomyelitis.

Semmes-Weinstein Monofilaments

One of the most widely used methods for measuring diabetic neuropathy is Semmes-Weinstein monofilaments, which measure pressure and touch sensation. It is a nylon filament attached to a handle that, when folded, applies a pressure of 10 g, regardless of the force with which it is applied on the skin of the patient. It is done twice, in three plantar points: hallux finger and heads of the first and fifth metatarsals, perpendicular to the skin and with uniform movements, exerting the sufficient force to bend the monofilament, during a time no longer of 1-2 seconds. The patient should answer affirmatively, if he perceives the pressure and to determine where he feels it; alternating with applications in which the patient will be questioned, but without pressure. If he does not respond to the contact in a particular area of the foot, the physician will continue with the sequence elsewhere on the foot. The patient is considered to be at risk of ulceration, if two out of three responses are incorrect.[20]

DIABETIC FOOT SYNDROME

It includes all those cutaneous manifestations that appear in the feet of diabetic patients such as dry skin, calluses, fissures and cracks, erosions and blisters, trophic ulcer, gangrene of the foot, by different mechanisms.

Many factors contribute to the development of diabetic foot, among which we can mention:
- Atherosclerotic ischemic occlusive vasculopathy of the arteries below the knee due to decreased perfusion of large vessels; as well as to microangiopathy with dysfunction of the small vessels.[21]
- *Skin and soft tissue:* The presence of intertrigo or onychomycosis, are considered risk factors for the development of foot ulcers.
- Progressive peripheral polyneuropathy with loss of protective sensation.
- Biomechanical alterations of the foot with increased pressure at the plantar level and longer duration of contact of the feet with the floor.[22]

In the early stages the foot is warm and well irrigated. Prior to loss of sensation, there may be numbness and pain with distribution in glove and sock. As the loss of sensation increases, a trauma that went unnoticed can cause blisters and ulcers in weight bearing points. An ulcer, however small, can cause considerable destruction of deep tissue and complicate with osteomyelitis.

The presence of DPN confers a high risk, since more than 50% are asymptomatic. More than 80% of the amputations recognize a previous injury or ulceration, generally not perceived by the patients, hence their early recognition is of paramount importance.[15]

From the dermatological point of view, we must examine the feet in search of the mentioned alterations: calluses, ulcers, deformities, etc.; inspect the shoes, recommend a visit to the podiatrist. At the same time, we should assess the presence of sensory neuropathy on the feet, reflexes, etc. which according to current recommendations, is suggested at the time of diagnosis of DM 2 and 5 years after the diagnosis of DM 1 and at least once a year.[15]

Among the preventive measures for the progression and consequent formation of the neuropathic ulcer, is the use of soft keratolytics to remove the calluses and to avoid the increase of pressure that they exert on the foot. The daily application of an emollient, to counteract the dryness of the skin, fissures and cracks, taking into account the cutaneous barrier dysfunction in diabetics, is another measure to be taken in mind.[23]

Also, the indication of an appropriate offloading and suitable footwear would be very opportune in this instance. In addition, educating the patient and getting him to perform a daily review of the foot and his footwear, are part of the therapeutic approach to diabetic foot syndrome. This could not be complete without emphasizing strict DM control.

Once the ulcer is formed, its debridement, offload the ulcerated area, application of local or systemic antibiotics if necessary, the use of stimulating factors for healing as various membranes and dressings, would be indicated.

When the alteration is so severe and compromises tissue viability, amputation may be an option, if it is not possible to restore blood flow through surgical procedures.[12]

REFERENCES

1. Gregg EW, Li Y, Wang J, et al. Changes in diabetes-related complications in the United States, 1990-2010. N Engl J Med. 2014;370(16):1514-23.
2. Singh VP, Bali A, Singh S, et al. Advanced Glycation End Products and Diabetic Complications. Korean J Physiol Pharmacol. 2014;18(1):1-14.
3. Crawford CL, Hardwicke P. Animal models of human diabetic polyneuropathy. JAMA. 2003;289(14):1779-80.
4. Park SY, Kim YA, Hong YH, et al. Up-regulation of the receptor for advanced glycation end products in the skin biopsy specimens of patients with severe diabetic neuropathy. J Clin Neurol. 2014;10(4):334-41.
5. Cohen MP, Ziyadeh FN, Chen S. Amadori-modified glycated serum proteins and accelerated atherosclerosis in diabetes: pathogenic and therapeutic implications. J Lab Clin Med. 2006;147(5):211-9.
6. Romero-Aroca P, Mendez-Marin I, Baget-Bernaldiz M, et al. Review of the relationship between renal and retinal microangiopathy in diabetes mellitus patients. Curr Diabetes Rev. 2010;6(2):88-101.
7. Conway BN, Aroda VR, Maynard JD, et al. Skin intrinsic fluorescence is associated with coronary artery disease in individuals with long duration of type 1 diabetes. Diabetes Care. 2012;35(11):2331-6.
8. Dalla Paola L, Faglia E. Treatment of diabetic foot ulcer: an overview strategies for clinical approach. Curr Diabetes Rev. 2006;2(4):431-47.

9. Donaghue KC, Chiarelli F, Trotta D, et al. Microvascular and macrovascular complications associated with diabetes in children and adolescents. Pediatr Diabetes. 2009;10 (Suppl 12):195-203.
10. Grassi W, Del Medico P. Diabetes mellitus. In: Grassi W, Del Medico P (Eds). Atlas of Capillaroscopy. Milan: EDRA-Medical Publishing & New Media; 2004. pp. 293-4.
11. Hosking SP, Bhatia R, Crock PA, et al. Non-invasive detection of microvascular changes in a paediatric and adolescent population with type 1 diabetes: a pilot cross-sectional study. BMC Endocr Disord. 2013;13:41.
12. Sehgal VN, Bhattacharya SN, Verma P. Juvenile, insulin-dependent diabetes mellitus, type 1-related dermatoses. J Eur Acad Dermatol Venereol. 2011;25(6): 625-36.
13. Pavlović MD, Milenković T, Dinić M, et al. The prevalence of cutaneous manifestations in young patients with type 1 diabetes. Diabetes Care. 2007;30(8):1964-7.
14. Ngo BT, Hayes KD, DiMiao DJ, et al. Manifestations of cutaneous diabetic microangiopathy. Am J Clin Dermatol. 2005;6(4):225-37.
15. Boulton AJ, Vinik AI, Arezzo JC, et al. Diabetic neuropathies: a statement by the American Diabetes Association. Diabetes Care. 2005;28(4):956-62.
16. Jin HY, Baek HS, Park TS. Morphologic Changes in Autonomic Nerves in Diabetic Autonomic Neuropathy. Diabetes Metab J. 2015;39(6):461-7.
17. Boada A. Skin lesions in the diabetic foot. Actas Dermosifiliogr. 2012;103(5):348-56.
18. Baselga Torres E, Torres-Padilla M. Manifestaciones cutáneas en niños con diabetes mellitus y obesidad. Actas Dermosifiliogr. 2014;105:546-57.
19. Vinik AI, Strotmeyer ES, Nakave AA, et al. Diabetic neuropathy in older adults. Clin Geriatr Med. 2008;24(3):407-35.
20. Feng Y, Schlösser FJ, Sumpio BE. The Semmes Weinstein monofilament examination is a significant predictor of the risk of foot ulceration and amputation in patients with diabetes mellitus. J Vasc Surg. 2011;53(1):220-6.
21. Chao CY, Cheing GL. Microvascular dysfunction in diabetic foot disease and ulceration. Diabetes Metab Res Rev. 2009;25(7):604-14.
22. Uçkay I, Gariani K, Pataky Z, et al. Diabetic foot infections: state-of-the-art. Diabetes Obes Metab. 2014;16(4):305-16.
23. Bristow I. Non-ulcerative skin pathologies of the diabetic foot. Diabetes Metab Res Rev. 2008;24 (Suppl 1):S84-9.

CHAPTER

11

Diabetes, Non-Enzymatic Glycation and Aging

Emilia Noemí Cohen Sabban, Denise Steiner

INTRODUCTION

Diabetes mellitus (DM) is a syndrome characterized by a chronic hyperglycemia state, which is responsible, among other manifestations, for premature and accelerated aging of both skin and internal organs. Non-enzymatic glycosylation (NEG), or glycation as it is now called, is a reaction that normally occurs during aging but accelerates in diabetes. In this chapter, we develop the NEG and its interrelationship, as a common pathogenic pathway, with diabetes and skin aging.

AGING

True or intrinsic aging is a status consisting of the accumulation of a series of defects in the metabolic pathways, which lead to a decrease in mitochondrial energy production. It is a multifactorial process, in which different mechanisms are involved simultaneously. Among others, genetics and the environment are part in progressive accumulation of damage at the cellular, tissue and organ levels, overtime, to disease and death.[1]

There are many theories about aging and the components that favor it with those that are generated as a result of normal metabolism, such as reactive oxygen species (ROS) or free radicals (FR), reducing sugars and NEG and its early and late products. In the last decades, much attention has been paid to the NEG as during the physiological aging, the advanced glycation end products (AGEs), progressively increases and accumulate in cartilage, collagen, pericardial fluid, skin, etc.[2]

Alterations are described in all three layers of skin, but during aging, changes in the collagen and elastin fibers, and the extracellular matrix (ECM) of the dermis in which they are embedded, are of particular importance. The ECM with age, undergoes modifications of the dry content and in particular of hyaluronic acid (HA). The amount of collagen per unit area of skin surface decreases approximately 1% per year throughout adult life and the remaining fibers are more disorganized and compact as well as more cross-linked. In addition, the concentrations of procollagen type I and III decrease, which is a proportional measure of collagen synthesis. All this is accompanied by an increase in the activity of collagenase, thus, over the years, the balance is clearly negative, less synthesis with more degradation of collagen. In females, the years immediately after menopause, correlate with a rapid deterioration of collagen levels, which sustains an estrogenic hormonal influence both in its synthesis and in its degradation.

Elastin fibers decrease in number and diameter, are fragmented by elastase activity and progressively increase both cross-linking and calcification. This leads to the loss of dermal elastic mesh which confers, among other things, mechanical protection.[3]

Skin functioning declines with age and processes that are decreased include cell turnover, barrier function, mechanical protection, wound repair, immune response, thermoregulation, sweat production, sebum and vitamin D and deoxyribonucleic acid (DNA) repair. Therefore, clinically aged skin has increased dryness and desquamation, increased laxity and wrinkles, thinning or atrophy, loss of brightness and a variety of benign tumors such as acrochordons, angiomas, seborrheic keratoses, etc.[4]

NON-ENZYMATIC GLYCATION

Maillard Reaction

Non-enzymatic glycation is a sugar reduction reaction that has been systematically studied since the beginning of the century (Maillard, 1912) from its application in the food industry to improve the appearance and taste of food. This chemical reaction is normally started in our body and increases progressively with aging and with processes related to glucose concentrations and oxidative stress. When there is a persistent excess of sugar, it binds to proteins, lipids and nucleic acids, forming a large number of early glycation products (Amadori) and advanced glycation end-products (AGEs), modifying the structure and function of biomolecules.[5,6]

From the chemical point of view, binding occurs between the primary amino groups of free amino acids, peptides, proteins, lipids and nucleic acids (mainly lysine and arginine), with the carbonyl group of reducing sugars, of which glucose is the most abundant in the body among others such as fructose, pentose, galactose, mannose and xylose. This reaction consists of three stages, (1) early, (2) intermediate and (3) late:
1. In the first step, unstable products, the Schiff bases, are formed by contact of reducing sugar with protein, lipids or nucleic acids, in a short time of hours.
2. In the intermediate step, in a period of days, by chemical rearrangement of the Schiff bases, more stable compounds, called Amadori products or early NEG products, are formed within which the glycosylated hemoglobin or hemoglobin A1c (HbA1c) is the best known. HbA1c is an early glycation product whose blood levels correlate with excess sugars, making it a standard parameter for the diagnosis and monitoring of DM. If there is a decrease in sugar concentrations in any of these two stages, the reactions are reversible.[7]

3. Finally, if Amadori products are accumulated, late Maillard's reaction, irreversible and slower, occurs over weeks, months, or years, in which by complex chemical rearrangements (reduction, condensation, oxidation and dehydration) and cross-linking, the advanced glycation end-products or AGEs are formed.[8] These compounds are insoluble, yellowish or brownish, some fluorescent, with different chemical structures: imidazole, pyrrole and others (imines, furans, pyridines, etc.).

Modified Amadori proteins and AGEs are structurally different; in addition, while AGEs exert their biological effects by binding to their specific receptor for AGE (RAGE), the modified Amadori proteins use other receptors.

The NEG triggers a cascade of inflammatory events, which alter cellular function. This is because the affected proteins do not reach their normal molecular conformation, modify their enzymatic activity, decrease its degradation and interfere with receptor recognition.[9]

Glycation of Collagen

A clear example of the modifications that NEG may produce in a protein, is the non-enzymatic glycation of collagen or collagen AGE.

Collagen (from the Greek *kolla*, glue and *geno*, produce) a central component of the connective tissue of almost all organs, is the adhesive of our body, holding it together and giving it elasticity and resistance to most tissues in which the mechanical function is essential, such as skin, cartilage, tendons and bones. Although it is a long-lived protein, not all body collagen is the same and its half-life varies according to its location, being 1–2 years in the bone, to about 10 years for the type I collagen in the skin.

It is the main supporting protein of the ECM, contains abundant residues of lysine, hydroxylysine and arginine that added to its slow turnover, make it an ideal target to accumulate sugars and to be more damaged by glycation. Collagen can thus interact with a large number of metabolites, particularly with glucose, to which is exposed in both, the vascular and extravascular spaces, and the glycation ends up damaging it throughout the body.[10]

Normal collagen has biological and biomechanical functions that are affected by glycation. The former is primarily related to the collagen-protein interaction and collagen-matrix cells. AGE-modified collagen at the level of specific amino acid groups could result in a dramatic change in intermolecular recognition, with proteoglycans, enzymes such as collagenase, and integrin. In turn, AGE-collagen undergoes alterations at its surface, that interfere with good cell-matrix interaction, which inhibits wound repair and exacerbates inflammation.[11]

On the other hand, the binding of glucose to the side chains of amino acids and subsequent reaction to form non-enzymatic intermolecular crosslinks, alter the biomechanical properties by physicochemical changes of the collagen molecule. Thus, by becoming a more rigid and less soluble molecule, the tissue is mechanically more fragile and less flexible. It also becomes more resistant to its degradation.[12] The alteration at the level of the physicochemical properties, in addition, is responsible for the yellowish color of the skin and the nails.

ADVANCED GLYCATION END-PRODUCTS AND THEIR RECEPTOR

Advanced Glycation End-Products (AGEs)

The AGEs form a heterogeneous group of compounds, whose sources may originate from an exogenous pathway or by endogenous formation.
- Via exogenous, through cigarette or meals. The heating of some foods promotes Maillard's reaction giving it the desired flavor, aroma and color. The more heat and the time of exposure to heat, the more quickly the reaction will occur. The Western diet is a huge source of AGEs, of which, 10% of what is ingested, goes into circulation and of these, 6.66% (2/3) is incorporated into tissues and 3.33% (1/3) is excreted in the urine. There is correlation between dietary AGEs and increased circulating endogenous levels of AGEs, regardless of the presence of DM or concomitant renal disease. AGEs from the exogenous pathway, like those from the endogenous pathway, act through the same receptor, RAGE.[12]
- Formation in vivo, there are three ways:
  1. The Maillard reaction or NEG that we already described.
  2. Glucose autoxidation and lipid peroxidation. It occurs with increasing oxidative stress, and α-dicarbonyl or oxoaldehyde derivatives such as glyoxaline, methylglyoxal (MGO) and 3-deoxyglucosones (3-DG) are formed, which can bind to extracellular proteins forming AGEs.
  3. The third is the path of polyols. In this, glucose is converted into sorbitol by the enzyme aldose reductase and then to fructose by sorbitol dehydrogenase, whose metabolites (fructose-3-phosphate) are converted to oxoaldehydes, which finally interact with amino acids forming AGEs.

Advanced glycation end products accumulate in and out of cells, in basement membrane proteins, in circulating proteins, and in structural proteins, particularly long-lived proteins such as collagen.[13] AGE-modified proteins can be rapidly degraded to free AGEs [imidazolone, N-ε-carboxymethyl-lysine (CML), etc.]. Some AGEs, on the other hand, can bridge free amino groups between neighboring proteins, forming intermolecular cross-links, making them more resistant to degradation by proteinases (e.g. collagen AGE and collagenase). As time goes by, the accumulation of AGEs at the tissue level increases, contributing to the senescence of many bodily organs including the skin. Among the most studied AGEs that are abundant in connective tissue is glucosepane, a lysine-arginine cross-linking,[14] which together with CML, pentosidine and pyrraline, and MGO, an α-oxoaldehyde, are used as biomarkers to detect in vivo formation of AGEs.[15]

The biological actions of AGEs are exerted by two mechanisms:
1. One independent of the recipient (damage to the protein structure and metabolism of the ECM).[16]
2. Another involving the specific receptor of AGEs, RAGE, whose binding activates the transduction pathways and promotes oxidative stress, the loading of glycol-oxidized products and the activation of cell lines, which will determine a greater tissue injury.[12]

Receptor of Advanced Glycation End-Products (RAGE)

The receptor of advanced glycation end-product (RAGE) is a transmembrane protein composed of three extracellular domains, the V-type and two C-type immunoglobulin domains, C1 and C2; a fourth transmembrane domain with anchor function and which in turn is connected to a fifth highly charged domain, which is a short cytosolic tail that mediates the interaction with molecules of the cytosol, acting as a signal of transduction. The binding of AGEs to RAGE occurs only with the V-type domain of the receptor, which is the one that has the properties to bind to the ligand.

Receptor for advanced glycation end product is expressed on the surface of epithelial cells, endothelial, immune system and central nervous system. In the skin, AGEs bind preferentially with elastin and collagen and interact with RAGE, which is expressed primarily in fibroblasts, dermal dendrocytes and keratinocytes, and to a lesser extent in endothelial and mononuclear cells.[17,6]

AGEs-RAGE Interaction, Inflammation and Oxidative Stress

The AGEs-RAGE interaction triggers different cascades of intracellular signaling that result in inflammation and oxidative stress, by activation of the protein kinase pathway on the one hand, and by NAD(P)H oxidase on the other.

Activation of protein kinase pathways [mitogen-activated protein kinases (MAPKs)] and that of phosphatidylinositol 3-kinase (PI3-K) in turn activates transcription factor NF-kappa B (NF-κB), which translocate to the nucleus to ultimately increase the expression of transcription genes for cytokines and proinflammatory factors such as interleukin-6 (IL-6) and tumor necrosis factor-α (TNF-α), and adhesion molecules as vascular cell adhesion molecule-1 (VCAM-1). Activation of NF-κB increases RAGE expression, generating a vicious circle by positive feedback, increasing the production of inflammation promoters.[18]

Increased expression and activation of NAD(P)H oxidase (a superoxide producing enzyme complex) due to the AGEs-RAGE interaction results in increased oxidative stress and ROS generation. ROS are highly reactive unstable molecules with an odd number of electrons, which enables them to interact with other molecules and thus form more free radicals (FR). At the same time, there are mechanisms of protection against ROS, which are enzymatic antioxidants [superoxide dismutase (SOD)] and non-enzymatic. It is said that there is oxidative stress, when the production of FR exceeds the antioxidant capacity of the organism. FR can be formed endogenously, through normal mitochondrial metabolism or exogenous influence, whose source comes from the environment (diet and drugs). Unfortunately, increased oxidative stress produced by NAD(P)H oxidase in response to the AGEs-RAGE interaction will activate the NF-κB, and so on. In conclusion, protein glycation then activates an inflammatory signaling cascade via AGEs-RAGE and stimulates the production of ROS.[19,12]

AGEs AND AGING

Serum levels of AGEs undergo transient increases and decreases that depend on both endogenous production and exogenous intake and their removal from the body. The latter, in turn, occurs in two ways: one is renal excretion, which under physiological conditions, eliminates the excess of AGEs; and the second is the enzymatic pathway (glyoxalase I and II, carbonyl reductase) responsible for detoxification and the system of counter regulation of the prooxidant effects of glycation.

Some authors have proposed that with age, as well as in certain pathological states, such as DM, there is an imbalance between synthesis and degradation, accumulating AGEs that impair the vascular endothelium, eyes, nervous system and other vital organs, as well as favor the development of chronic degenerative diseases, all proper to aging itself. Misbalance can be caused by an increase in endogenous production such as exogenous intake, and/or by decreased renal clearance.[20]

The increase in the serum concentration of AGEs, will impact at the tissue level due to its prooxidant and inflammatory effects. The greater the accumulation, the greater the functional deterioration of the different organs. For example, the loss of homeostasis at the connective tissue level of ECM reduces its ability to repair cellular damage and its ability to cope with repeated microinjuries from day to day, inherent in the passage of time.[21] In relation to its prooxidants effects, increasing FR also favors aging. If we add an exogenous source of FR as a diet rich in calories, FR and therefore aging increase. Physical exercise and restriction of ingestion can improve this impact, with the consequent reduction of oxidative stress and inflammatory markers.[22]

DIABETES MELLITUS

Diabetes Mellitus and Non-enzymatic Glycation

Persistently elevated glucose levels, for example in DM, produce structural and functional changes in plasma and tissue proteins (albumin, globulins, and fibrinogen) resulting in:
- Activation of platelets.
- Generation of oxygen free radicals (ROS).
- Deterioration of fibrinolysis.
- Deficiency in the regulation of the immune system.[23]

But these events, in turn, depend on the cellular type; those cells with greater expression of glucose transporter-1 (GLUT-1), will be exposed to higher concentrations of intracellular sugar and therefore to greater damage. As the higher glycemia, the greater the reaction, in DM there is more accumulation of these modified proteins, with an increase of Amadori products 1.5–3 times more than that found in nondiabetics.

Both modified Amadori proteins and AGEs resulting from NEG, one of the major pathways in the pathogenesis of the manifestations of DM, are linked to the development and progression of long-term complications of the disease. In skin biopsies of diabetic patients, a large number of AGEs were found, whose levels correlated directly with microangiopathy (retinopathy, nephropathy, and neuropathy). There are also studies that demonstrate their participation in the development of fibrosis or cutaneous thickening syndrome in DM, as well as skin aging. The limited joint mobility, which is one of the components of cutaneous thickening syndrome, is observed in both elderly and diabetic patients and is due to the accumulation of AGEs in the ECM collagen of the joint capsule, ligaments and a muscle tendon unit causing in collagen, the aforementioned changes.[20,9]

The NEG of structural and regulatory proteins induced by hyperglycemia, led to the description of DM as a disease characterized by accelerated chemical aging of long-lived tissue proteins leading to the formation of cataracts, atherosclerosis, etc.[24]

This has therapeutic implications because if we prevent the formation of Amadori-modified serum proteins or block their biological effects, we can reverse many of the cutaneous manifestations and serious complications of DM. Carnosine, an endogenous dipeptide that has antiglycation properties as well as metal ion and FR scavenger, partially due to its non-enzymatic binding with glycol-oxidized proteins, is a protective factor that can reduce protein glycation and its consequences.[25]

Diabetes Mellitus and Its Effects on the Skin

Diabetes mellitus produces changes in skin homeostasis either directly or indirectly through its complications, neuropathy and vasculopathy. In addition, partial or total insulin deficiency alters the role of insulin in the proliferation, differentiation and migration of keratinocytes, which results, among other consequences, in a cutaneous barrier dysfunction.[26] AGEs are also involved in the delay in wound healing that occurs in DM, probably related to vascular, neurological, and other changes, which accompany this pathology.[27] Other DM-induced skin changes include decreased sebaceous production, decreased skin elasticity and changes in pH. Yosipovitch et al. showed that in diabetics there was a large increase in cutaneous pH in flexural areas compared to nondiabetics, which partly explains the greater susceptibility to skin infections in these patients.[28]

NON-ENZYMATIC GLYCATION, DIABETES MELLITUS AND AGING

The NEG of proteins arouses a growing interest in the area of human health and medicine, as well as the role of AGEs, in the development of conditions related to age and diabetes. An example of this is NEG of SOD, a key enzyme in DNA repair and defense against ROS that pose a threat to biological systems because of the structural and functional genetic damage they produce. If the activity of SOD is blocked by glycation, the harmful effect of the FR is greater and therefore we also age more.[29]

There is a direct correlation between glycemia of ECM, aging and, for example, tissue fibrosis directly related to AGE-modified collagen. Glycation generates new molecular residues and induces cross-linking between macromolecules of dermal ECM. Therefore, glycation is responsible for the loss of elasticity and other physical properties of the dermis observed in patients with DM, similar to those found in chronological aging and photoaging. Clinically, the connective tissue is more rigid to touch with age and in DM, compared to healthy controls.[30]

In DM, direct exposure of some cell lines to high glucose concentrations and high levels of AGEs, increase ROS formation by activation of the enzyme NAD(P)H oxidase in concentration and time-dependent mode; parallel in DM there is a decrease in the antioxidant capacity by activation of the polyol pathway, which produces a depletion of NAD(P)H and inhibits NAD(P)H-dependent enzymes such as glutathione reductase. ROS are increased during glycooxidative stress via activated NF-κB, and participate in the pathogenesis of type 2 DM, aging, cardiovascular and neurodegenerative diseases, among others. Oxidative stress can, in turn, worsen the function of pancreatic cells and contribute as a result to DM, again generating a vicious circle.

Therefore, the glycation of proteins is accompanied by the generation of ROS by autoxidation of glucose and glycosylated proteins on the one hand, and via the interaction of AGEs with their receptor (RAGE) on the other hand, phenomena involved in the aging and in age-related diseases such as DM, cancer, Alzheimer's, etc.[31] Dyer et al. several years ago measured modified NEG collagen (early products like *fructose lysine*, and late as CML and pentosidine), in 39 patients with DM1 and 52 nondiabetic controls. The measurement of glycosylated collagen in the controls increased only 33% between the ages of 20 years and 85 years versus an increase up to 3 times higher in diabetic patients of the same age. By contrast, in controls and correlated with age, AGEs such as CML, pentosidine and the fluorescence increased fivefold, while in diabetics, they increased by up to twofold more than in controls. Therefore, the authors conclude that in both groups there was a strong correlation between AGEs (CML, pentosidine) and NEG-dependent collagen fluorescence by age, with an accelerated increase in DM.[32] These findings were confirmed in repeated subsequent studies, such as Sell et al. who found that a large amount of AGE-modified collagen may contribute to a number of structural dysfunctions and ECM cells observed in both senescence and diabetes.[14] Aging and diabetic tissues are accompanied by the characteristic yellowish color of the collagen matrix, which was attributed, according to experimental studies, to NEG with a consequent decrease in solubility and increased resistance to degradation by proteases as mentioned previously.[15]

Another point to consider in this common final pathway between DM and cutaneous aging is the alteration of the normal skin barrier and several of the defense mechanisms against infections (*see* Chapter 3: Cutaneous barrier and Diabetes).[33]

In conclusion, there are similarities between the gradual changes of the aged collagen and those of the diabetic patient, in whom an acceleration of the the collagen alterations is described, with the consequent premature aging. The biochemical abnormality common to cellular aging and to the development of some manifestations and chronic complications of diabetes is NEG and AGEs increased by chronic hyperglycemia of DM. The AGEs-RAGE interaction not only has proinflammatory action but also increases the oxidative stress, which determines more aging by generating more ROS and increasing the production of adhesion molecules and proinflammatory mediators.

In fact, all these processes are interconnected in such a way that, for example, DM increases oxidative stress and thus aging. Aging, on the other hand, increases the oxidative stress, mediators of inflammation and accumulation of AGEs, in which a closed circle of aging is established, e.g. AGEs, ROS, etc.

REFERENCES

1. Gkogkolou P, Böhm M. Advanced glycation end products. Key players in skin aging? Dermatoendocrinol. 2012;4(3):259-70.
2. Pageon H, Zucchi H, Rousset F, et al. Skin aging by glycation: lessons from the reconstructed skin model. Clin Chem Lab Med. 2014;52(1):169-74.
3. Cohen Sabban Emilia N. La glicosilación no enzimática: una vía común en la diabetes y el envejecimiento. Med Cutan Iber Lat Am. 2011;39(6):243-6.
4. Zouboulis CC, Makrantonaki E. Clinical aspects and molecular diagnostics of skin aging. Clin Dermatol. 2011;29(1):3-14.
5. Méndez JD, Xie J, Aguilar-Hernández M, et al. Trends in advanced glycation end products research in diabetes mellitus and its complications. Mol Cell Biochem. 2010;341(1-2):33-41.
6. Nedić O, Rattan SI, Grune T, et al. Molecular effects of advanced glycation end products on cell signalling pathways, ageing and pathophysiology. Free Radic Res. 2013;47(Suppl 1):28-38.
7. Juarez DT, Demaris KM, Goo R, et al. Significance of HbA1c and its measurement in the diagnosis of diabetes mellitus: US experience. Diabetes Metab Syndr Obes. 2014;7:487-94.
8. Ahmed N. Advanced glycation endproducts—role in pathology of diabetic complications. Diabetes Res Clin Pract. 2005;67(1):3-21.
9. Singh VP, Bali A, Singh N, et al. Advanced Glycation End Products and Diabetic Complications. Korean J Physiol Pharmacol. 2014;18(1):1-14.
10. Avery NC, Bailey AJ. The effects of the Maillard reaction on the physical properties and cell interactions of collagen. Pathol Biol (Paris). 2006;54(7):387-95.
11. Snedeker JG, Gautieri A. The role of collagen crosslinks in ageing and diabetes—the good, the bad, and the ugly. Muscles Ligaments Tendons J. 2014;4(3):303-8.
12. Luevano-Contreras C, Chapman-Novakofski K. Dietary advanced glycation end products and aging. Nutrients. 2010;2(12):1247-65.
13. Cárdenas-León M, Díaz-Díaz E, Argüelles-Medina R, et al. Glycation and protein crosslinking in the diabetes and ageing pathogenesis. Rev Invest Clin. 2009;61(6):505-20.
14. Sell DR, Biemel KM, Reihl O, et al. Glucosepane is a major protein cross-link of the senescent human extracellular matrix. Relationship with diabetes. J Biol Chem. 2005;280(13):12310-5.

15. Monnier VM, Mustata GT, Biemel KL, et al. Cross-linking of the extracellular matrix by the maillard reaction in aging and diabetes: an update on "a puzzle nearing resolution". Ann N Y Acad Sci. 2005;1043:533-44.
16. Conway BN, Aroda VR, Maynard JD, et al. Skin intrinsic fluorescence is associated with coronary artery disease in individuals with long duration of type 1 diabetes. Diabetes Care. 2012;35(11):2331-6.
17. Lohwasser C, Neureiter D, Weigle B, et al. The receptor for advanced glycation end products is highly expressed in the skin and upregulated by advanced glycation end products and tumor necrosis factor-alpha. J Invest Dermatol. 2006;126(2):291-9.
18. Park SY, Kim YA, Hong YH, et al. Up-regulation of the receptor for advanced glycation end products in the skin biopsy specimens of patients with severe diabetic neuropathy. J Clin Neurol. 2014;10(4):334-41.
19. Nowotny K, Jung T, Grune T, et al. Accumulation of modified proteins and aggregate formation in aging. Exp Gerontol. 2014;57:122-31.
20. Yamagishi S, Fukami K, Matsui T. Evaluation of tissue accumulation levels of advanced glycation end products by skin autofluorescence: A novel marker of vascular complications in high-risk patients for cardiovascular disease. Int J Cardiol. 2015;185:263-8.
21. Gautieri A, Redaelli A, Buehler MJ, et al. Age- and diabetes-related nonenzymatic crosslinks in collagen fibrils: candidate amino acids involved in Advanced Glycation End-products. Matrix Biol. 2014;34:89-95.
22. Bengmark S. Impact of nutrition on ageing and disease. Curr Opin Clin Nutr Metab Care. 2006;9(1):2-7.
23. Yamagishi S. Potential clinical utility of advanced glycation end product cross-link breakers in age- and diabetes-associated disorders. Rejuvenation Res. 2012;15(6):564-72.
24. Yamaoka H, Sasaki H, Yamasaki H, et al. Truncal pruritus of unknown origin may be a symptom of diabetic polyneuropathy. Diabetes Care. 2010;33(1):150-5.
25. Cohen MP, Ziyadeh FN, Chen S. Amadori-modified glycated serum proteins and accelerated atherosclerosis in diabetes: pathogenic and therapeutic implications. J Lab Clin Med. 2006;147(5):211-9.
26. Behm B, Schreml S, Landthaler M, et al. Skin signs in diabetes mellitus. J Eur Acad Dermatol Venereol. 2012;26(10):1203-11.
27. Peppa M, Stavroulakis P, Raptis SA. Advanced glycoxidation products and impaired diabetic wound healing. Wound Repair Regen. 2009;17(4):461-72.
28. Yosipovitch G, Tur E, Cohen O, et al. Skin surface pH in intertriginous areas in NIDDM patients. Possible correlation to candidal intertrigo. Diabetes Care. 1993 Apr;16(4):560-3.
29. Höhn A, Jung T, Grune T. Pathophysiological importance of aggregated damaged proteins. Free Radic Biol Med. 2014;71:70-89.
30. Piérard GE, Seité S, Hermanns-Lê T, et al. The skin landscape in diabetes mellitus. Focus on dermocosmetic management. Clin Cosmet Investig Dermatol. 2013;6:127-35.
31. Noordzij MJ, Mulder DJ, Oomen PH, et al. Skin autofluorescence and risk of micro- and macrovascular complications in patients with Type 2 diabetes mellitus-a multi-centre study. Diabet Med. 2012;29(12):1556-61.
32. Dyer DG, Dunn JA, Thorpe SR, et al. Accumulation of Maillard reaction products in skin collagen in diabetes and aging. J Clin Invest. 1993;91(6):2463-9.
33. Park HY, Kim JH, Jung M, et al. A long-standing hyperglycaemic condition impairs skin barrier by accelerating skin ageing process. Exp Dermatol. 2011;20(12):969-74.

CHAPTER 12

Nail Alterations in Diabetic Patients

Judith Dominguez-Cherit, Michelle Gatica-Torres

INTRODUCTION

The main function of nails in human beings is to provide protection to the distal part of the fingers and toes, including soft tissues, fingertips and the distal phalanges, and anatomic sites that are constantly exposed to trauma.

When evaluating nail alterations, the clinician should be familiarized with the nail apparatus anatomy and physiology. Having a clear knowledge of these two aspects makes it easier to obtain an accurate diagnosis and understand its possible causes. The nail apparatus consists of several structures, which can be altered under different circumstances; the nail folds (lateral and proximal), nail matrix (proximal and distal), nail bed, hyponychium and nail plate. The nail is a permeable structure, meaning that harmful substances can penetrate it. Moreover, when periungual folds or the cuticles have been damaged, an easy entry for bacteria, fungi and humidity is created. Although a complete review of nail anatomy and physiology is beyond the scope of this chapter, the reader should have these concepts clear before proceeding reading.

Systemic diseases can cause alterations on the nails, and diabetes mellitus is not the exception. In diabetic patients, apart from systemic factors, local and environmental factors are also important contributors to nail changes. Diabetes mellitus can be associated with a variety of clinically significant nail alterations, which can range in severity from mild to severe, and can involve different parts of the nail apparatus. Toenails are affected more frequently than fingernails. In order to analyze these changes, we will classify them as following, according to their etiology:
- Infectious nail disorders.
- Nail alterations secondary to altered biomechanics of the feet.
- Nail alterations induced by vascular abnormalities.
- Other nail findings in diabetic patients.

TERMINOLOGY

- *Leukonychia:* White discoloration of the nail. True leukonychia refers to the white coloration of the nail plate, while apparent leukonychia is caused by a white underlying bed.

- *Nail bed hyperkeratosis:* Thickening of the nail bed.
- *Onychogryphosis:* Thickening of a large and laterally curled nail.
- *Onycholysis:* Separation of the nail plate from the nail bed, more frequently on the distal free margin.
- *Pachyonychia:* Thickening of the nail plate.
- *Paronychia:* Inflammation of the nail folds.
- *Pincer nail:* Overcurvature of the transverse axis of the nail plate.
- *Splinter hemorrhages:* Small, linear, longitudinally-oriented hemorrhages that occur between the nail plate and the nail bed.
- *Terry nails:* Apparent leukonychia of the nail bed with a distal pink or brown band.

INFECTIOUS NAIL DISORDERS

Diabetic patients are more prone to develop infectious disease due to organism-specific factors and host factors; hyperglycemia, vascular insufficiency, sensory neuropathy, diabetes-induced immunosuppression, and skin and mucosal colonization with species of *Candida*[1,2] and *Staphylococcus aureus*. Given the proximity of the nail apparatus to the phalanges, there is a plausible risk of developing osteomyelitis, if an infection is not identified and treated on time.[3] Moreover, the risk of developing severe complications from cutaneous and nail apparatus infections is high, representing a leading cause of morbidity, disability and even mortality.

Onychomycosis

The most common nail disorder in diabetic patients is onychomycosis, affecting up to one-third of the patients.[3-7] Severe onychomycosis poses a serious issue given the risk of developing soft tissue infections, and it is considered a predisposing factor for foot ulcers[3-7] (Fig. 1).

Factors associated with toenail onychomycosis in this population include advanced age, male gender[8,9] and not washing the feet every day. A larger area of involvement of the nail plate is associated with a lower toe brachial index and it is considered a marker of subclinical atherosclerosis.[10] Thicker nails in onychomycosis directly correlate with higher hemoglobin A1C levels[11] (Fig. 2).

Subungual and distal involvement is seen in most of the cases, followed by a total dystrophic presentation. Dermatophytes, especially *Trichophyton rubrum*, account for most cases of onychomycosis; however, infections caused by molds and yeasts are seen more frequently than in the general population (Fig. 3).

High-risk patients, with sensory neuropathy and impaired circulation should receive treatment with oral antifungal therapy, physical debridement and proper education regarding foot inspection and care[4] (Fig. 4). Washing the feet every day should be encouraged as well as drying meticulously between the toes.[11]

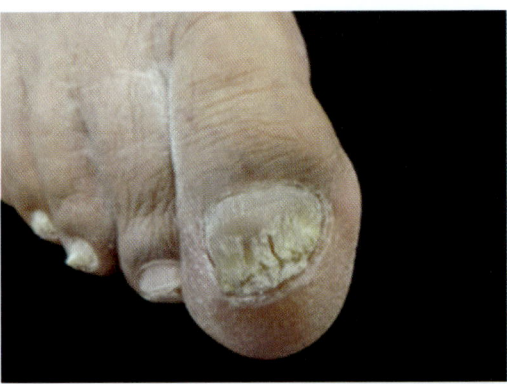

Fig. 1: Distal subungual onychomycosis of the first, third and fourth toes. Prominent pachyonychia and yellow discoloration with pulverization of the nail plate.

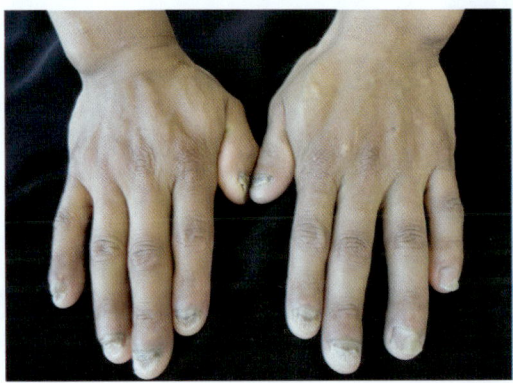

Fig. 2: Onychomycosis of the fingernails in a young patient with type 1 diabetes mellitus.

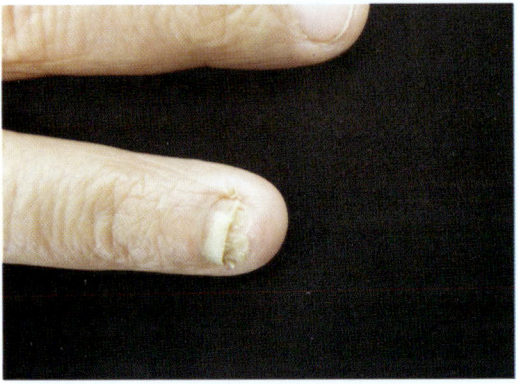

Fig. 3: Distal subungual onychomycosis. Onycholysis, yellow discoloration and subungual hyperkeratosis.

Paronychia

Paronychia is an acute or chronic inflammation of the periungual folds (Fig. 5). Patient with diabetes are at risk of developing chronic paronychia.[12]

Trauma to the cuticle or lateral and proximal nail folds allow penetration of irritating substances and moisture, bacteria and mainly *Candida* species. Prevention of paronychia should be encouraged by avoiding trimming of the cuticle, nail biting, keeping nails short and improving glycemic control.[13]

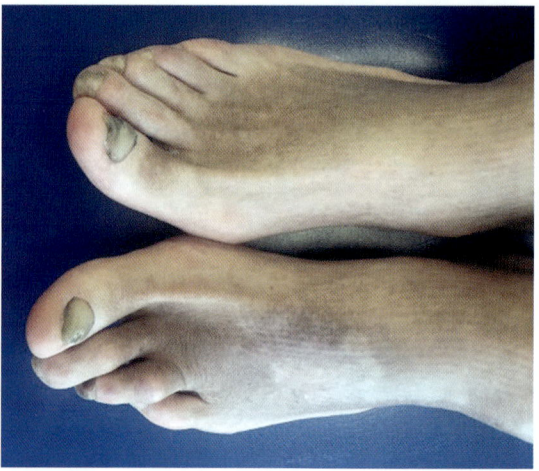

Fig. 4: A 58-year-old diabetic patient with long-standing diabetes mellitus and severe complications, with prominent deformity of the feet secondary to neuropathy and digital amputation. The nails are thick, with a yellow and green discoloration; there is onychomycosis and traumatic dystrophy of the nine toenails.

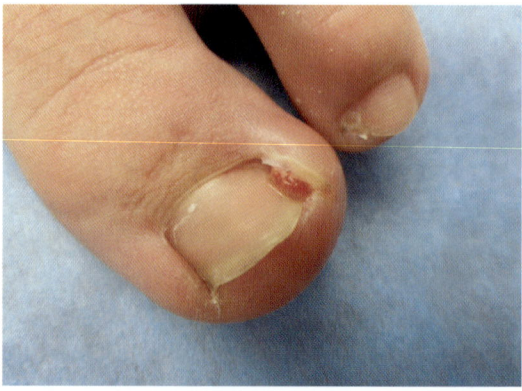

Fig. 5: Ingrown nail causing acute paronychia and granulation tissue on the lateral nail fold.

NAIL ALTERATIONS SECONDARY TO ALTERED BIOMECHANICS OF THE FEET

Foot deformities in the diabetic population are found in up to 50% of patients. It is closely related to a long-standing and a poorly controlled disease. The etiology of these deformities has not been elucidated. Several factors have been implicated, for instance, neuropathy, ischemia, muscle weakness, limited joint mobility and gait abnormalities.[14] Proprioceptive and protective abilities are lost as the disease progresses[15] culminating in chronic ulceration.

Nerve damage can induce nail changes. Motor and sensory loss can cause abnormally slow growth, fragility or yellow discoloration of the finger and toenails[16] (Figs. 4 and 6).

After an amputation is performed, the biomechanics of the foot changes dramatically due to muscular weakness, tendinous detachment and redistribution of pressure sites. Nails can suffer changes due to constant friction and trauma with adjacent toes or inappropriate shoes (Fig. 6). Onycholysis, pachyonychia, transverse and longitudinal overcurvature, yellow discoloration and frictional melanonychia are frequently encountered in patients with history of digital amputations.

NAIL ALTERATIONS INDUCED BY VASCULAR ABNORMALITIES

Diabetes mellitus causes severe changes in the vascular system, including microvascular and macrovascular damage. Both will end up having

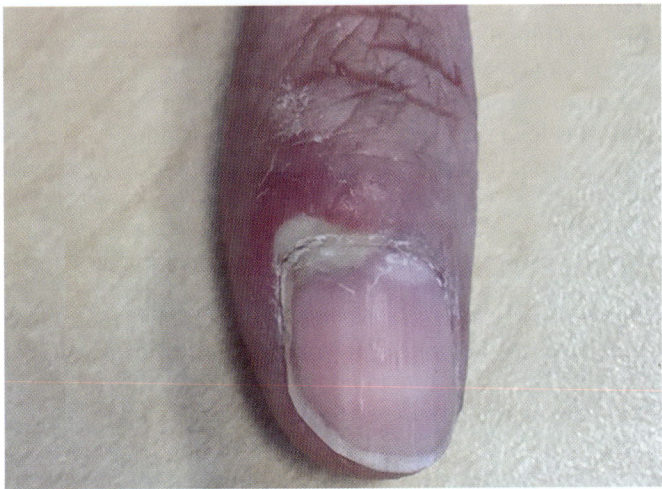

Fig. 6: Periungual abscess on the proximal and lateral nail folds that required drainage.

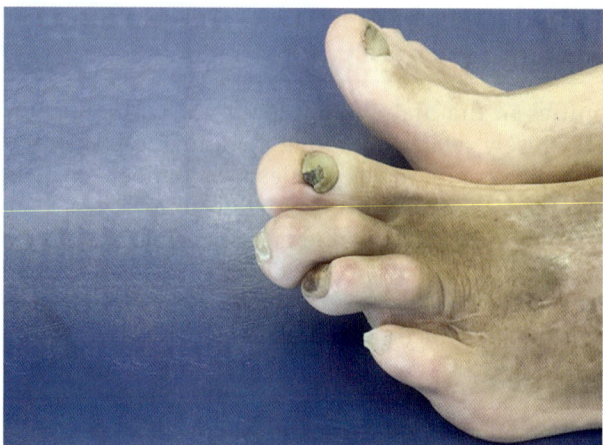

Fig. 7: This patient had history of diabetic foot that required a digit amputation. There is absence of the left fourth toe. The third toe is now constantly exposed to trauma, note the subungual hematoma.

manifestations on the nail apparatus. Vascular disease in diabetic patients has a complex pathophysiology including inflammation, hypercoagulability, atherosclerosis and alterations in endothelial and vascular smooth muscle cell function. Hyperglycemia decreases endothelium-derived nitric oxide and increases superoxide anion production, which then leads to the production of oxygen-derived free radicals and increases intracellular production of advanced glycation end products that then affect cellular function.[17] Patients with peripheral vascular disease have an increased risk for claudication, ischemic ulcers, gangrene, severe infections and amputations (Figs. 7 and 8).

Structural and functional abnormalities on capillaroscopic examination of the proximal nail fold have been reported on diabetic patients and may reflect the extent of microvascular involvement. The maximum increment percentage of flow velocity is lower, as well as the capillary response after reperfusion in induced ischemia, reflecting an abnormal capillary flow regulation and endothelial cells.[18,19]

OTHER NAIL FINDINGS IN DIABETIC PATIENTS

Patients with diabetes may exhibit a yellow discoloration of the nails, especially toenails, secondary to advanced glycosylation end products. Periungual erythema can also be found due to engorgement of postcapillary venules in the papillary dermis caused by increased viscosity of blood with stiff red blood cell membranes.[20]

Terry nails have been described in diabetes mellitus, presenting as leukonychia with a pink or brown band 0.5–3 mm wide on the distal part of the nail bed.[21]

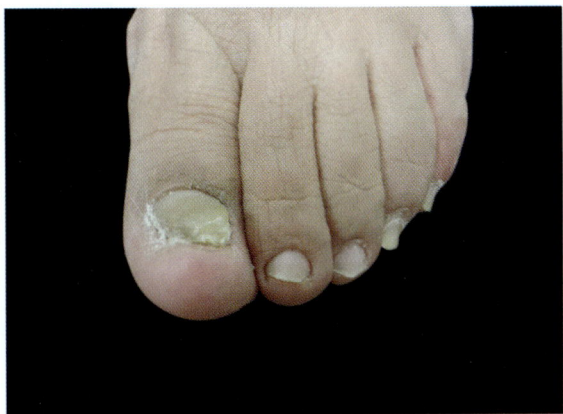

Fig. 8: Thickening of the nail plate and yellow discoloration. No evidence of onychomycosis is seen.

A common nail deformity in diabetic patients, particularly of advanced age is onychogryphosis. If onychogryphosis is not taken care of, patients can develop subungual gangrene due to increased pressure. In these patients, careful nail clipping and trimming should be advised.[22,23]

Given the presence of peripheral neuropathy, peripheral vascular disease and atherosclerosis, onychocryptosis can be a serious problem in patients with diabetes (Fig. 5). When nail deformities such as pincer nails, or a history of onychocryptosis is present, the possibility of performing surgical treatment, preferably with a chemical matricectomy, should be considered.

Splinter hemorrhages can also be found in about 10% of patients but are not specific of diabetes. When found on the distal portion of the nail plate, they are usually trauma induced.[24] Given the foot deformities and altered biomechanics after amputations, it is not rare to find subungual hematomas on the toenail (Figs. 9 to 12).

NAIL APPARATUS EVALUATION IN DIABETICS

A complete clinical history is needed. A past history of neuropathy or peripheral vascular disease should be addressed. On physical examination, the whole extremity should be examined. Vascular evaluation should at least include palpation of the dorsalis pedis pulse using the fingertips. Identify diabetic neuropathy symptoms and loss of protective sensation. If present, look for evidence of increased pressure, bony deformities, and muscle weakness.

All nails need to be carefully scanned. Abnormal size, shape, color, surface contour, texture and growth abnormalities should be noted.

Early identification of biomechanical faults is essential. Special footwear can be considered to redistribute pressure when biomechanical alterations are found, this will help prevent and diminish existent nail deformities.

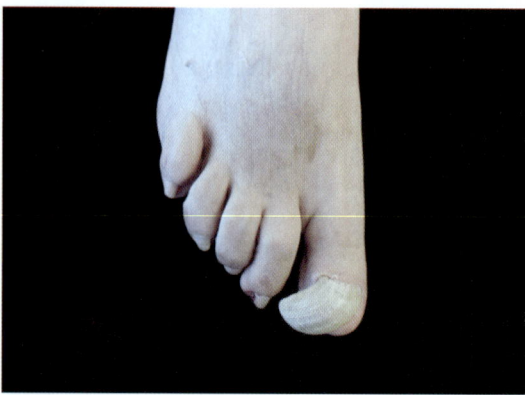

Fig. 9: Onychogryphosis. Hypertrophic nails resembling a ram's horn.

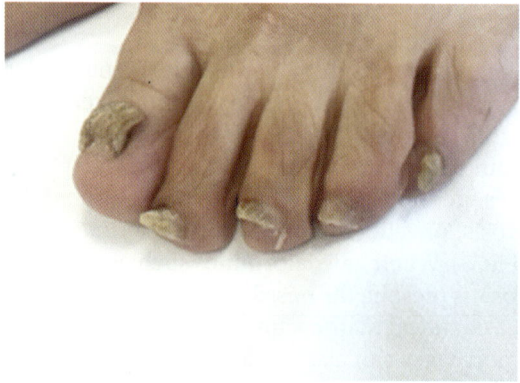

Fig. 10: Prominent nail deformity, nail thickening, yellow and brown discoloration. The nails have completely lost their normal axis growth.

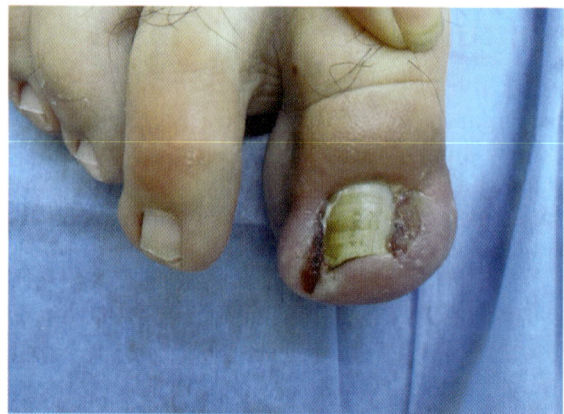

Fig. 11: Patient's recovery after chemical matricectomy.

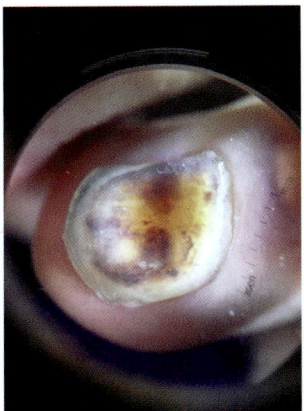

Fig. 12: Dermoscopic view of a subungual hematoma of a toenail. In this patient the third toe was longer than the second one, this causes continuous trauma to the second nail bed.

A mycological examination with a potassium hydroxide (KOH) examination should be performed to rule out a fungal infection when a nail dystrophy is present.

Clinicians in contact with diabetic patients should educate them in adequate nail and feet care. After adequate cleaning and drying of the feet, patients should cautiously examine the twenty nails every day. Rather than cutting the nails, filing to smoothen the nail border should be advised to avoid accidental cuts. It is important to encourage the patient to seek for early healthcare attention when minor cuts are encountered around the nails. Early detection of complications due to nail abnormalities leads to an optimal treatment, reducing morbidity in this population.

REFERENCES

1. Jautová J, Virágová S, Ondrasovic M, et al. Incidence of Candida species isolated from human skin and nails: a survey. Folia Microbiol (Praha). 2001;46:333-7.
2. Dorko E, Jautová J, Pilipcinec E, et al. Occurrence of Candida strains in cases of paronychia. Folia Microbiol (Praha). 2004;49:591-5.
3. Cox HA, Jones RO. Direct extension osteomyelitis secondary to chronic onychocryptosis. Three case reports. J Am Podiatr Med Assoc. 1995;85:321-4.
4. Rich P, Hare A. Onychomycosis in a special patient population: focus on the diabetic. Int J Dermatol. 1999;38 (Suppl 2):17-9.
5. Rich P. Onychomycosis and tinea pedis in patients with diabetes. J Am Acad Dermatol. 2000;43(5 Suppl):S130-4.
6. Rich P, Elewski B, Scher RK, et al. Diagnosis, clinical implications, and complications of onychomycosis. Semin Cutan Med Surg. 2013;32(2 Suppl 1):S5-8.
7. Rich P. Special patient populations: onychomycosis in the diabetic patient. J Am Acad Dermatol. 1996;35(3 Pt 2):S10-2.
8. Gupta AK, Humke S. The prevalence and management of onychomycosis in diabetic patients. Eur J Dermatol. 2000;10:379-84.

9. Gupta AK, Konnikov N, MacDonald P, et al. Prevalence and epidemiology of toenail onychomycosis in diabetic subjects: a multicentre survey. Br J Dermatol. 1998;139:665-71.
10. Onalan O, Adar A, Keles H, et al. Onychomycosis is associated with subclinical atherosclerosis in patients with diabetes. Vasa. 2015;44:59-64.
11. Takehara K, Oe M, Tsunemi Y, et al. Factors associated with presence and severity of toenail onychomycosis in patients with diabetes: a cross-sectional study. Int J Nurs Stud. 2011;48:1101-8.
12. Rockwell PG. Acute and chronic paronychia. Am Fam Physician. 2001;63:1113-6.
13. Rigopoulos D, Larios G, Gregoriou S, et al. Acute and chronic paronychia. Am Fam Physician. 2008;77:339-46.
14. Allan J, Munro W, Figgins E. Foot deformities within the diabetic foot and their influence on biomechanics: A review of the literature. Prosthet Orthot Int. 2015 Jul 24. pii: 0309364615592705. [Epub ahead of print]
15. Kim PJ. Biomechanics of the Diabetic Foot: Consideration in Limb Salvage. Adv Wound Care (New Rochelle). 2013;2:107-11.
16. Mann RJ, Burton JL. Nail dystrophy due to diabetic neuropathy. Br Med J (Clin Res Ed). 1982:15:1445.
17. Creager MA, Lüscher TF, Cosentino F, et al. Diabetes and vascular disease: pathophysiology, clinical consequences, and medical therapy: Part I. Circulation. 2003;108:1527-32.
18. Kaminska-Winciorek G, Deja G, Polańska J, et al. Diabetic microangiopathy in capillaroscopic examination of juveniles with diabetes type 1. Postepy Hig Med Dosw (Online). 2012;66:51-9.
19. Abi-Chahin TC, Hausen Mde A, Mansano-Marques CM, et al. Microvascular reactivity in type 1 diabetics. Arq Bras Endocrinol Metabol. 2009;53:741-6.
20. Huntley AC. Cutaneous manifestations of diabetes mellitus. Dermatol Clin. 1989;7:531-46.
21. Holzberg M, Walker HK. Terry's nails: revised definition and new correlations. Lancet. 1984;1:896-9.
22. Bernard O. Onychogryphosis and the involuted nail in diabetes mellitus. West Indian Med J. 2001;50 (Suppl 1):29-30.
23. Mohrenschlager M, Wicke-Wittenius K, Brockow K, et al. Onychogryphosis in elderly persons: an indicator of long-standing poor nursing care? Report of one case and review of the literature. Cutis. 2001;68:233-5.
24. Kilpatrick ZM, Greenberg PA, Sanford JP. Splinter Hemorrhages - Their Clinical Significance. Arch Intern Med. 1965;115(6):730-5.

CHAPTER 13

Ulcers and Wound Healing in Diabetics

Patricia Troielli, Lucrecia Juarez

INTRODUCTION

The number of patients who suffer from diabetes mellitus (DM) has increased from 153 million in 1980 to 383 million in 2014, according to the estimation of the World Health Organization. The global prevalence is of 9% in young adults over 18 years of age.[1-3] This assessment has significantly surpassed predictions and allowed this pathology to be categorized as epidemic.[4,5]

The increase has been attributed to modifications in lifestyles, as well as growth and ageing of the global population. There are variations within diverse regions related to genetic susceptibility as well as social, economic and cultural traits.

Considered as a chronic disease, it has a huge impact in the economy. In the United States America, the average medical expenditure for diabetics was 2.3 higher than for those that do not suffer from it.[6] Latin American countries have a high prevalence of diabetic patients, such as Mexico with an average of 14.4%.[2,7]

Patients with DM often develop lesions of the skin as a result from peripheric neuropathy, vascular complications and ischemia manifestations. Loss of sensation and alteration in scarring associated to this disease lead to ulcers in the feet and may extend to the amputation of limbs. There is higher morbility and increase in medical costs. The risk of developing ulcers in the feet reaches 25% throughout the lifespan of a diabetic patient and the recurrence lies between 50 and 70% within the next 5 years.[8] Over 60% of nontraumatic amputations in lower limbs occur in diabetic patients. The estimated cost in Europe for treating ulcers in a diabetic foot ranges from 4514 Euros for noninfected neuropathic ulcers to 16.835 Euros for infected ischemic ulcers.[9,10]

Comprehensive programs for the care of lower limbs which include risk assessment, education, preventive therapy and the intervention of specialized teams may reduce the lower-extremity amputation rate by more than 50%.[6,11]

This chapter will describe the process of wound healing and its alterations in diabetic patients as well as current strategies for diagnosis, treatment and prevention of ulcers.

CUTANEOUS WOUND HEALING

The healing of a skin wound is a dynamic process that involves interaction with the immune system, inflammatory mediators, endothelial cells, blood platelets and skin cells, keratinocytes and fibroblasts.[12-14] It develops in three stages that tend to overlap (Fig. 1).

Wound characteristics, ill-suited care and patient management, associated diseases, or topical/systemic treatments may delay the time of one or several of these stages.

Inflammation

The process of coagulation begins within 2 or 3 hours following the occurrence of a wound.

In the case of a wound of the skin with extravasation of blood, the first mechanism that arises depends on the activation of platelets that promote the development of fibrin plug. Proinflammatory mediators cytokines and growth factors are released and neutrophils and monocytes are recruited to the site of the wound. The normal development of inflammatory response is influenced by the proteinases activated by the injury, the release of reactive oxygen species (ROS) and the changes in the gradients of O_2 and pH in the site of the wound.

Several anti-inflammatory and anticoagulant drugs, acetylsalicylic acids, antagonists of thromboplastin or factor III extend this stage leading to impaired wound healing. The inflammatory stage continues for days with the recruitment of circulating cells, neutrophils and macrophages.

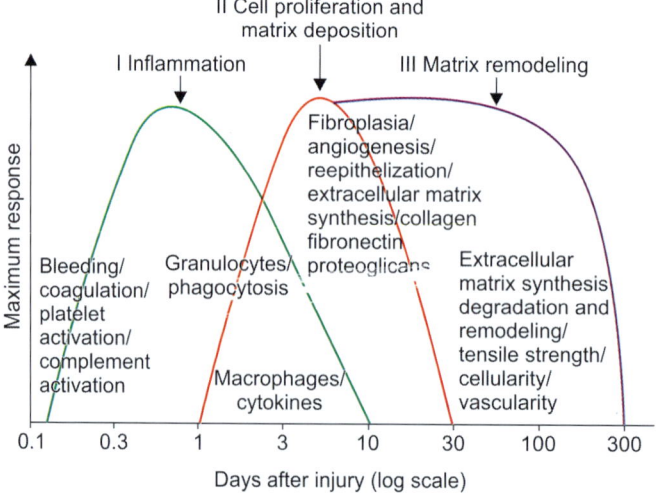

Fig. 1: Stages of wound healing.

> **BOX 1:** Major cytokines and factors in skin wound.
>
> Vascular endothelial growth factor (VEGF)
> Interleukin-1β (IL-1β)
> Interleukin-4 (IL-4)
> IL-1 antagonist receptor (a-rIL-1)
> Platelet-derived growth factor (PDGF)
> Epidermal growth factor (EGF)
> Keratinocyte growth factor-1 (KGF-1)
> Tumor necrosis factor-alpha (TNF-α)
> Transforming growth factor-beta (TGF-β)

The increase of cytokines interleukin-1 (IL-1), IL-6, tumor necrosis factor alpha (TNFα), chemokine production and the release of preformed mediators with activation of its cell receptors perform a main role at this stage. This is the onset of mechanisms and signals of cell repair.

Several cytokines and major factors of the wound healing are shown in Box 1.

This stage is clinically diagnosed by the sharp red and granular appearance at the wound bed. It represents the overlapping of neoangiogenesis and granulation mechanisms with formation and deposit of the components of extracellular matrix (ECM). Research carried out on neoangiogenesis showed that hypoxia is one of the major factors delaying healing. Mammalian target of rapamycin (mTOR), which does not play any role during normoxia, may do so during angiogenesis and proliferation induced by hypoxia. Therapeutic blockage with mTOR inhibitors, such as rapamycin or sirolimus, has proven antiangiogenic and antiproliferative activity. Long-term research on similar drugs could accelerate the wound healing process in the future.[15]

Proliferation

Macrophages derived from monocytes found at the site of the wound are activated in the presence of IL-4 from T-cell type Th2. IL-4 triggers changes in the macrophages phenotype specific to the wound. This promotes production of proinflammatory cytokines and growth factors inducing hyperproliferation and increase of fibroblastic activity. The macrophage is the main cell at this stage and starts up the proliferation.

Long-term treatment with nonsteroidal anti-inflammatory drugs may interfere with the activity of the macrophages and delay the cutaneous wound repair.

This stage brings nonstop activation and proliferation of different types of cells, migration and formation of new vessels, angiogenesis, and deposit of ECM. The initial fibrin plug is replaced by fibronectin, effective substrate for the reepithelialization of the wound by keratinocytes.

Healing time depends on the adequate interaction between inflammatory cytokines and receptors, such as transforming growth factor beta-1 from keratinocytes resulting in strong paracrine stimulus of proliferation of fibroblasts and the balance between receptors and antagonists (e.g. IL-1r /a-IL1r) sustaining inflammatory homeostasis.

Various types of adhesion molecules are involved in recruiting inflammatory cells to the skin. The intercellular adhesion molecule 1 (ICAM-1) and its ligands allow for the adhesion of the ECM ligands integrin *a6 β4* and the movement of keratinocytes for differentiation in a new epidermis.

Remodeling

The last stage of the wound healing involves remodeling and scar tissue formation which may take months and up to 2 years. This is due to collagen deposit, components of ECM and their degradation from metalloproteinases. It is featured by the contraction of the scar throughout the months and the stability of the wound tensile strength over time. It is at this stage when functional and cosmetic integrity of the skin is reestablished.

WOUND HEALING IN DIABETES MELLITUS

Multiple factors can lead to impaired wound healing in diabetic patients. Skin fails to heal because nerve and vascular dysfunction affect intimately the cutaneous homeostasis.

As a result of these dysfunctions, there is prolonged proinflammatory response in the wound and strong evidence of a crucial involvement of nerve during cutaneous wound healing.

Effects of Hyperglycemia

Hyperglycemia is correlated to a slower healing rate in diabetic patients, especially those with lower limb neuropathic ulcers and peripheral arterial disease.

This slowing down in healing is secondary to the inhibition of proliferation with increase in the differentiation of skin keratinocytes, production of ROS associated with the decrease in endogen antioxidants and formation of advanced glycosylation end-products (AGEs).[9,16,17]

These AGEs accumulation in nerves can produce structural and functional alterations of the peripheral nerves.

Oxidative Stress

Recent studies of lymphocytes in diabetic patients confirmed the relationship between the increase in oxidative stress and apoptosis detected in these cells. The clinical outcome is delay in healing and increases the potential of infection in these patients.[18,19]

Apoptosis

Apoptosis deregulation, as a response to hyperglycemia, is in every cell type.

This affects the repair of each target organ and it is the main cause for diabetic foot wounds. It precedes neuropathy and peripheral vascular disease.

Evidence shows that deregulation in apoptosis of the immune cells determines a bad outcome in the process of wound healing, especially in the resolution of inflammation and final stages of proliferation in chronic diabetic wounds.

Lymphocyte apoptosis in diabetic wounds is initiated by the increase in ROS which determines the expression of proapoptotic proteins, such as caspases, Fas and Bax, and the decrease in antiapoptotic proteins, such as genes from B-cell lymphoma (BCL-2).

In addition, connexins are proteins of the intercellular GAP unions and are upregulated after a wound, allowing for the passage of inflammatory and proapoptotic signals from one cell to another. Diabetic wounds have shown an increase in connexins Cx26, Cx30.3, Cx31.1 and Cx43 compared to nondiabetic wounds.[19]

Neuropeptides

Neuropeptides play an important role in the process of wound healing in diabetics. These are released in normal skin by the autonomous nervous system as well as cells such as keratinocytes, endothelial cells, fibroblasts, epidermic dendritic cells and Langerhans cells. These molecules may induce activation of immune cell system (neutrophils, macrophages, antigen-presenting dendritic cells and lymphocytes) acting as a proinflammatory mediators.

In contrast, several neuropeptides Y, nerve growth factor, calcitonin gene-related peptide, and substance P levels are decreased in the skin of patients with diabetic neuropathy affecting the neurovascular response to injury.[20]

Vasodilatation, perception of pain, and function of the sebaceous and sweat glands are affected and the skin becomes dry and susceptible to fissures, tearing and infections.

Tissue repair in diabetic patients involves another aspect that is reinnervation and the cutaneous regenerative rate decreases similarly in patients irrespective of neuropathy.

Antimicrobial Peptides

It has been reported that diabetic patients have lower levels of antimicrobial peptides (AMPs) at the ulcers which contribute to the impairment of wound healing and facilitate secondary infections.

Antimicrobial peptides are small molecules involved in the innate immunity through direct killing of microorganism and are present in healthy skin surface.

They have also proinflammatory and proangiogenic properties.

The AMPs, human beta-defensin (HBD) and cathelicidin play an important role during the healing processes such as activation of dermal fibroblasts and

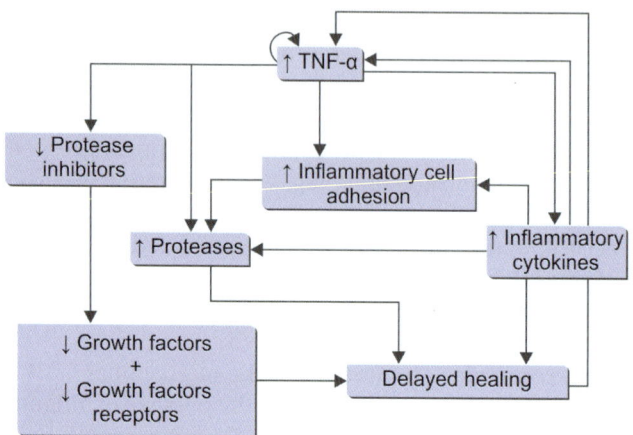

Fig. 2: Role of tumor necrosis factor-alpha (TNF-α) in chronic wounds.

keratinocytes by HBD and angiogenesis and keratinocytes migration by the cathelicidin peptide named LL-37.

Several studies demonstrated that biopsies from diabetic foot ulcers have low or none expression of LL-37 peptide which is directly associated to delayed healing.

Tumor Necrosis Factor-alpha

Excess of TNFα could be the promoter of a proinflammatory environment set in a chronic wound. Substantial inflammation, increase in proteolytic activity and diminished levels of growth factors generate an inadequate situation for healing. This means less mythogenic potential when compared to acute wounds[21] (Fig. 2).

Bone Marrow Precursors

Endothelial progenitor cells (EPCs) derived from bone marrow play an important role in the neovascularization process in response to hypoxia as seen in diabetic wounds with alterations in peripheral blood circulation.

Endothelial progenitor cells in bone marrow respond to ischemia, recruiting by cytokine gradient from the affected areas where they participate in the neovascularization. These progenitor cells are moved from the bone marrow into the blood flow by activation of endothelial nitric oxide synthase (eNOS) enzyme, after the release of vascular endothelial growth factor (VEGF) by macrophages, fibroblasts and epithelial cells.

In skin, the recruiting of EPCs to the wound site depends on the overregulation of the stromal cell-derived factor-1 alpha (SDF-1α) induced by hypoxia.

In diabetic wounds liberation and recruitment of EPCs are diminished. There is less VEGF and nitric oxide (NO) and SDF-1α (Fig. 3).

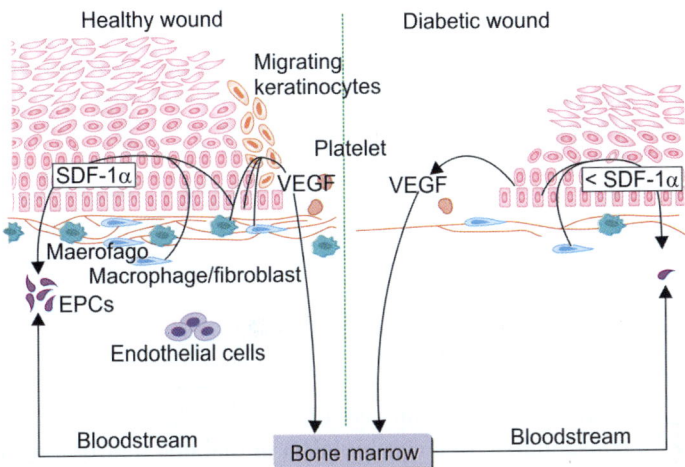

Fig. 3: Mechanisms of wound healing in healthy people versus people with diabetes.[18]
(SDF-1α: Stromal cell-derived factor-1 alpha; EPCs: Endothelial progenitor cells; VEGFE: Vascular endothelial growth factor).

These findings have therapeutic significance for the use of hyperbaric oxygen (HO), increase the production of NO in the marrow mobilizing EPCs. However, when this therapy is applied to diabetics, the results have been varied.

It is currently known that these different responses are caused by less production of SDF-1α in diabetic patients. When SDF-1α is administered together with HO, EPCs may be effectively recruited to the wound site.[15,22,23]

MOLECULAR BASES FOR DEBRIDEMENT

Molecular study of skin biopsies from diabetic patients have shown pathogenic markers related to delayed healing. Two of them, c-myc and the nuclear β-catenin are overexpressed in the hyperkeratosis area at the edge of the ulcer and there is a diminished expression and abnormal siting of the receptor of epidermal growth factor (rEGF). This indicates inhibition of migration of keratinocytes and change in fibroblast phenotype.[22]

In the adjacent skin of the ulcer, cells show normal phenotypes and are able to become active and respond to the administration of growth factors and cellular treatment.

Studies on fluids taken from diabetic lower limb ulcers show increased levels of metalloproteinases as compared to nondiabetic wound fluids.[8]

These types of molecular markers may be used in the near future to guide debridement.

BIOMECHANIC ALTERATIONS

The skin of diabetics has different biomechanic properties when compared to nondiabetic persons. There is less elasticity, tensile strength, and collagen deposit due to failure in regulation of collagen synthesis at posttranscriptional level.

These defects in tissue integrity predate the occurrence of a wound and make diabetic patients more prone to wounds regardless of neuropathy or vascular dysfunction.[24]

PREVENTION AND TREATMENT OF ULCERS IN DIABETICS

Diabetic patient run a potential risk of amputation in every lower limb wound as a consequence of a combination of diabetic neuropathy, arterial insufficiency and local trauma.

The diabetic foot ulcers allow microorganisms to gain access to a tissue that can lead to sepsis and occasionally may require amputation of the limb. Thus, treatment and prevention of ulcers in a diabetic foot must be known and applied by healthcare professionals.

Treatment of Ulcers in Diabetic Patients (Flowchart 1)

Diagnosis

First step in the treatment of foot ulcers is etiological diagnosis. Neuropathic ulcers correspond to 60% of all cases while purely ischemic and neuroischemic rate at 15% each, respectively.[25]

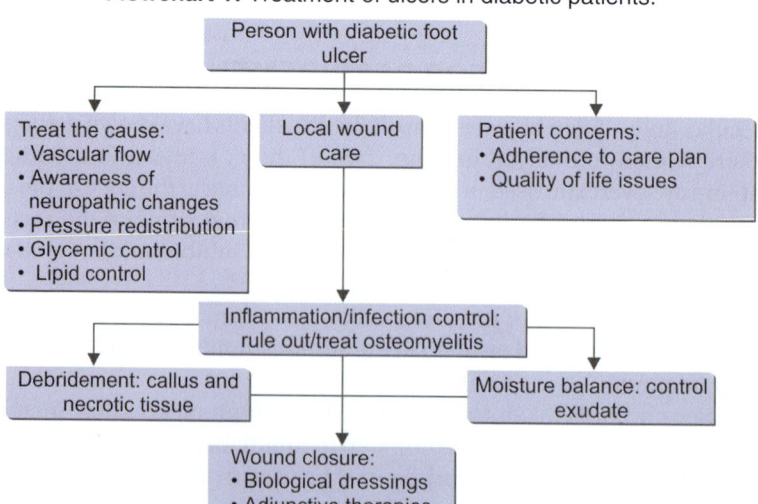

Flowchart 1: Treatment of ulcers in diabetic patients.

Loss of sensitivity (loss of protection sensation) leads to ulceration in high pressure sites. Autonomic neuropathy might increase the possibility of skin rupture.

Ischemic ulcers are small. Pain while resting is the main symptom. The pain is due to lower tensor gradient when lying which triggers deficient distal vascular circulation. When arterial occlusive disease is suspected, it must be confirmed and treated in order to reach successful treatment.

The localization and clinical manifestation guide the differential diagnosis (Table 1).

Offloading

Areas that might experience increase in pressure must be evaluated in order to prescribe offloading methods. Clinical manifestations are callus formation, especially hemorrhagic callus, blisters or macerated skin. During physical examination, limited dorsiflexion of hallux (<30°) is a common finding, as well as prominent metatarsal heads and other plantar bony prominences. Charcot fractures are a common finding in X-rays.

Offloading of the affected area may prevent ulcers and in patients with ulcers, the relief from pressure is fundamental to promote healing.

All patients with risk factors for amputation must be advised in the use of protective footwear[26] (Box 2).

Infection Control

It is of vital importance to remove necrotic and/or devitalized tissue either by mechanical, biological or autolytic means to avoid bacterial growth.

If infection is suspected in a debrided ulcer or if epithelialization from the margin is not progressing within 2 weeks of debridement and initiation of

TABLE 1: Types of ulcers in diabetic foot.

Types	Localization	Clinical features
Neuropathic ulcer	First and fifth metatarsal (acral areas) Calcaneus (posterior end)	Painless ulcer with perilesional rounded callus and loss of sensation. Good blood perfusion and peripheral pulses preserved.
Neuroischemic ulcer	Hallux Fifth metatarsal (lateral surface) Heel	Laterodigital dry necrosis can progress to ulceration with drainage of infected content. Pain according to the degree of neuropathic involvement. Deficit or absence of tibial pulse and altered sensation by prior neuropathy.
Ischemic ulcer	Distal areas of the digits Heel	Small well-defined ulcer with necrosis or crust, pale, shiny skin Deficit or absence of tibial pulse

> **BOX 2:** Risk factors related to ulcers or amputation.
>
> Previous amputation
> Foot ulcer history
> Peripheral neuropathy
> Foot deformity
> Peripheral vascular disease
> Visual impairment
> Diabetes nephropathy (especially dialysis patients)
> Inadequate glycemic control
> Smoking

offloading therapy, it is important to make bacterial wound cultures. Cultures should be performed to isolate both aerobic and anaerobic bacteria and preferably in tissue biopsy.[27,28]

If more than 10^6 CFU/g or hemolytic Streptococcus β are found, topical antibiotics must be administered if the infection compromises only granular tissue, otherwise systemic antibiotics must be prescribed.

Cellulitis around the ulcer must be treated with systemic antibiotics for Gram-positive germs.

In order to dispel any doubt about osteomyelitis, diagnostic imaging and adequate cultures should be taken. If diagnosis is confirmed, the affected bone must be removed and systemic antibiotics must be administered for 2–4 weeks.

Wound Bed Preparation

The aim is to facilitate the endogen process of healing and/or enhance positive results of other therapeutic measures.

It is important to carry out comprehensive clinical tests on patients. Reconsider factors that challenge wound healing, such as systemic diseases and medicines, abnormalities in nutrition, tissue perfusion and oxygenation. Optimizing glucose control improves healing.

After the initial debridement, maintenance debridement (surgical, enzymatic, mechanical, biological or autolytic) must be an ongoing process. As a rule, sharp surgical debridement is preferred for diabetic ulcers. Cleanse wound initially and at each dressing change using a neutral, nonirritating and nontoxic solution (such as saline solution). Accomplish with minimal trauma. Antiseptics become toxic for granular tissue.

If ulcer does not reduce by 40% or more after 4 weeks of therapy, reevaluate and consider other treatments.

Dressing

Dressing should keep the area around the wound moist, allow for swabbing, protect the surrounding skin, and ease the pain. Dressing should be held firmly in place and minimize friction. Choose cost/benefit options according to the etiology of the ulcer and ease of use.[26,29-32]

TABLE 2: Dressings commonly used in ulcers.

Product	Advantages	Disadvantages	Indications
Gauzes	Inexpensive Accessible	Drying Poor barrier High frequency of change	Packing deep wounds (Use as moist wound healing)
Films	Moisture-retentive Protects from contamination Semiocclusive Transparent	No absorption Fluid trapping	Wounds with minimal exudate
Hydrogels	Moisture-retentive Pain relief	May overhydrate	Dry wounds Painful wounds
Hydrocolloids	Absorbent Protects from contamination Long wear time	Opaque Fluid trapping Malodorous discharge	Wounds with light to moderate exudate
Alginates and Hydrofibers	Highly absorbent Hemostatic	Fibrous debris	Wounds with moderate to heavy exudate Filling cavities Hemostasis

Table 2 shows advantages, disadvantages and indications for dressings that are most popularly applied.

Surgery

In diabetic patients, Achilles tendon lengthening by surgery has been shown to decrease pressure in the forefoot where most ulcers are located. This technique improves flexibility and has its benefits on heel ulcers. Patients with ischemia should undergo revascularization surgery.

Adjuvant Agents

- Platelet-derived growth factor-BB that is derived from platelets is useful when applied topically in neuropathic ulcers (Becaplermin is prescribed in neuropathic uniparental disomy in normal blood flow).
- Delivery of fibroblasts through devices in absorbable net
- Delivery of fibroblasts and keratinocytes in collagen type I matrix
- Systemic hyperbaric oxygen therapy reduces the number of amputations in patients with ischemic ulcers.[10,28]

Prevention of Ulcers in Diabetic Patients

Identifying the complications that might arise from diabetes before the appearance of ulcers should be an absolute priority in prevention.

- *Blood pressure deficiency*: Limb pulse, rate arm/ankle, rate arm/foot, echo Doppler color, transcutaneous oxygen pressure
- *Neuropathy (Semmes-Weinstein monofilament 10 g):* Clinical examination of lower limbs, look for presence of deformities in feet and alterations in sensitivity (pain, touch, vibration) in both limbs.
- *Laboratory*: Values of HbA1c are related to risk in developing a diabetic ulcer and delay in healing.[33]

Examination of Feet

Annual checkups are recommended (high-risk patients more often).

Looking for anatomical deformities, dry skin, fissures, calluses, corns, plantar warts, diseased nails, ingrown toenails, fungal infections, alterations in sensitivity and blood pressure deficiency. Shoes should conform to needs.[11] Check for calluses, mainly those with hemorrhage as they signal the onset of a wound and ulceration of feet. Getting rid of calluses decreases the pressure on the sole.

Onycomycosis affects one-third of patients with diabetes and the afflicted nails host bacteria that may cause skin infections. These nails must be treated.

Care of the Feet

Proper hygiene, care of nails and daily inspection. Adequate shoes with protection and/or padding if there is risk of ulcers.

Education

Patients, doctors and health workers, who care for them, should be taught about care of the feet. The end result will be to identify those patients at risk of developing diabetic feet[34-36] (Table 3).

SUMMARY

The aims in caring for the chronic ulcer in a diabetic foot are the following:
- Treatment of the associated infection
- Revascularization when recommended and possible

TABLE 3: Modified risk classification of diabetic foot by IWGDF (International Working Group on the Diabetic Foot); the greater the group, the higher the risk.

Criteria	Description
Group 0	Without peripheral neuropathy Without peripheral occlusive arterial disease
Group 1	Peripheral neuropathy
Group 2	Peripheral occlusive arterial disease
Group 3	History of ulceration
Group 4	History of amputation

- Lowering pressure in order to minimize trauma at site of an ulcer
- Wound management to promote scarring.

Main principles in treatment of wounds are the most basic:
- Regular inspection
- Cleansing hygiene
- Debridement
- Protection of scar tissue from harmful environmental factors.

REFERENCES

1. World Health Organization. (2015). Diabetes Fact Sheet n 312. January 2015 www.who.int
2. Diabetes atlas 2014 update. International Diabetes Federation. www.idf.org
3. Danaei G, Finucane MM, Lu Y, et al. National, regional, and global trends in fasting plasma glucose and diabetes prevalence since 1980: systematic analysis of health examination surveys and epidemiological studies with 370 country-years and 2·7 million participants. Lancet. 2011;378:31-40.
4. King H, Aubert RE, Herman WH. Global burden of diabetes, 1995-2025: prevalence, numerical estimates, and projections. Diabetes Care. 1998;21:1414-31.
5. Zimmet P, Alberti KG, Shaw J. Global and societal implications of the diabetes epidemic. Nature. 2001;414:782-7.
6. Centers for Disease Control and Prevention. National diabetes fact sheet: national estimates and general information on diabetes and prediabetes in the United States, 2011. Atlanta, GA: U.S. Department of Health and Human Services, Centers for Disease Control and Prevention, 2011.
7. Guzmán JR, Lyra R, Aguilar-Salinas CA, et al. Treatment of type 2 diabetes in Latin America: a consensus statement by the medical associations of 17 Latin American countries. Rev Panam Salud Publica. 2010;28(6):463-71.
8. Alavi A, Sibbald RG, Mayer D, et al. Diabetic foot ulcers: Part I. Pathophysiology and prevention. J Am Acad Dermatol. 2014;70:1.e1-18.
9. Boulton AJ, Vileikyte L, Ragnarson-Tennvall G, et al. The global burden of diabetic foot disease. Lancet. 2005;366:1719-24.
10. Prompers L, Huijberts M, Schaper N, et al. Resource utilisation and costs associated with the treatment of diabetic foot ulcers. Prospective data from the Eurodiale Study. Diabetologia. 2008;51(10):1826-34.
11. Ndip A, Ebah L, Mbako A. Neuropathic diabetic foot ulcers – evidence-to-practice. Int J Gen Med. 2012;5:129-34.
12. Steed D, Attinger C, Brem H, et al. Guidelines for the prevention of diabetic ulcers. Wound Rep Reg. 2008;16:169-74.
13. Schreml S, Szeimies RM, Prantl L, et al. Wound healing in the 21st century. J Am Acad Dermatol. 2010;63:866-81.
14. Troielli PA, et al, Curación de heridas. Act Terap Dermatol. 1995;18:43-51.
15. Gallagher KA, Liu ZJ, Xiao M, et al. Diabetic impairments in NO-mediated endothelial progenitor cell mobilization and homing are reversed by hyperoxia and SDF-1 alpha. J Clin Invest. 2007;117(5):1249-59.
16. Spravchikov N, Sizyakov G, Gartsbein M, et al. Glucose effects on skin keratinocytes: implications for diabetes skin complications. Diabetes. 2001 Jul;50(7):1627-35.
17. Velander P, Theopold C, Hirsch T, et al. Impaired wound healing in an acute diabetic pig model and the effects of local hyperglycemia Wound Repair Regen. 2008;16:288-93.

18. Arya AK, Pokharia D, Tripathi K. Relationship between oxidative stress and apoptotic markers in lymphocytes of diabetic patients with chronic non healing wound. Diabetes Res Clin Pract. 2011;94:377-84.
19. Arya AK, Tripathi R, Kumar S, et al. Recent advances on the association of apoptosis in chronic non healing diabetic wound. World J Diabetes. 2014;5:756-62.
20. da Silva L, Carvalho E, Cruz MT. Role of neuropeptides in skin inflammation and its involvement in diabetic wound healing. Expert Opin Biol Ther. 2010;10(10): 1427-39.
21. Weinstein D, Kirsner RS. Refractory ulcers: The role of tumor necrosis factor-alpha. J Am Acad Dermatol. 2010;63:146-54.
22. Brem H, Tomic-Canic M. Cellular and molecular basis of wound healing in diabetes. J Clin Invest. 2007;117:1219-22.
23. Liu ZJ, Velazquez OC. Hyperoxia, endothelial progenitor cell mobilization, and diabetic wound healing. Antioxid Redox Signal. 2008;10:1869-82.
24. Bermudez D, Herdrich BJ, Xu J, et al. Impaired Biomechanical Properties of Diabetic Skin. Am J Pathol. 2011;178:2215-23.
25. Margolis DJ, Allen-Taylor L, Hoffstad O, et al. Diabetic neuropathic foot ulcers: the association of wound size, wound duration, and wound grade on healing. Diabetes Care. 2002;25:1835-9.
26. American Diabetes Association. Standards of medical care in diabetes. Diabetes Care. 2011;34(Suppl 1):S11-61.
27. National Institute for Health and Clinical Excellence (2011). Clinical Guideline 119. Diabetic foot problems: Inpatient management of diabetic foot problems. [online] Available from https://www.nice.org.uk/guidance/cg119?unl id=6622543172015122693533. [Accessed January 2017]
28. Steed D, Attinger C, Colaizzi T, et al. Guidelines for the treatment of diabetic ulcers. Wound Repair Regen. 2006;14:680-92.
29. Fonder M, Lazarus GS, Cowan DA, et al. Treating the chronic wound: A practical approach to the care of nonhealing wounds and wound care dressings. J Am Acad Dermatol. 2008;58:185-206.
30. Skórkowska-Telichowska K, Czemplik M, Kulma A, et al. The local treatment and available dressings designed for chronic wounds. J Am Acad Dermatol. 2013 Apr;68(4):e117-26.
31. Alavi A, Sibbald RG, Mayer D, et al. Diabetic foot ulcers. Part II. Management. J Am Acad Dermatol. 2014;70:21.e1-24.
32. Hinchliffe RJ, Valk GD, Apelqvist J, et al. Specific guidelines on wound and wound-bed management. Diabetes Metab Res Rev. 2008;24(Suppl 1):S188-9.
33. Christman AL, Selvin E, Margolis DJ, et al. Hemoglobin A1c is a predictor of healing rate in diabetic wounds. J Invest Dermatol. 2011;131(10):2121-7.
34. Lavery LA, Peters EJ, Williams JR, et al. Reevaluating the way we classify the diabetic foot. Restructuring the diabetic foot risk classification system of the International Working Group on the Diabetic Foot. Diabetes Care. 2008;31:154-6.
35. Nather A, Siok Bee C, Keng Lin W, et al. Value of team approach combined with clinical pathway for diabetic foot problems: a clinical evaluation. Diabet Foot Ankle. 2010;1:5731.
36. Orsted HL, Searles GE, Trowell H, et al. Best practice recommendations for the prevention, diagnosis, and treatment of diabetic foot ulcers: update 2006. Adv Skin Wound Care. 2007;20:655-69.

CHAPTER
14

Multidisciplinary Approach in Managing Wound Healing

Anahi Belatti, Noelia Capellato, Maria Gala Santini Araujo

INTRODUCTION

It is a well-established fact that diabetic patients with feet injuries have a higher risk of amputations and death compared with the general population.[1] The therapeutic approach of diabetic foot should be interdisciplinary, calling for multiple medical specialties.[2] The identification and correction of the metabolic, neuropathic, ischemic and infectious components are essential for each patient, as well as a jointly approach which considers first the patient as a whole, secondly the affected limb and finally the particular wound.

Successful treatment requires a correct initial assessment that stands as the first step to identify the patient's pathological components.

METABOLIC COMPONENT

Sustained hyperglycemia in diabetic patients with poor metabolic control generates nonenzymatic glycosylation of proteins and non-advanced glycosylation products primarily responsible for tissue alterations in these patients.[3]

From the point of view of management, it is important to consider the need for insulin therapy when dealing with diabetic foot ulcers, given that this hormone is a pro-metabolic hormone and its deficiency commits the trophic responses of the patients. It is demonstrated that insulin plays a key role in keratinocyte differentiation and proliferation, and hence its deficiency leads to impaired healing among other complications.[4]

VASCULAR COMPONENT

Vascular alteration in diabetic patients is usually both macro- and microvascular,[5] and 85% of diabetic foot lesions is caused by neuroischemia.[6] The medical team, regardless which medical specialty, should recognize the character of urgency on a limb with critical ischemia and therefore act quickly to avoid amputation of the limb or part of it.

When examining a diabetic patient, palpation of pulses complemented with an arterial Doppler scan should never be missed. The addition of an ankle-brachial index measurement, which is a long-term prognosis vascular marker,[6] is of aid in spite of some limitations occurring when there is nonocclusive calcification of the arterial wall, known as Monckeberg sclerosis. This condition is not rare in these patients.[7]

Vascular assessment by a specialist in the field is required in order to determine if the patient may be submitted to a vascular intervention given that the gold standard for the management of ischemic patients with diabetic foot is the revascularization of the limb.[8]

In the last 15 years, the increasing use of endovascular therapy (angioplasty), which allows reaching distal territories, has improved the chances of successful revascularization in patients with critical limb ischemia. This practice is considered less risky than conventional bypass, particularly in patients with associated comorbidities, risk factors and poor life expectancy, as in most diabetic patients.[9]

INFECTIOUS COMPONENT

Infections delay healing processes[10] and can threaten the affected limb and the patient's life. As in other chronic wounds, cutaneous infections in diabetic foot must be suspected when clinical manifestations of delayed healing occur, or when an increase in the size or pain associated to the wound and changes in the exudate or color are observed, among others.

Critical colonization of a wound increases not only the metabolic requirements of cells included within, but also neutrophil chemotaxis and oxygen consumption by bacterial colonies in the biofilm that generate the detention of normal healing processes and favor tissue destruction.[10]

It is important to underline that infectious processes often occur without major systemic repercussion. Therefore, it is considered essential to reach an accurate etiological diagnosis with a correct tissue biopsy for culture, that is to say, biopsy per gram of tissue. A germ concentration higher than 10^6 allows the diagnoses of wound infection.[11]

For the management of this condition and according to the characteristics of the patient and the wound in particular, one must take into account the rational use of antiseptics, the debridement that allows mechanical removal of the biofilm and tissue sampling, and the use of local antibiotics, bacteriostatic dressings and systemic antibiotics as indicated in each case.

There is no laboratory data in critical colonization suggesting infection, whereas in osteomyelitis, we can find increased levels of erythrocyte sedimentation rate or reactive C protein.[12]

Diagnostic medical imaging is a useful tool for the diagnosis of foreign bodies, abscesses, collections and the presence of osteomyelitis that may be negatively contributing to the healing of a particular wound.

NEUROPATHIC COMPONENT

Although infections and ischemia are frequent and serious complications of diabetic foot, neuropathy is the most prevalent. Peripheral neuropathy is present in almost 80% of patients with diabetic foot ulcers and represents the main risk factor for the development of wounds at this level.[13] This component is considered mixed because it affects both motor and sensory and autonomic systems. We will give special attention to this throughout the chapter.

Sensory neuropathy causes loss of protective foot sensitivity. Thus, mechanical, chemical or thermal injuries go unnoticed and traumatic skin injuries may appear generating ulcers.

Autonomic neuropathy (neurovegetative) is responsible for anhydrosis and cutaneous atrophy[14] that leads to xerosis and thinning of the skin with subsequent formation of fissures and hyperkeratosis. These phenomena lead to skin breakdown, which is considered a pre-ulcerative condition and often represents the gateway for bacteria or fungi that will produce local or systemic infections.

Motor neuropathy is closely related to various disorders of the foot shape and its support. This is why fundamentals of prevention and treatment of diabetic foot are based on downloading and prevention of excessive pressure, with the correct use of templates, shoes according to each patient's need, and total contact casts, among other elements for the redistribution of pressures.

A foot with these structural alterations will be subject to continuous rubbing of the footwear (often wrongly adapted) and the repetitive stress associated with gait on an insensitive limb with support abnormalities. Together with dry skin and fissures, the result is the development of traumatic injuries, calluses and hyperkeratosis with subsequent ulceration.

All these changes acting jointly determine the appearance of skin lesions in the forefoot sole on the metatarsal heads and the hallux interphalangeal joint area more frequently.

The loss of skin barrier integrity in a diabetic foot, due to either a superficial erosion caused by interdigital mycotic intertrigo, a blister, a callus or an ulcer, should make us think in all the aforementioned pathogenic components acting together.

This is why we point out that avoiding weight bearing is to a diabetic foot what rotation and pressure management is to the prevention of pressure ulcers.

The strategy of comprehensive assessment is dynamic. While taking into account several distinct components, it is important to identify the stage in which the ulcer is and to develop an ability to choose the best treatment at all times.

In short, the interdisciplinary management of diabetic foot should include the assessment of risk factors, vascular evaluation with revascularization whenever necessary or possible, control of infections, management of weight bearing, a proper skincare and a local treatment of the wound.

LOCAL APPROACH TO WOUND HEALING

It is well known that wound healing implies a sequence of regulated molecular and cellular events that aim to restore the integrity of the damaged tissue.[15]

The three sequential phases of normal healing in a wound are: 1) Hemostasis and inflammation, 2) Proliferation, and 3) Repair. They are regulated by multiple growth factors that are vital for the differentiation, proliferation and metabolism of the cells within the wound.[15] These growth factors are polypeptides that control the healing process by binding to specific receptors, thereby stimulating cell mitosis within the wound.

Diabetic patients alter these healing processes, and the latest studies[16] have demonstrated that they have local deficiency of growth factors, less polymorphonuclear activity and reduced expression of the extracellular matrix (receptor glycosylation of the fibroblast growth factor, which is involved in the angiogenesis, proliferation of fibroblasts and keratinocytes). Furthermore, there is insufficient formation of granulation tissue due to inadequate fibroblast functionality.[17,18]

After a comprehensive evaluation of the patient, and considering the existing alterations in the normal wound healing process of a diabetic foot, wounds can be subdivided according to their closure as shown in Flowchart 1.

- *Healable ulcers:* Ulcers located on a limb with adequate blood oxygen supply in a patient with controlled disease and good chances of wound closure
- *Non-healable ulcers:* Ulcers that lack adequate arterial blood supply and will not be able to heal unless local arterial circulation is restored. In this case, dry wound healing with antiseptics on the necrotic tissue would be an adequate treatment until the final vascular treatment is defined.
- *Maintenance ulcers:* Ulcers with adequate vascular arterial supply but with other factors that may impair healing such as anemia, malnutrition, significant immunosuppression, lack of adherence to treatment due to psychosocial reasons, etc. All these variables are reversible and healing will only be possible if the aforementioned factors are corrected.[19]

Flowchart 1: Wounds in patients with diabetic foot.

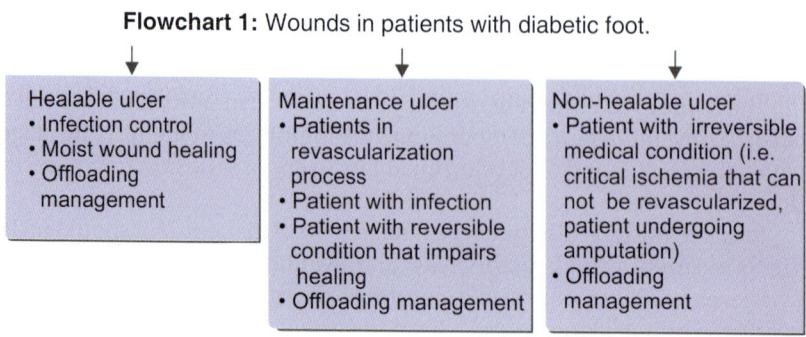

In relation to the management of ulcers with no healing capacity due to compromised arterial supply or in maintenance ulcers pending revascularization, both active surgical debridement and the use of products that preserve the moisture balance of the wound (moist wound healing) are contraindicated because they can worsen the clinical manifestations. In such cases, the purpose of medical treatment is to prevent infection and enlargement of the wounds with everyday antiseptics, avoid local humidity, and provide maintenance treatment with dessication of the necrotic tissue.

The current paradigm of wound healing follows the idea of nontraumatic tissue management in order to keep cellular vitality in the wound bed and avoid maneuvers of excessive rubbing or profuse and abrasive washes.[20,21] In order to pursue this paradigm, two basic concepts for local management of wounds arise:
1. Avoidance of classic antiseptics
2. Moist wound healing.[22]

OFFLOADING

The proposed strategy to provide an integral treatment of diabetic foot ulcers during the orthopedic examination includes a proper assessment of the axes and overload prevention.

Orthotic insoles are essential to avoid ulcers. The physician who provides an appropriate offloading will enable a good and quick closure of the latter. A weight-bearing ulcer is not a well-treated ulcer.

There are different useful approaches, depending on the location of the ulcer. If it is located on the dorsal part of the foot, other types of footwear will be required rather than a plantar one. In the literature, a systematic review[23] supports the use of nonremovable devices as the most reliable method for treating neuropathic plantar ulcers.

Types of Offloading Devices

Total Contact Cast

This method is considered the gold standard[24] for plantar ulcer treatment. However, it is used only in 1.7% of worldwide centers, according to some reports.[25] Most healing clinics do not have a healthcare professional or technician available to apply a total contact cast. Moreover, the implementation of the technique is time-consuming and the learning period is long.

Advantages:
- Transfers 30% of the leg's load directly to plaster walls
- Decreases 28% of forefoot pressures.

Disadvantages:[26]
- Sometimes, the cast slides along the leg causing thigh lacerations in the edges during knee bending.
- If the cast is applied too tight over the finger level, it may cause pressure lesions.

- If the cast layers are applied too lightly in overweight patients, the material may collapse.
- Placing the cast improperly using finger pressure may cause dents that in turn generate pressure on the skin.
- If the foot has insufficient dorsiflexion, improperly increased loads may be generated (Fig. 1).

Irremovable Pneumatic Boots

These boots are irremovable pneumatic walking braces, which are used with protective inner soles and "locked" by seals placed by the physician to improve patient's adherence to treatment.

Removable Boots

Within this group, there are specific pneumatic braces ideally used for diabetic patients (Fig. 2). They can be used with protective inner soles or felted foam dressings adapted to each patient's ulcer.

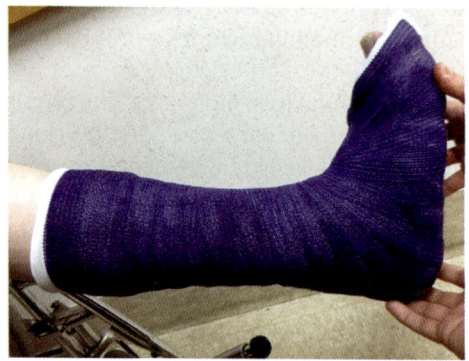

Fig. 1: Total contact cast.

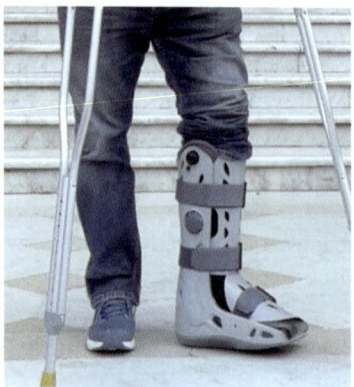

Fig. 2: Removable boots.

Advantage:
- The wounds that require frequent administration of topical products may be inspected as often as necessary for this purpose.

Disadvantages:
- Statistical studies confirm that patients do most of their daily activities without the boot in 72% of cases.[26] This fact reinforces the importance of patient education as the mainstay of ulcer treatment.
- Due to high costs and lack of health insurance coverage, the use of these kinds of devices only reaches to 15.2%.[25]

Healing Sandals, Half-shoes, Inner-soles and Therapeutic Shoes

There are many types of offloading sandals. Some of them have several types of wedges in order to prevent overloading different parts of the foot (Figs. 3A to C).

Compared to total contact casts and removable pneumatic boots, the use of sandals takes more time to heal the ulcers and the closure rate is less.[27] They can be used along with inner soles like, for instance, honeycomb-type soles, where cells are released into the ulcer area for relief of selective pressures, or three-density insoles in which the offload discharge is tailored by the physician to fit the ulcer. Custom-made insoles may be used too. These same inner soles may be used in pneumatic boots as well as in sandals (Figs. 4A to C). When using a healing sandal, physicians should be aware that it is important to prevent contralateral foot lesions with proper footwear.

Padded Adhesive Felts and Foams

The felt is cut to support the areas around the ulcer so as to keep it pressure free. Then, a layer of foam could be applied on top of the felt. The wound dressing material may be used in place of the foam over the ulcer site taking care that it is not as thick as the protective felt. A hypoallergenic fabric tape is used to secure the edges of the dressing.

There are few published studies with scarce results addressing the offload method over the total contact cast. It requires serial cures, nursing, and family and patient training for padding techniques.

When performing offloading with felts, it is necessary to consider the "edge effect",[28] which may increase the shear and pressure on the periphery of the wound. Discharges need to be performed by personnel with biomechanical knowledge to avoid overload of other areas.

Modified Usual Footwear

There is evidence that this method (which is not ideal but is widely used due to lack of resources or lack of patient acceptance of proper devices that truly offload pressure) might be useful for ulcers located on the dorsal part of the foot.[25] This is another example of why educating and negotiating with the patient is essential for the healing of diabetic foot ulcers. Crutches, walking sticks, walkers and wheelchairs may also be used to decrease pressure. However, when using these devices, physicians must take into account that:

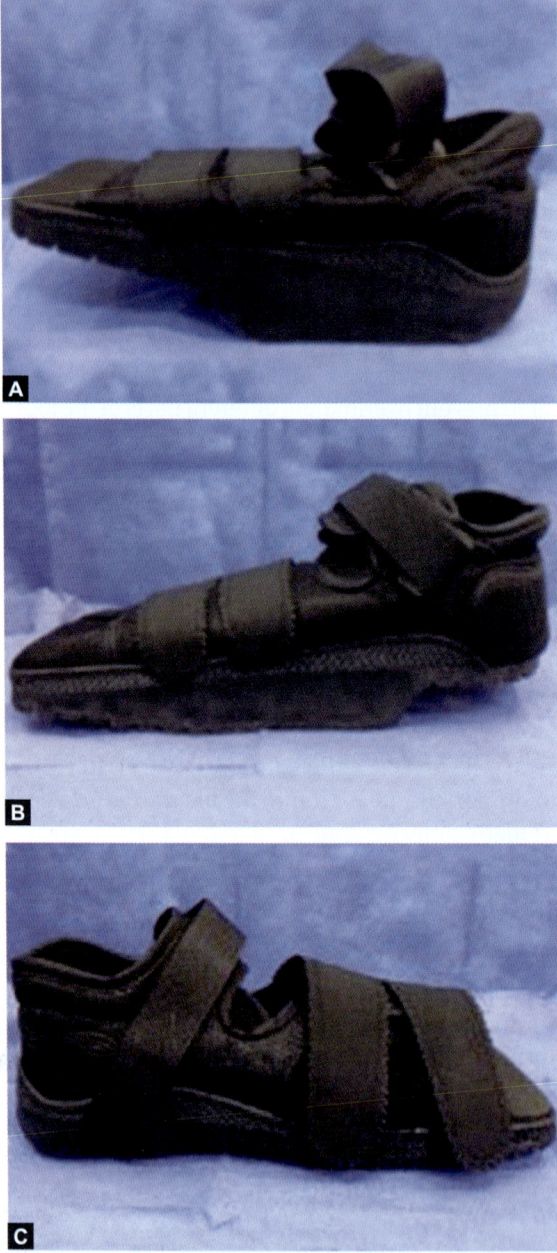

Figs. 3A to C: Sandals. (A) Forefoot offloading; (B) Hindfoot offloading; (C) Regular healing sandal.

- Diabetic patients need to be monitored for nerve compression injuries to the arms when using crutches
- Crutches must be measured correctly in order to determine the proper length

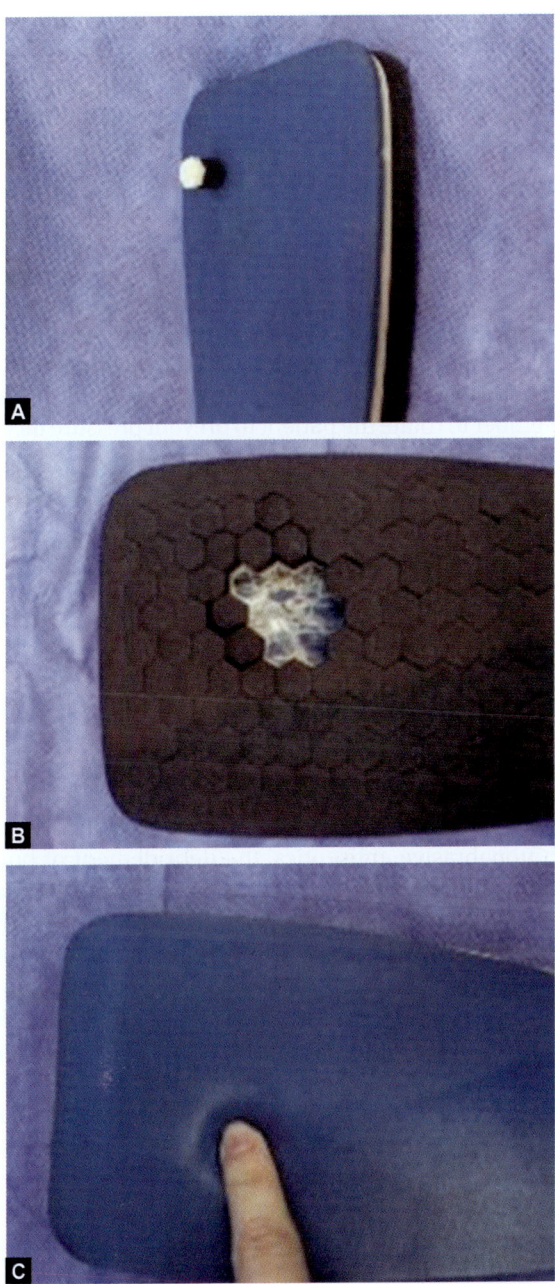

Figs. 4A to C: (A) Inner sole for sandal or removable boot use; (B and C) The offloading is tailored by the specialist.

- When a wheelchair was chosen, take care that the patient does not place the foot for rest over the Achilles tendon as well as any other sensitive part of the body to avoid a pressure ulcer.

FOOTWEAR AFTER HEALING

Footwear with proper insoles for plantar forefoot ulcers is essential to avoid recurrence and prevent new ulcerations. The shoes need extra depth in order to adapt the inner sole. Also, the shoe box should be sufficiently high and wide.

The shoes should not have seams that may cause friction inside. The materials of the inner soles must be soft and adapted to the contour of the patient's foot.

OFFLOADING THE ULCERATED PATIENT IN HOSPITAL

It is important to protect not only the ulcerated area but also to prevent new ulcers. Pay attention to the heel support or the sides of the foot when the patient is in bed. Remember to rotate the patient to prevent pressure ulcers. Check the shoes that are used to move around the hospital room.

ASSESSMENT PRIOR TO TREATMENT

- Localization, size and depth of the wound
- Characteristics of the wound bed (necrotic, fibrinous, granulating, etc.)
- General looks and amount of the exudate
- Perilesional area (erythema, maceration, hyperkeratosis, etc.)
- Ischemic and neuropathic pain.

LOCAL TREATMENT

For a proper local wound management, we should be able to provide a correct cleaning with nonabrasive antiseptics, the debridement of both callus and devitalized tissue of the wound bed, and the control of infections and moisture balance of the wound.

The ideal solutions for cleaning wounds in diabetic foot must have low cytotoxicity levels. Isotonic saline solution meets this condition and is indicated in all diabetic foot wounds. Soaps and classic antiseptics should be avoided as they change the pH of the wound bed, interfering with cell proliferation and generating cytotoxicity.[20-22]

There are low-toxicity antiseptics, such as those containing biguanides or chlorhexidine at low concentration, that have proven to be safe and effective in nontraumatic cleaning of chronic wounds.[21]

For local wound assessment, the acronym TIME is used (Flowchart 2 and Figs. 5A to D).

Debridement

Diabetic foot ulcer debridement has a relevant role and should be done only if the limb has an adequate blood supply, discarding ischemia.[29] This procedure is associated with higher healing rates, as it promotes removal of necrotic tissue, biofilm and allows wound granulation.[29]

Flowchart 2: Local wound assessment.

T	Tissue • Evaluation of the tissue in the wound bed	Action Debridement
I	Infection–inflammation	Action Bacterial load management Perilesional eczema control
M	Moisture	Action Exudate control
E	Epithelialization	Action Promote closure

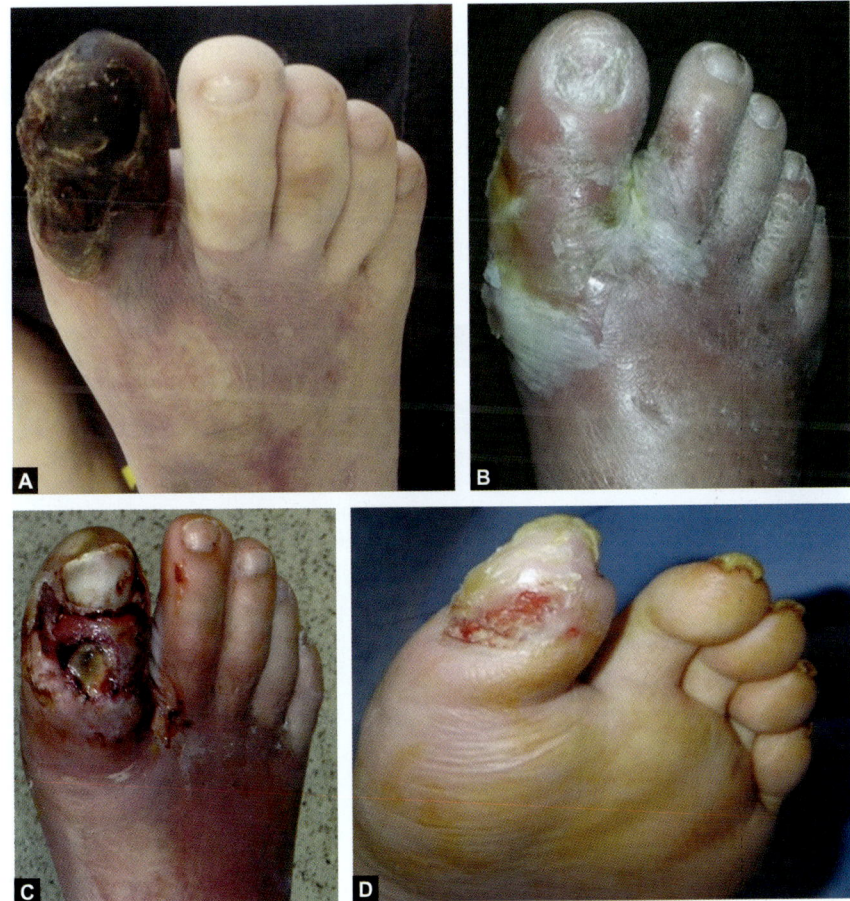

Figs. 5A to D: (A) Debridement of the tissue in the wound bed; (B) Management of bacterial load; (C) Management of the exudate; (D) Epithelization.

In the office, when a neuropathic diabetic foot is present, it is important to debride existing helomas in order to reduce injury-leading frictional forces, and also reduce plantar pressure at specific points which, as a consequence, decreases the risk of neuropathic ulcers. It has been shown that keratinocytes located in the edge of a hyperkeratotic wound have less proliferative and migration capacity. In the epidermis of these lesions, there are less receptors for epidermal growth factor, reducing keratinocyte response[30] (Table 1).

Management of Infection-inflammation

Every patient with diabetic foot injuries should be monitored by an infectious disease specialist. More than half of the patients with diabetes develop soft tissue infections,[22] usually multi-bacterial, which generate high rates of hospitalization and frequent amputations. Clinically, skin, soft tissue and bone infections in the diabetic foot overlap, lacking in most cases' systemic symptoms. This is the reason why high suspicion is required.[11]

Apart from the aforementioned debridement, the main goal in local management of diabetic foot injuries is to reduce bacterial load. For this purpose, there are new nonabrasive antiseptics containing surfactants, low doses of chlorhexidine, biguanides and hexamidine. A cadexomer iodine product is also available in different presentations, providing moisture balance with antimicrobial action by sustained release of iodine while a desloughing action is provided by the cadexomer matrix.[31]

TABLE 1: Types of debridement.

Method	Surgical debridement	Enzymatic debridement	Autolytic debridement	Biologic debridement
Indications	Extensive necrotic areas Infections	Necrotic and slough wound bed	Necrotic and dry wound bed Cavitated ulcers Bone exposure	Necrotic wound bed Infected wound lesions
Characteristics	• Nonselective • Reactivation of a chronic wound • Painful • Fast results	• Selective • Not painful • Slow result	• Selective • Not painful • Slow result	• Selective • Can be painful • Intermediate result
		Contraindicated in tendon exposure		Contraindicated in vessels or organ exposure
Methods	• Scalpel • Curettage	• Collagenase • Papain	• Hydrogels	• Steril larvae (*Lucilia sericata*)

A precise indication for etiological diagnoses of a local soft tissue infection consists in taking a sample for culture per gram of tissue, given that swab culture aspiration biopsy samples are less specific in identifying the causative organism.[11]

The use of topical antibiotics is indicated in cases of critical colonization for short periods not exceeding 15 days. Within the topical antibiotic therapy spectrum, we may find fusidic acid 2% and silver sulfadiazine. The use of mupirocin 2% should be spared and reserved only for the treatment of colonization by methicillin-resistant *Staphylococcus aureus*.[22]

A positive semiological "probe to bone" sign orients us to the diagnosis of osteomyelitis in most cases.[32] However, magnetic resonance imaging is recommended, bearing in mind that the final diagnosis should involve microbiological and anatomopathological studies of bone biopsy in order to assess and correlate the different results.[33] An elevated erythrocyte sedimentation rate and C-reactive protein levels represent extra information that, although not specific, is considered valuable.[12] An antibiogram is necessary for specific antibiotic treatment selection.

Wound Moisture Control

Diabetic foot ulcers are rarely exudative lesions. However, certain complications predispose to excessive moisture in the wound area, such as infection (wet gangrene) and critical ischemia in which the patient puts down the limb in an antalgic position generating edema and exudate. In these circumstances, the treatment aims to target the underlying causes and the preservation of the perilesional area using barrier films.

Epithelization

In order to achieve epithelization, we must ensure that granulation in the bottom of the wound reaches the surface, filling the defect. This serves as a scaffolding used by keratinocytes to grow towards the center of the wound favoring its closure.

A dressing provides the wound a protective barrier that helps maintain stable pH levels, moisture balance and temperature according to the homeostasis of the wound.

There are numerous products available in the market to promote moist wound healing, therefore ensuring granulation of wounds; the most versatile in the opinion of the authors is calcium alginate as it promotes cell migration, has a bacteriostatic effect, is biodegradable and can be used to fill wound defects including undermining and tunneling (Fig. 6).

Once the wound becomes superficial, the epithelization phase begins, which can be supported by multiple dressings (meeting the goals established by the paradigm of moist wound healing), allowing the newly synthetized keratinocytes to inhibit a nontraumatic wound bed. These include collagen patches, maltodextrin, lyophilized hyaluronic acid and extra-thin hydrocolloid patches, among others (Table 2).

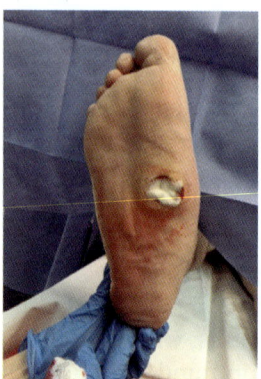

Fig. 6: Use of alginate in a diabetic ulcer.

TABLE 2: Dressings and their actions.	
Product	Main action
Hydrogel	Low exudate Debridement
Hydrocolloid	Low exudate Granulation Epithelization
Alginate	Moderate exudate Granulation Hemostasis
Hydrofiber	High exudate Granulation
Maltodextrin	Low exudate Granulation Epithelization
Hyaluronic acid	Moderate exudate Granulation Epithelization
Collagenase	Debridement Granulation Epithelization

In brief, choosing a dressing will depend on the wound size, depth, amount of exudate, associated pain and infectious status, following the outlines established by the acronym "TIME" (*see* dressings and main functions).

ADVANCED WOUND THERAPIES

These methods should be considered when wounds show no progress (despite having ruled out causes that could be contributing to an impaired healing and after an integral patient assessment), and also in patients with tendon, bone and/or joint exposure. It is important because these situations require quick reparation.

Multiple studies have demonstrated that advanced wound therapy used in a timely fashion and associated with a correct local management promotes healing in diabetic foot.[34]

The treatments considered as advanced wound therapies nowadays are the following:
- Autologous skin grafts
- Growth factors
- Negative pressure therapy
- Matrices or scaffolds
- Hyperbaric chamber.

Growth Factors

These are biologically active polypeptides that have the ability to alter the cell signal transduction cascade in the wound.
- *Becaplermin* is a recombinant human platelet growth factor. It is considered the only non-sterile topical gel approved by the FDA for treatment of diabetic foot free from vascular component.[35] It is used daily on the wound bed and requires cold chain.
  It has been demonstrated that it improves healing rates compared to standard treatment.[35] Although there are some reports of increased cancer mortality with the use of more than three tubes, other studies with follow-ups for over 6 years have not found statistically significant results.[36]
- *Recombinant human epidermal growth factor* is available in lyophilized form for intralesional or perilesional use. This product promotes granulation. It is indicated with good results for neuropathic or ischemic (Wagner grade 3-4) diabetic foot.[37,38] Note that it is contraindicated in unstable cardiac disease, diabetic ketoacidosis and history of malignancy, and its use should not exceed 8 weeks.

Platelet-rich Plasma

Currently, platelet-rich plasma is a widespread technique due to the ease of sample collection and for being a relatively cheap resource. It is a platelet concentrate superior to baseline within a limited volume of plasma. This hemoderivative has multiple growth factors contained in the platelet alpha granules, being the most relevant: transforming growth factor beta (TGF-beta), platelet-derived growth factor (PDGF), insulin-like growth factor 1 (IGF-1), fibroblast growth factor (FGF), epidermal growth factor (EGF), vascular endothelial growth factor (VEGF), and endothelial cell growth factor (ECGF).[39-43]

These factors increase cell migration, proliferation of stem cells and fibroblasts, stimulate the collagen synthesis, the angiogenesis and modulate chronic inflammation due to chemotactic faculties over macrophages.[39-43]

Negative Pressure Systems

Negative pressure devices transfer a subatmospheric pressure to the wound, promoting granulation, cell proliferation, and stimulating angiogenesis and control of the exudate.[44]

Its use in diabetic foot ulcers has shown benefits with higher cure rates than those observed with conventional cure, achieving granulation tissue faster than the average, being very useful to cover areas with bone or tendon exposure. It is also useful for surgical dehiscence of the stump.[31]

There are multiple technologies available ranging from institutional devices to modern models for ambulatory use. In recent years, a hybrid between a dressing and a negative pressure system of even easier applicability was designed.

Hyperbaric Oxygen

Hyperbaric oxygen involves the exposure to 100% oxygen. The hyperbaric environment in which the body is located is subjected to pressures greater than or equal to 1.4 atm during a stipulated time. Under these physical effects, it is possible to increase free oxygen transport in the plasma,[31] and the arrival of the flow will be directly proportional to the extent of collateral vasculature developed by the patient at the time of treatment. For monitoring purposes, oxygen transcutaneous oximetry assesses the results before and after each session.

According to evidence-based medicine, the hyperbaric oxygen requires better methodological quality studies to achieve categorical conclusions. Nevertheless, up to this day, multiple expert groups suggest this therapy for cases such as patients with diabetic foot ulcers due to vascular components, adjunct therapy to revascularization, patients that cannot be revascularized, and patients with infectious complications and osteomyelitis.[45]

Skin Substitutes

In recent years, the industry has developed skin substitutes, scaffolds or skin equivalents which may be cellular or acellular and promote wound healing in different ways. These can be epidermal, dermal or combined, derived from animals (pig, cattle), human, synthetic or compounds. Some of them are permanent and become integrated to the wound, and others serve as cover and need to be removed.[46] They have the objective to temporarily or permanently replace the structure and function of the skin, and showed a decrease in cure time rates, reducing the contraction and retraction of the wound, improving the function, and lowering morbidity compared to other invasive treatments such as grafts.

Scaffolds are fibrous matrices composed of hyaluronic acid, collagen or fibronectin and can be acellular. In contact with the wound bed, they nurture from it, filling their fibrous cells/compartments with liquid matrix. The endogenous cells are then integrated to the matrix regenerating the tissue through cell infiltration and neovascularization.

There are also cellular matrices containing living cells such as keratinocytes and fibroblasts inside the matrix. These can be autologous, allogeneic or of other species.[46] It is essential to note that the choice of the matrix will be determined by the availability and the characteristics of the wound bed, which should be in optimal conditions to receive it. In all cases, a nontraumatic cleaning of the wound should be performed and then place the matrix in an ideal wound bed, a granulating and vital one, preserving adequate moisture to avoid drying. Critical colonization and local infection must be resolved before the application.

CONCLUSION

In the management of diabetic foot ulcers the understanding of the pathophysiological factors that lead to injury is considered essential in order to solve them with a comprehensive approach.

These patients have pathological conditions that require the intervention of an interdisciplinary team composed of nutritionists, dermatologists, orthopedic surgeons, endocrinologists, vascular surgeons, cardiologists, infectologists, podiatrists, nurses, orthotic professionals and prosthetists, working together with systematic guidelines and developing a transdisciplinary language.

The education of healthcare providers and patients, as well as prevention together with early detection and effective multidisciplinary management of diabetic foot ulcers, are the clues to reduce the severity of complications and the rate of amputation in diabetic foot.

REFERENCES

1. Girach A, Manner D, Porta M. Diabetic microvascular complications: can patients at risk be identified? A review. Int J Clin Pract. 2006;60:1471-83.
2. Center for Diseases Control and Prevention. National diabetes fact sheet: national estimates and general information on diabetes and prediabetes in the United States. 2011.
3. Cohen Sabban E. La glicosilación no enzimática: una vía común en la diabetes y el envejecimiento. Med Cutan Iber Lat Am. 2011;39:243-6.
4. Dandona P, Aljada A, Mohanty P. The anti-inflammatory and potential anti-atherogenic effect of insulin: a new paradigm. Diabetologia. 2002;45:924-30.
5. Boyko EJ, Ahroni JH, Davignon D, et al. Diagnostic utility of the history and physical examination for peripheral vascular disease among patients with diabetes mellitus. J Clin Epidemiol. 1997;50:659-68.
6. Snyder RJ. Controversies regarding vascular disease in the patient with diabetes: a review of the literature. Ostomy Wound Manage. 2007;53:40-8.
7. Libby P. Patogenia de la Ateroesclerosis. In: Harrison. Principios de Medicina Interna Interamericana de España, 15th edition. Madrid: McGraw-Hill Education; 2001.

8. Alexandrescu V-A, Hubermont G, Philips Y, et al. Selective primary angioplasty following an angiosome model of reperfusion in the treatment of Wagner 1-4 diabetic foot lesions: practice in a multidisciplinary diabetic limb service. J Endovasc Ther. 2008;15:580-93.
9. Bedriñana-Gómez M, Quevedo-Rojas E, Rojas-Salinas G, et al. Tratamiento endovascular de angioplastia comparado con angioplastia más colocación de prótesis endovascular metálica en pacientes con pie diabético. Rev Peru Radiol. 2011;15:30-7.
10. Williams DT, Hilton JR, Harding KG. Diagnosing foot infection in diabetes. Clin Infect Dis. 2004;39 (Suppl 2):S83-6.
11. NICE. Diabetic Foot Problems. Inpatient management of diabetic foot problems. (Clinical guideline 119). London: NICE; 2011.
12. Karr JC. The diagnosis of osteomyelitis in diabetes using erythrocyte sedimentation rate. J Am Podiatr Med Assoc. 2002;92:314.
13. Costa Gil J, Fuente G. Diabetes Mellitus: visión latinoamericana. Rio de Janeiro: Guanabara Coogan; 2009.
14. Vinik AI, Freeman R, Erbas T. Diabetic autonomic neuropathy. Semin Neurol. 2003;23:365-72.
15. Park JE, Barbul A. Understanding the role of immune regulation in wound healing. Am J Surg. 2004;187:11S-16S.
16. Jeffcoate WJ, Price P, Harding KG, et al. Wound healing and treatments for people with diabetic foot ulcers. Diabetes Metab Res Rev. 2004;20 (Suppl 1):S78-89.
17. Jude EB, Blakytny R, Bulmer J, et al. Transforming growth factor-beta 1, 2, 3 and receptor type I and II in diabetic foot ulcers. Diabet Med. 2002;19:440-7.
18. Lobmann R, Ambrosch A, Schultz G, et al. Expression of matrix-metalloproteinases and their inhibitors in the wounds of diabetic and non-diabetic patients. Diabetologia. 2002;45:1011-6.
19. Lavery LA, Peters EJG, Williams JR, et al. Reevaluating the way we classify the diabetic foot: restructuring the diabetic foot risk classification system of the International Working Group on the Diabetic Foot. Diabetes Care. 2008;31:154-6.
20. Fernandez R, Griffiths R. Water for wound cleansing. Cochrane database Syst Rev. 2012;2:CD003861.
21. Witkowski JA, Parish LC. Wound cleansers. Clin Dermatol. 1996;14:89-93.
22. Alavi A, Sibbald RG, Mayer D, et al. Diabetic foot ulcers: Part II. Management. J Am Acad Dermatol. 2014;70:21.e1-24; quiz 45-6.
23. Bus SA, van Deursen RW, Armstrong DG, et al. Footwear and offloading interventions to prevent and heal foot ulcers and reduce plantar pressure in patients with diabetes: a systematic review. Diabetes Metab Res Rev. 2015;32 (Suppl 1):99-118.
24. Centers for Disease Control and Prevention (CDC). Lower extremity amputation episodes among persons with diabetes—New Mexico, 2000. MMWR Morb Mortal Wkly Rep. 2003;52:66-8.
25. Lewis J, Lipp A. Pressure-relieving interventions for treating diabetic foot ulcers. Cochrane database Syst Rev. 2013;1:CD002302.
26. Robins H. Offloading the diabetic foot ulcer: podiatry. Wound Heal South Africa. 2008;1:18-20.
27. Boulton J, Cavanagh P, Rayman G. The Foot in Diabetes, 4th edition. Chichester: John Wiley & Sons, Ltd.; 2006.
28. Armstrong DG, Athanasiou KA. The edge effect: how and why wounds grow in size and depth. Clin Podiatr Med Surg. 1998;15:105-8.

29. Steed DL, Donohoe D, Webster MW, et al. Effect of extensive debridement and treatment on the healing of diabetic foot ulcers. Diabetic Ulcer Study Group. J Am Coll Surg. 1996;183:61-4.
30. Lebrun E, Tomic-Canic M, Kirsner RS. The role of surgical debridement in healing of diabetic foot ulcers. Wound Repair Regen. 2010;18:433-8.
31. Contreras Ruiz J. Abordaje y manejo de las heridas. Intersistemas Editores; 2013.
32. Grayson ML, Gibbons GW, Balogh K, et al. Probing to bone in infected pedal ulcers. A clinical sign of underlying osteomyelitis in diabetic patients. JAMA. 1995;273:721-3.
33. Khodaee M, Lombardo D, Montgomery LC, et al. Clinical Inquiry: what's the best test for underlying osteomyelitis in patients with diabetic foot ulcers? J Fam Pract. 2015;64:309-10, 321.
34. Kirsner RS, Warriner R, Michela M, et al. Advanced biological therapies for diabetic foot ulcers. Arch Dermatol. 2010;146:857-62.
35. Gilligan AM, Waycaster CR, Motley TA. Cost-effectiveness of becaplermin gel on wound healing of diabetic foot ulcers. Wound Repair Regen. 2015;23:353-60.
36. Berlanga-Acosta J, Gavilondo-Cowley J, Barco-Herrera DG del, et al. Epidermal Growth Factor (EGF) and Platelet-Derived Growth Factor (PDGF) as Tissue Healing Agents: Clarifying Concerns about their Possible Role in Malignant Transformation and Tumor Progression. J Carcinog Mutagen. 2011;02:115.
37. Yera-Alos IB, Alonso-Carbonell L, Valenzuela-Silva CM, et al. Active post-marketing surveillance of the intralesional administration of human recombinant epidermal growth factor in diabetic foot ulcers. BMC Pharmacol Toxicol. 2013;14:44.
38. Fernández-Montequín JI, Betancourt BY, Leyva-Gonzalez G, et al. Intralesional administration of epidermal growth factor-based formulation (Heberprot-P) in chronic diabetic foot ulcer: treatment up to complete wound closure. Int Wound J. 2009;6:67-72.
39. Knighton DR, Ciresi KF, Fiegel VD, et al. Classification and treatment of chronic nonhealing wounds. Successful treatment with autologous platelet-derived wound healing factors (PDWHF). Ann Surg. 1986;204:322-30.
40. Steed DL, Goslen JB, Holloway GA, et al. Randomized prospective double-blind trial in healing chronic diabetic foot ulcers. CT-102 activated platelet supernatant, topical versus placebo. Diabetes Care. 1992;15:1598-604.
41. Krupski WC, Reilly LM, Perez S, et al. A prospective randomized trial of autologous platelet-derived wound healing factors for treatment of chronic nonhealing wounds: a preliminary report. J Vasc Surg. 1991;14:526-32; discussion 532-6.
42. Baró Pazos F, Alonso Verduras C, Lopez S. Ministerio de Sanidad-servicios sociales e igualdad de España-Informe de la Agencia Española de Medicamentos y Productos Sanitarios sobre el uso de Plasma Rico en Plaquetas. 2013;1-5.
43. Anitua E, Sánchez M, Orive G, et al. The potential impact of the preparation rich in growth factors (PRGF) in different medical fields. Biomaterials. 2007;28: 4551-60.
44. Nain PS, Uppal SK, Garg R, et al. Role of negative pressure wound therapy in healing of diabetic foot ulcers. J Surg Tech Case Rep. 2011;3:17-22.
45. Löndahl M, Katzman P, Nilsson A, et al. Hyperbaric oxygen therapy facilitates healing of chronic foot ulcers in patients with diabetes. Diabetes Care. 2010;33: 998-1003.
46. Debels H, Hamdi M, Abberton K, et al. Dermal matrices and bioengineered skin substitutes: a critical review of current options. Plast Reconstr Surg Glob Open. 2015;3:e284.

Index

Note: Page numbers followed by *f* and *t* indicate figures and tables respectively.

A

Acanthosis nigricans (AN) 73
  benign 75*t*
  generalized 76*t*
  malignant 74*t*
Achilles tendon 65
Acquired immune deficiency syndrome (AIDS) 2
Acquired perforating collagenosis 131
Adhesive capsulitis 53
Adrenal failure 117
Advanced glycation end-products (AGEs) 12, 170
AGEs and aging 172
AGEs-RAGE interaction, inflammation and oxidative stress 171
Aging 167
Alteration of neutrophil mobility 32
American diabetes association (ADA) 2
Antimicrobial peptides 191
Argentine diabetes society 2
Arterial ulcer 152*t*
Association of insulin resistance 2
Atherosclerosis 12
Autoimmune diseases 5
Autoimmune thyroid disease 117
Autoimmunity in diabetes 5

B

Bacterial infections in diabetics 92
  corynebacterium minutissimum 100
  diagnostic evaluation of skin and soft tissue infections 98
  normal skin flora and pathogens 93
  Pseudomonas aeruginosa 101
    ecthyma gangrenosum 101
    malignant otitis externa 101
    onychomycosis 101
  Staphylococcus aureus and beta-hemolytic streptococci 94
  erysipelas 96
  furuncles 97
  impetigo 96
  necrotizing fasciitis 98
  treatment 99
    carriage status 99
    systemic antibiotics 99
    tissue debridement, drainage and wound care 99
    topical treatment 99
Biomechanic alterations 194
B lymphocytes 4
Bullous pemphigoid produced by incretins 145*t*

C

Capillaroscopic alterations 58
Capillaroscopy: periungual erythema 155*t*
Carotenoids 47
Carpal tunnel syndrome 53
Cerebrovascular disease 65
Charcot arthropathy 53
Charcot neuroarthropathy 162*t*
Chronic hyperglycemia 12
Circumscribed pigmentation 137
Class II molecules 4
Clinical signs for limited joint mobility (LJM) 64*f*
Collagen patches 213
Complications of diabetes 11
Cutaneous barrier 15
  alterations in cutaneous barrier in diabetics 22
    alterations of permeability 22
    dermocosmetic management 22
  antioxidants and sunscreens 25
  physiology 15

antimicrobial barrier 20
antioxidant barrier 20
permeability barrier 18
ultraviolet barrier 22
pruritus 26
psychosocial stress 27
topical treatment with lipids 24
  nonphysiological lipids 24
  physiological lipids 24
topical treatment with urea 25
Cutaneous biopsy 65
Cutaneous manifestations 11
Cutaneous manifestations due to diabetic neuropathy 158
  autonomic neuropathy 162
  motor neuropathy 163
  Semmes-Weinstein monofilaments 164
  sensory neuropathy 163
Cutaneous manifestations due to diabetic vasculopathy 149
Cutaneous manifestations induced by antidiabetic treatment 137
  insulin analogues 142
  insulin therapy 137
    insulin allergy 137
    lipodystrophies 139
  non-insulin therapy 142
    non-insulin hypoglycemic agents 142
Cutaneous markers 13
Cutaneous markers of diabetes mellitus 38*f*
Cutaneous necrosis 152*t*
Cutaneous wound healing 188
  inflammation 188
  proliferation 189
  remodeling 190
  stages 188*t*
Cutis rhomboidalis 108*t*
Cystic fibrosis 2

D

Dendritic cells 4
Deoxyribonucleic acid (DNA) 168
Dermatoses related to diabetes 105
  immunological mechanism 117
    bullous pemphigoid 120
    vitiligo 117
  metabolic mechanism 106
    acrochordons 116
    eruptive xanthomas 109

    migratory necrolytic erythema 111
    porphyria cutanea tarda 106
    pruritus 113
  mixed metabolic immunological mechanism 123
    psoriasis 123
  unknown mechanism 126
    acquired perforating dermatosis 131
    Kaposi's sarcoma 130
Dermoepidermal junction 129
Dermoepidermal thickening 58
Diabetes mellitus 1
  classification 2
  diagnosis 1
Diabetes mellitus and its effects on the skin 173
Diabetes mellitus and non-enzymatic glycation 172
Diabetes mellitus diagnostic criteria 2
Diabetic blister 44
Diabetic dermopathy 42
Diabetic foot syndrome 164
Diabetic scleredema 66
Dupuytren's contracture 64

E

Ehlers-Danlos syndrome 131
Epidermal growth factor 215
Eruptive xanthomas 110*t*
Erythematous erosions 85
Erythematous nodules 32*t*
Extracellular matrix 189
Extra-thin hydrocolloid patches 213

F

Fasting hyperglycemia 3
Fibroblast growth factor 215
Finger pebbles 55*t*
Follicle-stimulating hormone 78
Fungal infections in diabetics 83
  candidal infections 83
    intertriginous candidiasis 84
    vulvovaginitis 84
  dermatophytic infections 85
  infections caused by zygomycetes 86
Fungal structures in mucormycosis biopsy 89*t*

G

Gamma-aminobutyric acid (GABA) 5
Generalized granuloma annulare 38
Gestational diabetes mellitus (GDM) 2, 8
Glutamic acid decarboxylase antibodies (GADA) 5

H

Hallux interphalangeal joint 203
Hashimoto's thyroiditis 73
Hepatitis B virus 41
Hepatitis C virus 41
High blood viscosity 12
Histopathology of
    finger pebbles 57t
    necrobiosis lipoidica 35t
HLA genes 4
Human beta-defensin 191
Human immunodeficiency virus 41
Human leukocyte 5f
Human leukocyte antigen (HLA) 4
Huntley's papules 54
Hyperglycemic crisis 2

I

Immune system 4
Impaired fasting glucose (IFG) 1
Impaired glucose tolerance (IGT) 1
Indirect immunofluorescence (IFA) 5
Insulin 78
Insulin deficiency 2
Insulin receptor (IR) 11
Insulin resistance 78
    types 80f
Insulin sensitizing agents 81
Intercellular lipids of corneal cells 47
Interphalangeal joint 55t
Islet antigen-2 (IA-2) 5

K

Kaposi's sarcoma 131t
Keratotic papules 137
Koebner phenomenon 124, 132

L

Latent autoimmune diabetes in adults (LADA) 9
Lichen planus 129t
Limited joint mobility 58
Lipoatrophy 140t
Lipohypertrophy 140
Loss of autoregulation of vessels 12
Luteinizing hormone 78
Lymphedema 130
Lymphocyte apoptosis in diabetic wounds 191
Lyophilized hyaluronic acid 213

M

Macroangiopathy 12
Macrovascular disease 65
Maculopapular exanthema 143t
Maillard's reaction 170
Malar hypertrichosis 107t
Maturity-onset diabetes of the young (MODY) 2
Mediterranean region 130
Metabolic syndrome 78
Metacarpophalangeal joints 59
Methyltestosterone 73
Microangiopathy 12
Molecular bases for debridement 193
Mucoral on Sabouraud dextrose agar 87t
Multidisciplinary approach in managing wound healing 201
    advanced wound therapies 214
        growth factors 215
        hyperbaric oxygen 216
        negative pressure systems 216
        platelet-rich plasma 215
        skin substitutes 216
    footwear after healing 210
        debridement 210
        epithelization 213
        management of infection-inflammation 212
        wound moisture control 213
    infectious component 202
    local approach to wound healing 204
        healable ulcers 204
        maintenance ulcers 204
        non-healable ulcers 204

local treatment 210
metabolic component 201
neuropathic component 203
   autonomic neuropathy 203
   motor neuropathy 203
   sensory neuropathy 203
offloading devices 205
   healing sandals, half-shoes, inner-soles and therapeutic shoes 207
   irremovable pneumatic boots 206
   modified usual footwear 207
   padded adhesive felts and foams 207
   removable boots 206
   total contact cast 205
vascular component 201
Multifunctional hormone 11

N

Nail alterations in diabetic patients 177
   altered biomechanics of the feet 181
   infectious nail disorders 178
      onychomycosis 178
      paronychia 180
   terminology 177
      leukonychia 177
      nail bed hyperkeratosis 178
      onychogryphosis 178
      onycholysis 178
      pachyonychia 178
      paronychia 178
      pincer nail 178
      splinter hemorrhages 178
      terry nails 178
   vascular abnormalities 181
Nail apparatus evaluation in diabetics 183
Necrobiosis lipoidica 31
Nerve conduction velocity (NCV) 65
Neuropathic foot 159t
Nodular elastoidosis 108t
Nodules of necrobiosis lipoidica 33t
Non-enzymatic glycation 168
   glycation of collagen 169
   Maillard reaction 168
Non-enzymatic glycation, diabetes mellitus and aging 173
Nonenzymatic glycation (NEG) 32
Nonenzymatic glycation (NEG) of proteins 12

O

Ocre dermatitis 155t
Oral glucose tolerance test 1f
Organ transplantation 2
Osteomyelitis 154t

P

Pancreatic deficiency of insulin secretion 3
Pancreatic β-cells 2
Perforating folliculitis 131
Periungual region 55t
Photodynamic therapy (PDT) 37
Pigmentary purpura 156t
Plantar erythema 161t
Plaque of necrobiosis lipoidica 35t
Platelet adhesion 12
Platelet aggregation 32
Platelet-derived growth factor 215
Prayer sign 60t
Pseudohyphae and yeast 84t
Psoriasis 125t
Psychogenic diseases 113
Purpura, infectious 137

R

Radiobinding assay (RBA) 5
Raynaud's phenomenon 58
Receptor of advanced glycation end-products (RAGE) 171
Reflex of the Achilles tendon 115
Reflex sympathetic dystrophy 53

S

Sabouraud dextrose agar 84
Semmes-Weinstein monofilament 164, 198
Sensory peripheral neuropathy 115
Sjörgen's syndrome 73
Skin manifestations in diabetes mellitus (DM) 13f
   classification 13f
Skin-thickening syndrome 53

T

Tabletop sign 64
Tiny papules 55t

Tortuous vessel 155*t*
Truncal pruritus of unknown origin 115
Tumoral necrosis factor alpha 37
Type 1 diabetes mellitus 3
    autoimmunity 5
    genetic determinism 4
Type 2 diabetes mellitus 7

U

Ulcers in diabetics 194
    care of the feet 198
        education 198
    examination of feet 198
    prevention 197
        blood pressure deficiency 198
        laboratory 198
        neuropathy 198
    treatment 194
        adjuvant agents 197
        diagnosis 194
        dressing 196
        infection control 195
        offloading 195
        surgery 197
        wound bed preparation 196
Uroporphyrinogen decarboxylase 106

V

Vascular complications of diabetes 12
Vascular endothelial growth factor 215
Vascular foot 152*t*
Vascular occlusion 32
Vascular ulcers 152*t*
Verhoeff-van Gieson staining 132
Visceral obesity 80
Von Willebrand factor 12

W

Waxy skin 58
Wet gangrene 213
Wound healing in diabetes mellitus 190
    effects of hyperglycemia 190
        antimicrobial peptides 191
        apoptosis 190
        bone marrow precursors 192
        neuropeptides 191
        oxidative stress 190
        tumor necrosis factor-alpha 192
    mechanisms of wound healing 193*t*

X

Xanthelasmas 111*t*
Xanthosis 47
Xerosis 159*t*

Y

Yellow skin 47

Z

Zinc transporter-8 islet 5

Praise for *Good Kids*

"*Good Kids* is a deeply profound, paradigm-shifting love letter to anyone who grew up believing they had to earn love by being "good." With warm compassion, clinical wisdom, and tender vulnerability, Maggie Nick guides us back to the truth all "Good Kids" needed to know: that we have always been inherently lovable and worthy. This book is a compassionate guide for the cycle-breakers who are ready to heal the shame we've carried for too long so we can raise children who know deep in their bones that they are seen, safe, and unconditionally loved. If you're reparenting yourself while raising your kids, *Good Kids* is an absolute must-read."

Shelly Robinson, Founder, Raising Yourself

"THIS is the kind of book that I wish people had recommended to me before I became a Mom! Maggie Nick balances clinical expertise and personal experience in an approachable way that makes the healing work involved in parenting feel doable, no matter where you are in your journey. Whether you are already a parent or planning on becoming one, I cannot recommend this book enough. To put it simply, it makes SO much about reparenting yourself while parenting your own children "make sense" and it makes you feel less alone in the process. I will be a better parent as a result of what I have learned in *Good Kids* and I am forever grateful."

Logan Cooper, LMHC, Licensed Therapist

"Maggie Nick's *Good Kids* is an invaluable guide for anyone learning to parent in the aftermath of trauma. With honesty and compassion, Maggie illuminates the struggle of raising children without having been given a healthy blueprint yourself. This book not only offers practical guidance for nurturing children toward authenticity and fulfilment, but also shows us how parenting can become a pathway back to our own healing. *Good Kids* is both a roadmap for reparenting ourselves and a gentle companion for raising the next generation with more love, presence, and wholeness."

Katie McKenna, accredited psychotherapist and co-author of the international bestseller *You're Not The Problem*

"As a reformed good kid and parent, *Good Kids* is THE exclusive guide you need for how to break perfectionism cycles. As a therapist, I cannot wait to share this with clients."

> Amanda White, LPC, Therapist, Author of *Not Drinking Tonight*,
> Founder, Therapy For Women

"As a therapist and mother, I know how many of us learned to survive childhood by quieting our needs, managing other people's emotions, and performing for love. Maggie Nick writes with such honesty and compassion that you can't help but feel both seen and understood. This book transforms the pain of the 'good kid' narrative into a path of healing, reminding us that authenticity is reclaimable and cycle breaking is within reach."

> Bryana Kappadakunnel, LMFT, Therapist, Author of *Parent Yourself First*
> and Founder of Conscious Mommy